Handbook of Cardiovascular Magnetic Resonance Imaging

Handbook of Cardiovascular Magnetic Resonance Imaging

Editor: Ray Abbott

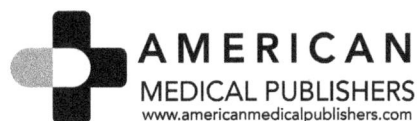

AMERICAN
MEDICAL PUBLISHERS
www.americanmedicalpublishers.com

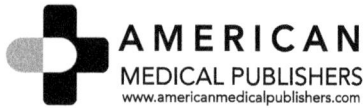

AMERICAN
MEDICAL PUBLISHERS
www.americanmedicalpublishers.com

Cataloging-in-Publication Data

Handbook of cardiovascular magnetic resonance imaging / edited by Ray Abbott.
   p. cm.
Includes bibliographical references and index.
ISBN 978-1-63927-073-6
   1. Cardiovascular system--Magnetic resonance imaging. 2. Magnetic resonance imaging. 3. Diagnostic imaging.
   4. Cardiovascular system--Diseases--Diagnosis--Equipment and supplies. I. Abbott, Ray.
RC670.5.M33 H36 2022
616.107 548--dc23

© American Medical Publishers, 2022

American Medical Publishers,
41 Flatbush Avenue,
1st Floor, New York,
NY 11217, USA

ISBN 978-1-63927-073-6 (Hardback)

Contents

Permissions

List of Contributors

Index

Preface

I am honored to present to you this unique book which encompasses the most up-to-date data in the field. I was extremely pleased to get this opportunity of editing the work of experts from across the globe. I have also written papers in this field and researched the various aspects revolving around the progress of the discipline. I have tried to unify my knowledge along with that of stalwarts from every corner of the world, to produce a text which not only benefits the readers but also facilitates the growth of the field.

The medical imaging technology that is used for the non-invasive assessment of the function and structure of the cardiovascular system is referred to as cardiovascular magnetic resonance imaging (CMR). This imaging technique is helpful in evidence-based diagnostic and therapeutic pathways in cardiovascular disease. The applications of cardiovascular MRI include the assessment of myocardial ischemia and viability, myocarditis, iron overload, congenital heart disease and vascular disease. CMR study includes a few techniques of imaging such as cine imaging for heart function, 4D flow CMR, adenosine for perfusion, etc. This book presents the complex subject of cardiovascular magnetic resonance imaging in the most comprehensible and easy to understand language. It presents researches and studies performed by experts across the globe. The book will help the readers in keeping pace with the rapid changes in this field.

Finally, I would like to thank all the contributing authors for their valuable time and contributions. This book would not have been possible without their efforts. I would also like to thank my friends and family for their constant support.

Editor

Comparative cost-effectiveness analyses of cardiovascular magnetic resonance and coronary angiography combined with fractional flow reserve for the diagnosis of coronary artery disease

Karine Moschetti[1,2]*, David Favre[1], Christophe Pinget[1,2], Guenter Pilz[3], Steffen E Petersen[4], Anja Wagner[5], Jean-Blaise Wasserfallen[1,2] and Juerg Schwitter[6]

Abstract

Background: According to recent guidelines, patients with coronary artery disease (CAD) should undergo revascularization if significant myocardial ischemia is present. Both, cardiovascular magnetic resonance (CMR) and fractional flow reserve (FFR) allow for a reliable ischemia assessment and in combination with anatomical information provided by invasive coronary angiography (CXA), such a work-up sets the basis for a decision to revascularize or not. The cost-effectiveness ratio of these two strategies is compared.

Methods: Strategy 1) CMR to assess ischemia followed by CXA in ischemia-positive patients (CMR + CXA), Strategy 2) CXA followed by FFR in angiographically positive stenoses (CXA + FFR). The costs, evaluated from the third party payer perspective in Switzerland, Germany, the United Kingdom (UK), and the United States (US), included public prices of the different outpatient procedures and costs induced by procedural complications and by diagnostic errors. The effectiveness criterion was the correct identification of hemodynamically significant coronary lesion(s) (= significant CAD) complemented by full anatomical information. Test performances were derived from the published literature. Cost-effectiveness ratios for both strategies were compared for hypothetical cohorts with different pretest likelihood of significant CAD.

Results: CMR + CXA and CXA + FFR were equally cost-effective at a pretest likelihood of CAD of 62% in Switzerland, 65% in Germany, 83% in the UK, and 82% in the US with costs of CHF 5'794, € 1'517, £ 2'680, and $ 2'179 per patient correctly diagnosed. Below these thresholds, CMR + CXA showed lower costs per patient correctly diagnosed than CXA + FFR.

Conclusions: The CMR + CXA strategy is more cost-effective than CXA + FFR below a CAD prevalence of 62%, 65%, 83%, and 82% for the Swiss, the German, the UK, and the US health care systems, respectively. These findings may help to optimize resource utilization in the diagnosis of CAD.

Keywords: Cost-effectiveness analysis, Coronary artery disease, Cardiovascular magnetic resonance, Coronary angiography, Fractional flow reserve, Decision making

* Correspondence: karine.moschetti@chuv.ch
[1]Institute of Health Economics and Management (IEMS), University of Lausanne, Route de Chavannes 31, VIDY, 1015 Lausanne, Switzerland
[2]Technology Assessment Unit (UET), University Hospital (CHUV), Lausanne, Switzerland
Full list of author information is available at the end of the article

Background

In many countries, cardiovascular diseases are the leading cause of morbidity and also of loss of quality of life. In particular, coronary artery disease (CAD) constitutes a major public health problem. In Europe the total costs of CAD and stroke were estimated at 49 billion Euros in the year 2008 [1] and for the United States these costs were estimated as high as 156 billion dollars [2]. It is well established that patients with no evidence of myocardial ischemia have low cardiac events rates, even when invasive coronary angiography (CXA) demonstrates lesions of intermediate severity [3,4]. In addition, patients without ischemia can be treated safely with medical therapy [5,6] thereby reducing the total costs of patient management [7]. On the other hand, randomized trials e.g. in diabetic patients demonstrated a survival benefit of patients with ischemia being treated by revascularization versus medical treatment alone [8]. Accordingly, recent guidelines recommend to revascularize patients if a relevant burden of myocardial ischemia is present (i.e. proximal vessel(s)) with a positive fractional flow reserve (FFR) and/or >10% of myocardium ischemic [9] or ≥2 ischemic segments in cardiovascular magnetic resonance (CMR) perfusion examinations [10].

Nevertheless, neither vessel anatomy nor presence or absence of ischemia is the factor that will exclusively decide on revascularizations. Symptoms, co-morbidities and other factors have to be taken into account before a treatment decision is made. Thus, the current analysis was undertaken to assess the cost-effectiveness to acquire information (significant ischemia and full anatomical information) relevant for decision making, but did not include the costs for all information needed to manage patients with CAD. Also, we do not know whether a large ischemia burden is directly related to adverse effects, whether it represents a marker of higher risk for occlusion of a severe stenosis that causes ischemia, or whether more severe ischaemia is simply a marker of more extensive atherosclerosis and more vulnerable plaques that go along with a worse outcome. Large trials such as ISCHEMIA and others [11] will hopefully improve our knowledge in a near future on how to treat ischemic patients. Despite this current lack of a detailed understanding of the underlying mechanisms that link ischemia to outcome, current guidelines recommend an ischemia-based approach for decision making in patients with CAD. Therefore, the aim of the current study was to assess the cost-effectiveness of two diagnostic strategies that are ischemia-based and provide both full anatomical and functional evaluation of CAD, which are the basis for a revascularization procedure.

A variety of new imaging techniques allow for such a combined anatomical and functional assessment of CAD, and as a result, the selection of the optimum test becomes more and more challenging. The choice of cardiovascular imaging techniques should consider both, their clinical benefits for the patients as well as the costs and cost-effectiveness compared to others. Invasive coronary angiography (CXA) remains the reference for the morphological assessment of CAD and it is often used in daily practice as a first line test, e.g. in patients with a positive treadmill test. While this strategy is not recommended by current guidelines, the advent of the FFR measurement to assess the hemodynamic significance of coronary artery stenoses [12] may even increase the attractivity to use invasive CXA as a first line test, as it can be easily combined with FFR in case of intermediate stenoses. Also, the FFR results were highly predictive for patient outcome [13,14] and the combination of CXA with FFR was more cost-effective than a CXA-only approach for the treatment of CAD [15]. Accordingly, recent guidelines recommend using FFR to correctly identify lesions that should undergo percutaneous coronary interventions (PCI) [9]. However, the invasive nature and radiation exposure of CXA and FFR limit their usefulness in a screening process [16]. Considering the fact that CXA is still extensively used in many industrialized countries as an early step in the work-up of suspected CAD [17,18], and further considering that FFR is recommended in recent guidelines, the combination of CXA + FFR was one diagnostic strategy to be assessed in the current study with respect to its cost-effectiveness.

As an alternative to the FFR measurement, perfusion CMR has emerged as a robust non-invasive technique for the evaluation of myocardial ischemia [19-22]. Furthermore, recent studies demonstrated the excellent prognosis of patients with known or suspected CAD, when perfusion-CMR was normal [23-25]. Accordingly, in the present study, the cost-effectiveness of a combination of CMR + CXA was compared with that of a CXA + FFR strategy.

In the current economic context, the health care systems have to be economically sustainable while preserving high quality medical standards. Consequently, in the following study we estimated the costs of the two different strategies relative to their effectiveness to 1) correctly diagnose the presence of relevant ischemia (= significant CAD) and 2) to yield full anatomical information of the coronary vasculature in case of ischemia. In particular, the cost-effectiveness of the two strategies was compared when applied to patient populations with varying CAD pre-test probabilities. Strategy 1 consists of a CMR examination to assess ischemia followed by CXA in ischemia-positive patients (CMR + CXA). This strategy yields complete information on myocardial ischemia and coronary anatomy. Strategy 2 consists of a CXA in all patients followed by a FFR test in patients with intermediate stenoses on CXA (CXA + FFR). Finally, the cost-effectiveness ratios of the two strategies were calculated for the health care systems in Switzerland, Germany, the United Kingdom, and the United States.

Methods

Using a mathematical model, we compared the cost-effectiveness of 2 algorithms for diagnosing the presence of hemodynamically significant coronary lesion(s) (= significant CAD) for hypothetical patient cohorts characterized by different pretest likelihood of CAD (P_{isch}): 1) A perfusion CMR to assess myocardial ischemia before referring positive patients to CXA and 2) A CXA combined with an FFR in patients with angiographically positive stenoses (see also Figure 1).

Model characteristics

The model is based on Bayes' theorem and consequently assesses cost-effectiveness ratios of strategies in hypothetical patient cohorts with different pretest likelihoods of disease [26]. The mathematical model was initially suggested by Paterson and co-workers [27] and was later on applied by others [28-30]. The simulation approach

has the advantage to allow the evaluation of diagnostic algorithms for patients with different pretest likelihoods of CAD regardless of currently accepted and applied clinical strategies to detect CAD. In order to determine the pretest likelihood of CAD in patients, the same testing procedures would precede both strategies, i.e. CMR + CXA and CXA + FFR, implying the same costs for both strategies. Therefore, these "upstream" costs need not to be considered in the model. Similarly, once a treatment decision is made, based on either diagnostic strategy the same treatment costs will occur and therefore, these "downstream" costs were not considered either in the model. No ethics approval was obtained for this study as it is based on simulation model calculations and therefore no patients data from our institution were required. Calculations were performed with Microsoft Office Excel 2007 software.

Cost-effectiveness analysis
Definition of effectiveness

In the present study, the criterion of effectiveness is the ability to accurately identify those patients with one or more hemodynamically significant coronary lesion(s) (=significant

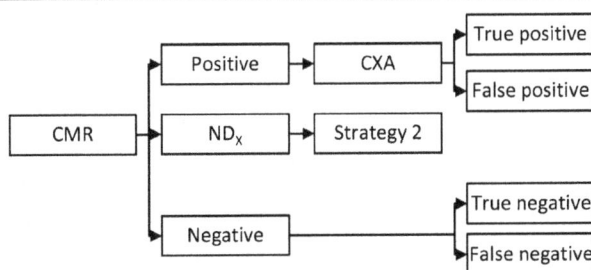

Strategy 1 (CMR+CXA) involves a perfusion CMR to assess myocardial ischemia (P_{isch}) before referring positive patients to coronary angiography (CXA). This latter test either confirms or rejects the CMR diagnosis and adds anatomical information in true positive patients which is required for the final diagnosis. Patients with non diagnostic CMR (NDx) cross over to strategy 2. False-negative patients due to diagnostic errors are at risk for complications (e.g. myocardial infarction) due to the undetected and thus in-correctly treated CAD.

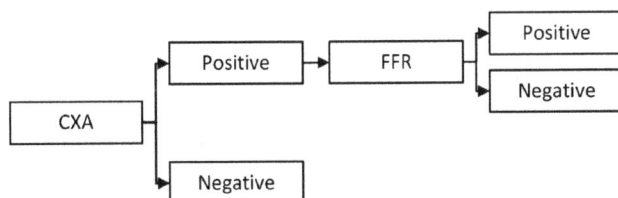

In strategy 2 (CXA+FFR), a CXA is performed in all patients and is combined with an FFR test in patients with angiographically positive stenoses, i.e. ≥50% diameter reduction.

Figure 1 Decision tree for CAD diagnosis including strategy 1 and strategy 2 used to design the model.

CAD), combined with the complete anatomical information on the coronary arteries. These patients with a relevant ischemia burden are the primary candidates for revascularizations according the most recent guidelines [10]. This ischemia burden is defined in the newest guidelines as a positive FFR of proximal coronary vessels [9,10] or by ≥ 2 segments with ischemia on perfusion-CMR [10]. The effectiveness criterion for strategy 1 is achieved by a positive perfusion-CMR study (≥ 2 segments ischemic, see also Table 1), which is complemented by a complete anatomical information provided by a CXA examination in patients positive for ischemia. For strategy 2, the effectiveness criterion is achieved by the detection of a stenosis $\geq 50\%$ in CXA combined with an FFR ≤ 0.75 (= significant CAD). By assumption, invasive CXA and FFR were the reference tests with an assumed 100% diagnostic accuracy (Table 1). For the calculation of hemodynamically significant lesions by the CMR + CXA strategy, per-patient sensitivities (Sn_{CMR} = 0.88) and specificities (Sp_{CMR} = 0.90) were considered as determined by Rieber et al. who compared ischemia on CMR (i.e. ≥ 2 segment positive) versus FFR ≤ 0.75 as the reference for ischemia [31]. Cost-effectiveness is defined as the costs per effect which is calculated as the ratio between the total costs and the number of patients correctly diagnosed as having one or more hemodynamically significant coronary lesion(s) (true positive). Also, the costs of complications in patients with a false negative diagnosis are included in the cost-effectiveness ratio.

In this study, the objective of the analysis was to compare cost-effectiveness ratios from the third party payer perspective and not to assess the general impact of CAD detection on the society welfare.

Table 1 Test performance parameters used in the effectiveness calculations

Abbreviation	Description	Parameter value
Test to yield anatomical information (= detection of diameter reduction $\geq 50\%$)		
Sn_{CXA}	Sensitivity of CXA	1
Sp_{CXA}	Specificity of CXA	1
Sn_{FFR}	Sensitivity of FFR	1
Sp_{FFR}	Specificity of FFR	1
R_{CXA}	Rate of complications with invasive CXA	0.0005 [27]
Test to yield ischemia information (=detection of myocardial ischemia)		
Sn_{CMR}	Sensitivity of CMR (≥ 2 segments positive vs FFR ≤ 0.75)	0.88 [31]
Sp_{CMR}	Specificity of CMR (≥ 2 segments positive vs FFR ≤ 0.75)	0.90 [31]
NDx	Non diagnostic rate for CMR	0.05 [32]
R_F	Rate of complications per 10-year follow-up period for patients with CAD and false-negative tests	0.15 [27]

When performing cost-effectiveness analysis, a wide variety of factors and parameters related to the costs and the performances of the tests have to be considered. The model must be able to take into account the costs associated with false-positive results (i.e. costs of unnecessary diagnostic tests or treatments) as well as the costs associated with false negative results (i.e. costs of complications because of inappropriate management of the disease). To this end, data from the published literature on the performances of tests (sensitivities, specificities and rate of nondiagnostic examinations) and the complication rates were used (Table 1).

To appropriately model strategy 2 (CXA + FFR), the portion of patients with diameter stenoses $\geq 50\%$ on CXA having ischemia in FFR must be known. In other words, the relationship between the probability of stenoses $\geq 50\%$ on CXA (P_{sten}) and the probability of having ischemia on FFR (P_{isch}) must be known. In order to assess this relationship, we used published data from 5 recent articles (see Additional file 1: Section A1 for details).

Definition of costs and calculations of the costs per effect

The costs of a diagnostic strategy consist of first-line test costs and subsequent costs. The first-line test costs are the fees (F_t) for the CMR and CXA tests. Subsequent costs were costs of additional tests (i.e. in case of nondiagnostic CMR or unnecessary diagnostic tests in case of false-positive results), costs of major complications induced by the diagnostic procedure or resulting from mis-diagnosis of a patient (e.g. as false negative patients are at risk to have complications per 10-years follow-up because of inappropriate management of the disease). Due to the non-invasive nature of CMR and recent results showing that no severe complications occurred in >17,000 CMR examinations (i.e. 7 mild reactions in >7,200 stress CMR examinations) in the EuroCMR registry [33] and in large multicenter trials [19], we assumed that CMR is not associated with direct procedure-related major complications. As an anaphylactic shock is extremely rare and may occur after administration of both MR- and CXA-related contrast media, this complication was not considered in the analysis. We assumed that a potential complication associated with either a diagnostic CXA or an untreated hemodynamically significant lesion (i.e. false negatives) is a myocardial infarction (MI). Costs for this complication (hereafter C) included medical costs associated with the complications and accounted for a PCI, a hospital stay of one week, and a rehabilitation period of 4 weeks. The risk of developing malignancies induced by radiation exposure was not incorporated into the model. Future complications-related costs were discounted annually at a rate of 3% [34].

The total costs of a diagnostic algorithm were calculated as the sum of direct costs and subsequent costs multiplied by the respective number of patients. The cost-effectiveness ratios were calculated for patient cohorts with different pretest likelihoods ranging from 10% to 100%.

The cost-effectiveness ratios were calculated as follows:

$$\text{Cost} - \text{effectiveness Ratio} = \frac{\text{Direct cost} + \text{subsequent costs}}{\text{effectiveness}}$$

Calculations of the direct and subsequent costs and the detailed equations are presented in the Additional file 1: Section A2.

Evaluation of the costs in each country

The analyses were conducted from the third party payer perspective in 4 countries. We used 2012 and 2013 costs data in Swiss Francs (CHF) for Switzerland, in Euros (€) for Germany, in Pounds (£) for the United Kingdom (UK), and in American Dollars (US $) for the United States. The Additional file 2 provides a brief description on how the costs were derived for each country.

Sensitivity analysis

Due to the uncertainty of the data used and the numerous assumptions (parameter values) made in these calculations, a sensitivity analysis was performed to test the robustness of the model. Thus, the model was re-run with 1) changes in the costs of the tests and of the complications, 2) changes in the rates of complications associated with CXA, 3) changes in the accuracy of the CMR

test, and 4) change in the threshold of FFR to detect ischemia (<0.75 vs <0.80; regarding the method used refer to Additional file 1). In order to understand the impact of each parameter in the model they were changed one by one in the repeated calculations (for details, see the figures related to the sensitivity analyses in the Results section).

Results

Effect of the pretest likelihood of significant CAD on effectiveness and on costs of the two strategies

Figure 2 shows the effect of the pretest likelihood of significant CAD on effectiveness. The proportion of patients with CAD for whom a correct diagnosis is made by the CMR-based strategy depends on its sensitivity, specificity, and the rate of non-diagnostic CMR examinations (Additional file 1: Section A2). As CXA and FFR are assumed to be the reference with 100% accuracy, its advantage compared to CMR increases as P_{isch} increases. We derived that the difference between the 2 strategies slightly decreases with an increase of the rate of patients with non-diagnostic CMR tests (NDx). In the model, the NDx patients after CMR are oriented to strategy 2 in order to achieve 100% accuracy in these cross-over patients.

Figure 3 shows the effect of pretest likelihood of significant CAD on cost (example for the Swiss health care system). The cost per patient tested increases with increasing pre-test likelihood of significant CAD for both strategies. The costs for CXA + FFR slightly increase as the need for FFR increases with increasing

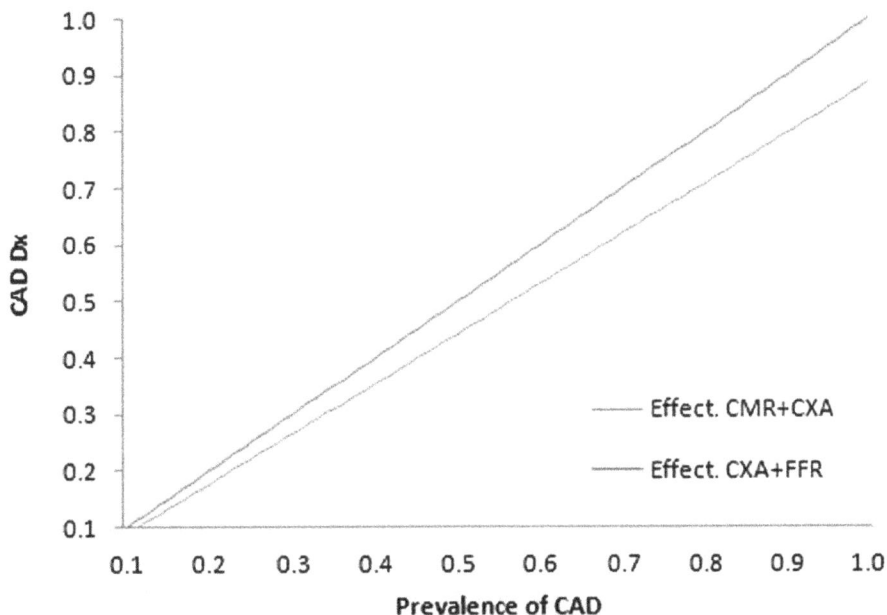

Figure 2 Example for the Swiss health care system: Proportion of patients with suspected CAD correctly diagnosed (CAD Dx) by the CMR + CXA and CXA + FFR strategies in relation to pre-test likelihood of significant CAD (P_{isch}).

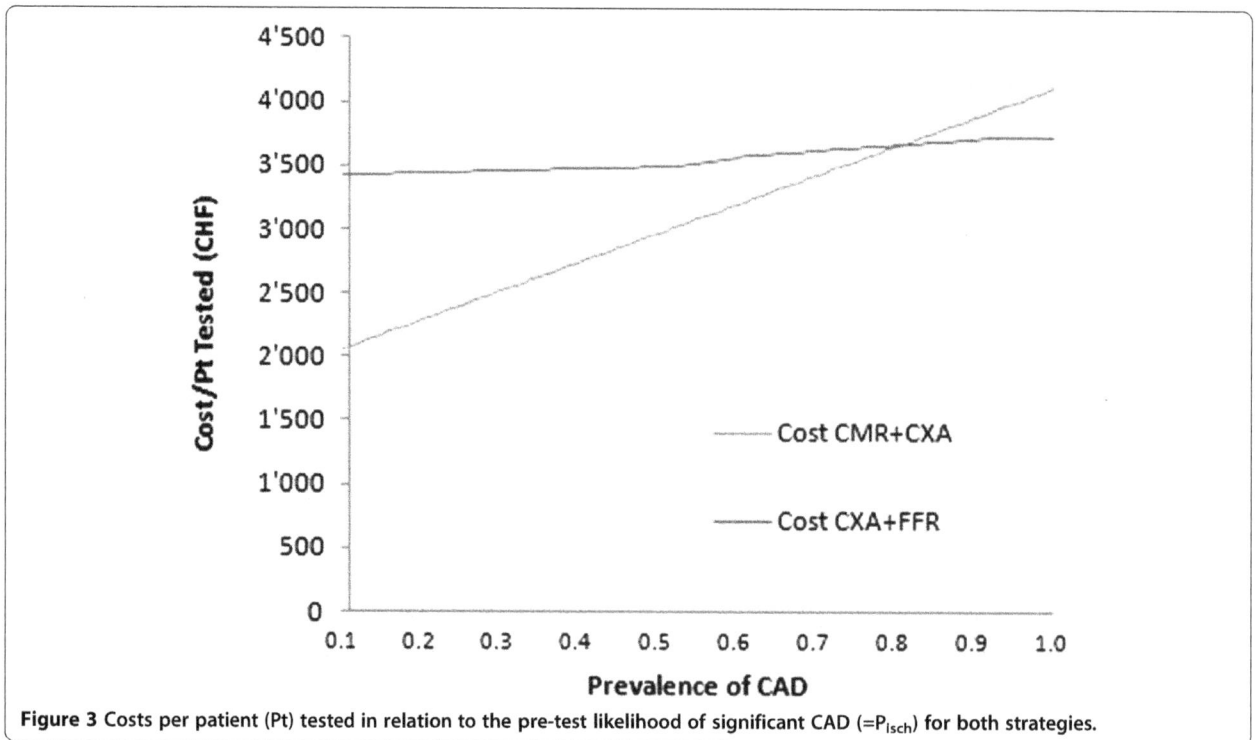

Figure 3 Costs per patient (Pt) tested in relation to the pre-test likelihood of significant CAD (=P_{isch}) for both strategies.

prevalence of significant CAD. For the CMR + CXA strategy the costs increase steeply with increasing pre-test likelihood of significant CAD, since patients positive for ischemia on CMR have to undergo CXA. The two strategies are equally costly for a prevalence of significant CAD of 0.87 (Figure 4). The value for such a crossing point, within the range of P_{isch} (0 – 1.0) depends on the relative costs of the tests and the accuracy of the CMR test (NDx and Sn_{CMR} and Sp_{CMR}) (see formulas of costs).

When CXA is considered as inpatient test, the cost per patient tested with strategy 1 (CMR + CXA) is lower than the cost per patient tested with strategy 2 (CXA + FFR) at any level of pre-test-likelihood of CAD.

Comparison of the cost per effect and of cost-effectiveness for the two strategies

Figure 4 shows the cost per effect, i.e. the cost per patient correctly diagnosed for significant CAD at various levels of CAD prevalence in the 4 countries. We observe that the cost per effect decreases hyperbolically for both strategies as the pretest likelihood increases. The hyperbolic relationship between the prevalence of significant CAD and the costs per patient correctly diagnosed shows the high cost per effect in the patient population with low prevalence of significant CAD (= low P_{isch} values). The costs per effect at low values of P_{isch} are higher for strategy 2 (CX + FFR) than for strategy 1 (CMR + CXA).

By assuming that all tests are outpatient tests, both strategies are equally cost-effective at a pretest likelihood of 62% in Switzerland, 65% in Germany, 83% in the UK, and 82% in the United States with costs of CHF 5,794, € 1,517, £ 2,680, and $ 2,179 per patient correctly diagnosed, respectively. Below this threshold, CMR + CXA shows lower costs per patient correctly diagnosed than CXA + FFR. When the CXA test is performed as an inpatient examination, the crossing point of the two curves shifts towards the right to a prevalence of significant CAD of 77% with costs of CHF 6,819 in Switzerland, to 90% with costs of € 2'847 in Germany, to 93% with costs of £ 4,633 in the UK, and to 94% with costs of $ 3,849 in the US.

Sensitivity analyses

Following a reduction of the sensitivity of the CMR examination by 10% the crossing point shifted to the left by 16, 20, 14, and 30 percentage points for the Swiss, the German, the UK, and the US health care systems, respectively. An increase of the CMR sensitivity by 10% shifted the crossing point to the right by 15, 19, and 12 percentage points for the Swiss, the German, and the UK health care systems, respectively. There is no crossing point for P_{isch} <1 for the US health care system (Figures 5, 6, 7 and 8), i.e. the costs of the CMR strategy are lower than those of the CXA strategy in the US system irrespectively of the pre-test likelihood of CAD.

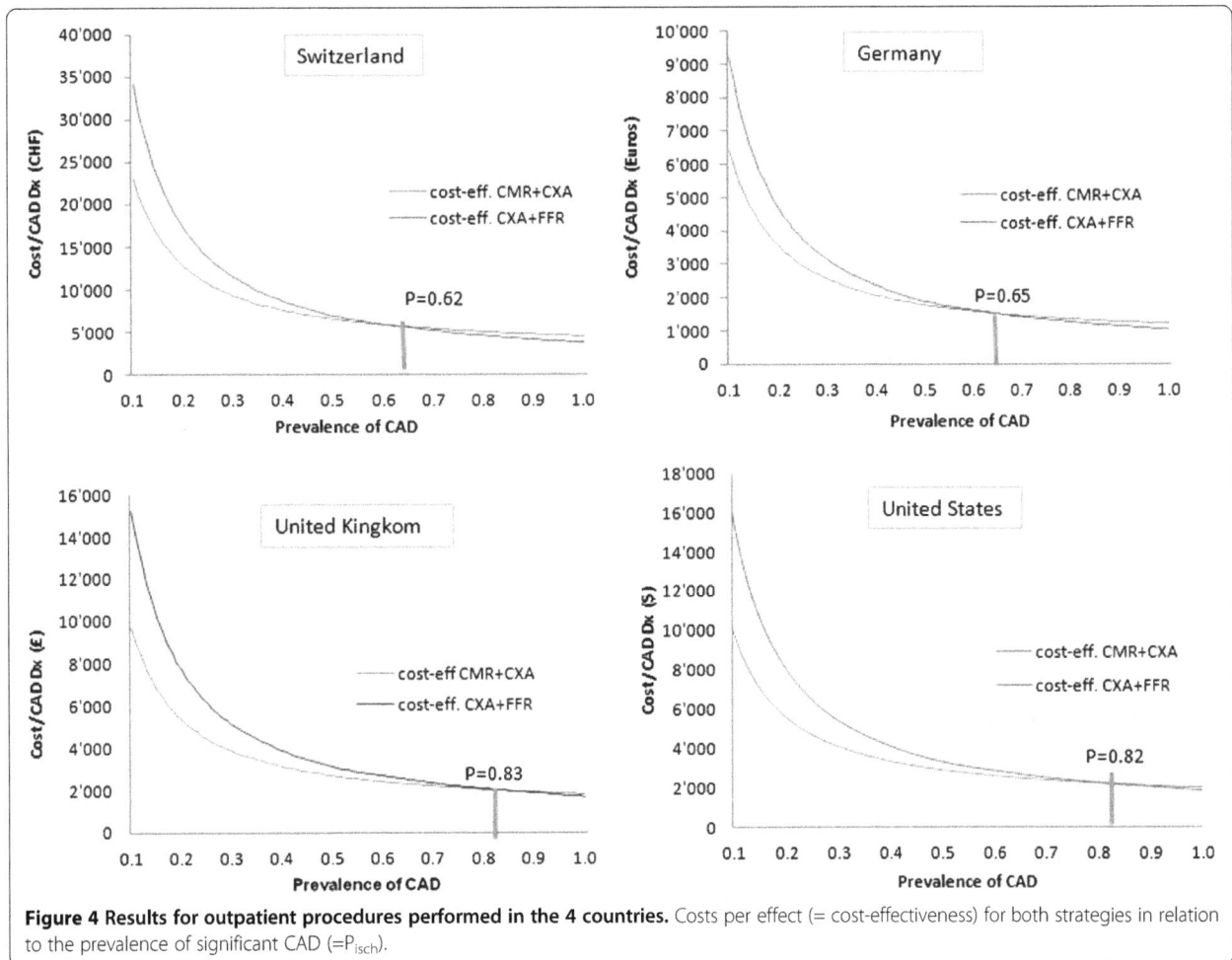

Figure 4 Results for outpatient procedures performed in the 4 countries. Costs per effect (= cost-effectiveness) for both strategies in relation to the prevalence of significant CAD (=P$_{isch}$).

Changing the specificity of CMR had a minor influence on the crossing point for all health care systems assessed. This was also the case for the other variables tested in the sensitivity analysis except the complications rate. The sensitivity analysis shows that the rate for complications caused by mis-diagnosed CAD, i.e. a lack of detecting CAD, is associated with relevant cost-effectiveness changes at least in the US system. If the rate of complications in false-negative patients by CMR is doubled the crossing point is shifted to the left by 10, 12, 6, and 23 percentage points in the Swiss, German, UK, and US systems, respectively.

An increase of the FFR threshold to <0.80 did not substantially influence the cost-effectiveness results as shown in (Figures 5, 6, 7 and 8). The crossing point shifted to the left by 2 or 3 percentage points for the 4 health care systems.

Discussion

The main findings of this study can be summarized as follows: 1) In all four health care systems analyzed, the cost effectiveness ratio decreases hyperbolically for both diagnostic strategies with an increasing prevalence of hemodynamically significant coronary lesions, i.e. with an increasing prevalence of significant CAD. 2) The increase in the cost-effectiveness for strategy 2, i.e. CXA + FFR, with increasing prevalence of significant CAD is more pronounced than that of the primarily non-invasive CMR + CXA strategy, implying that there is a threshold value of CAD prevalence where strategy 2 becomes more cost-effective than strategy 1. and 3) The crossing point indicating an equal cost-effectiveness for the 2 strategies varied for the 4 countries examined. In Switzerland, strategy 1, i.e. CMR + CXA, is more cost-effective than strategy 2 below a CAD prevalence of 62%. In the German, UK, and US health care systems, a higher cost-effectiveness for CMR + CXA is given for a CAD prevalence below 65%, 83%, and 82%, respectively.

CAD prevalence for optimum cost-effectiveness of various strategies and current utilization of resources

Current clinical practice guidelines recommend proceeding to PCI only, if relevant myocardial ischemia in symptomatic patients is present [9,10]. Therefore, it appears

Swiss context	Standard Value	Prev of CAD where both strategies are equally cost-effective	New value (-10% for fees)	Prev of CAD where both strategies are equally cost-effective	Cost value in CHF at the crossing point	New value (+10% for fees)	Prev of CAD where both strategies are equally cost-effective	Cost value in CHF at the crossing point
Fee for FFR	1'212		1'091	0.556	6'155	1'334	0.669	5'552
Fee for CMR in CHF	1'420		1'278	0.698	5'186	1'562	0.518	6'743
Fee for CXA (outpatient) in CHF	2'508		2'257	0.557	5'875	2'759	0.654	5'886
Costs for complications	23'083		20'778	0.628	5'709	25'396	0.605	5'899
		P$_{isch}$ =0.619 (CHF 5'794)	if all (above) new cost values are considered P$_{isch}$ = 0.619 at a cost per effect of CHF 5'215			if all above new cost values are considered P$_{isch}$ = 0.619 at a cost per effect of CHF 6'372		
	Standard Value		New value	Prev of CAD where both strategies are equally cost-effective	Cost value in CHF at the crossing point	New value	Prev of CAD where both strategies are equally cost-effective	Cost value in CHF at the crossing point
Accuracy CMR (NonDx)	0.05		0.03	0.634	5'660	0.10	0.560	6'300
Sensitivity CMR	0.88		0.80	0.456	7'634	0.96	0.776	4'709
Specificity CMR	0.9		0.84	0.573	6'179	0.96	0.646	5'562
Risk associated with CXA (R$_{CXA}$)	0.0005		0.001	0.620	5'800	-	-	-
Risk of complications per 10-year follow-up for patients with CAD & false negative results	0.15		0.10	0.654	5'503	0.30	0.514	6'799
FFR threshold	0.75		0.80	0.584	5'984	-	-	-

Figure 5 Sensitivity analysis: Switzerland.

reasonable to incorporate FFR testing or perfusion CMR for ischemia assessment into models that assess the cost-effectiveness of various strategies suggested for a CAD work-up. Moreover, an FFR-guided PCI approach was shown to be more cost-effective than a simple anatomy-guided, i.e. CXA-based PCI approach [7]. The current results show for all four health care systems assessed, that the pre-test likelihood of CAD is a major factor that influences the cost-effectiveness of a CAD work-up. This is in line with the fact that benefits from diagnostic tests

German context	Standard Value	Prev of CAD where both strategies are equally cost-effective	New value (-10% for fees)	Prev of CAD where both strategies are equally cost-effective	Cost value in € at the crossing point	New value (+10% for fees)	Prev of CAD where both strategies are equally cost-effective	Cost value in € at the crossing point
Fee for FFR in €	397		358	0.563	1'647	437	0.720	1'429
Fee for CMR in €	410		369	0.746	1'336	451	0.521	1'822
Fee for CXA (outpatient) in €	626		563	0.594	1'527	689	0.682	1'538
Costs for complications	5'976		5'378	0.659	1'492	6'574	0.635	1'542
		P$_{isch}$ = 0.647 (€ 1'517)	if all (above) new cost values are considered P$_{isch}$ = 0.647 at a cost per effect of Euros 1'364			if all above new cost values are considered P$_{isch}$ = 0.647 at a cost per effect of Euros 1'669		
	Standard Value		New value	Prev of CAD where both strategies are equally cost-effective	Cost value in € at the crossing point	New value	Prev of CAD where both strategies are equally cost-effective	Cost value in € at the crossing point
Accuracy CMR (NonDx)	0.05		0.03	0.667	1'476	0.10	0.580	1'665
Sensitivity CMR	0.88		0.80	0.455	2'075	0.96	0.838	1'206
Specificity CMR	0.90		0.84	0.612	1'594	0.96	0.675	1'461
Risk associated with CXA (R$_{CXA}$)	0.0005		0.001	0.649	1'518	-	-	-
Risk of complications per 10-year follow-up for patients with CAD & false negative results	0.15		0.10	0.689	1'434	0.30	0.523	1'814
FFR threshold	0.75		0.80	0.624	1'549			

Figure 6 Sensitivity analysis: Germany.

UK context	Standard Value	Prev of CAD where both strategies are equally cost-effective	New value (-10% for fees)	Prev of CAD where both strategies are equally cost-effective	Cost value in £ at the crossing point	New value (+10% for fees)	Prev of CAD where both strategies are equally cost-effective	Cost value in £ at the crossing point
Fee for FFR in £	631		568	0.748	2'556	694	0.909	2'813
Fee for CMR in £	600		540	0.922	2'718	660	0.731	2'642
Fee for CXA (outpatient) in £	1'053		948	0.801	2'501	1'158	0.845	2'858
Costs for complications	3'806		3'425	0.832	2'683	4'187	0.820	2'678
		Pisch =0.827 (£ 2'680)	if all (above) new cost values are considered Pisch = 0.827 at a cost per effect of £ 2'413			if all above new cost values are considered Pisch = 0.827 at a cost per effect of £ 2'948		
	Standard Value		New value	Prev of CAD where both strategies are equally cost-effective	Cost value in £ at the crossing point	New value	Prev of CAD where both strategies are equally cost-effective	Cost value in £ at the crossing point
Accuracy CMR (NonDx)	0.05		0.03	0.846	2'688	0.10	0.773	2'660
Sensitivity CMR	0.88		0.80	0.682	2'624	0.96	0.954	2'126
Specificity CMR	0.90		0.84	0.808	2'673	0.96	0.841	2'686
Risk associated with CXA (Rcxa)	0.0005		0.001	0.835	2'686	-	-	-
Risk of complications per 10-year follow-up for patients with CAD & false negative results	0.15		0.10	0.848	2'689	0.30	0.767	2'657
FFR threshold	0.75		0.80	0.809	2'809	-	-	-

Figure 7 Sensitivity analysis: The United Kingdom.

US context	Standard Value	Prev of CAD where both strategies are equally cost-effective	New value (-10% for fees)	Prev of CAD where both strategies are equally cost-effective	Cost value in € at the crossing point	New value (+10% for fees)	Prev of CAD where both strategies are equally cost-effective	Cost value in € at the crossing point
Fee for FFR in $	888		799	0.702	2'370	976	0.917	2'078
Fee for CMR in $	634		571	0.915	1'986	697	0.723	2'424
Fee for CXA (outpatient) in $	929		836	0.798	2'112	1'022	0.836	2'252
Costs for complications	19'105		17'195	0.850	2'110	21'016	0.790	2'248
		Pisch= 0.820 ($ 2'179)	if all (above) new cost values are considered PCAD = 0.820 at a cost per effect of $ 1'962			if all (above) new cost values are considered PCAD = 0.820 at a cost per effect of $ 2'396		
	Standard Value		New value	Prev of CAD where both strategies are equally cost-effective	Cost value in € at the crossing point	New value	Prev of CAD where both strategies are equally cost-effective	Cost value in € at the crossing point
Accuracy for CMR (NonDx)	0.05		0.03	0.839	2'135	0.10	0.765	2'308
Sensibility CMR	0.88		0.80	0.517	3'194	0.96	No crossing point for P<1	
Specificity CMR	0.9		0.84	0.803	2'216	0.96	0.833	2'149
Risk associated with CXA (RCXA)	0.0005		0.001	0.821	2'186	X	X	X
Risk of complications per 10-year follow-up for patients with CAD & false negative results	0.15		0.1	0.934	1'951	0.3	0.587	2'886
FFR threshold	0.75		0.80	0.795	2'211			

Figure 8 Sensitivity analysis: The United States.

depend on its performance but also on the prevalence of the disease within the evaluated population [35]. According to the current analyses a non-invasive CMR-guided approach is cost-effective for patients with an intermediate pre-test likelihood of disease, which is in line with most guidelines defining intermediate pre-test probabilities as 20-80%. Interestingly, in the US 62% of elective CXA examinations performed in a large sample of approximately 400,000 patients were found to be negative for CAD (stenoses <50% diameter reduction) [18], indicating that in the US the pre-test probability of CAD in daily routine is as low as ~38% which is substantially lower than the calculated threshold of 82%. Similarly, in the UK more than 58% of CXA examinations did not result in PCI or CABG procedures [36] indicating that currently, the pre-test likelihood of significant CAD of patients referred for CXA of 42% is substantially lower than 83% calculated for the UK. In the German health care system, the optimum pre-test likelihood of CAD for a CMR-based strategy is below 65%. However, in 2008, only 43% of patients after CXA were revascularized [17], indicating that an invasive approach was applied in a patient population with a relatively low CAD prevalence of approximately 43%. Finally, in Switzerland, the theoretical threshold for a directly invasive strategy is at 62% CAD prevalence. The portion of normal CXA studies ranged between 55% to 66% over the last 3 years [37], which translates into an approximated pre-test likelihood of significant CAD of 34-45% in Switzerland, thus, again still lower than the prevalence for a calculated optimal cost-effectiveness.

A cost analysis was recently performed based on the data of the German sample of the European CMR registry [38]. Cost savings of 50% were calculated between a CMR strategy and an outpatient invasive CXA strategy which is in line with the fact, that the pre-test probability of CAD in this cohort was 27%, i.e. well below the 65% level. The cost savings for this cohort reported in 2012 would be even higher considering that for these calculations costs for FFR were not yet included. Recently, a cost-effectiveness analysis for UK was performed based on the CE-MARC data [39]. For the prevalence of CAD of 39% in CE-MARC [22], the diagnostic strategy based on CMR (preceded or not by a treadmill test) followed by CXA in case of ischemia on CMR was the most cost-effective strategy of all tested. This finding is well in line with the current calculations which suggest cost-effectiveness for the MR-based approach below a CAD prevalence of 83%. In this context, it should be noted, that in the current study the threshold in favor of a CMR-guided work-up compared cost-effectiveness versus an outpatient CXA + FFR strategy. If inpatient CXA is included into the model, the crossing point shifts towards 77% for Switzerland, and is >90% for Germany, the UK and the US. This indicates that the

inpatient CXA + FFR procedures can only compete with non-invasive CMR + CXA for very high rates of CAD prevalence. This result is of even greater importance if we note that in-patient CXA is performed in approximately 67% [40,41], 40% [36], and 88% [42], in the US, the UK, and the German system, respectively.

Testing for ischemia by invasive *vs* non-invasive techniques

For the current analyses, the FFR technique was assumed to represent the gold standard. The assumption appears justified in the light of a rapidly increasing number of studies confirming the high prognostic value of FFR-guided PCI [5,6,12-14].

At a first glance, a Sn_{CMR} of 88% for ischemia detection (and of $Sn_{CMR} = 80\%$ in the sensitivity analysis) may appear relatively high. However, similar and even higher performances were reported with Sn_{CMR}/Sp_{CMR} of 82%/94% [43] and Sn_{CMR}/Sp_{CMR} of 91%/94% [44]. Importantly, it should be taken into account that these Sn_{CMR} for ischemia detection compare with an ischemia test, i.e. FFR. When lower sensitivities of CMR for ischemia detection are reported, they typically compare perfusion-CMR with coronary anatomy. FFR is generally accepted as a useful tool to guide treatment in CAD patients, as it discriminates patients at risk for complications (FFR-positive) versus those with minimal risk (FFR-negative). In FFR-positive patients, complication rates (death and non-fatal MI) were 3.2%-11.1%/y versus 0.7-7.3%/y in FFR-negative patients [5,6]. In a recent registry-based FFR study, MI in the FFR non-ischemia group was ~1%/y vs ~1.9%/y in the ischemia group [12]. For perfusion CMR, similar discriminative power was observed in approximately 1,700 patients of the EuroCMR registry, with complications rates of 2.7%/y in CMR-positive patients, i.e. in patients with ischemia, versus 0.7%/y in CMR-negative patients [24]. Thus, with this evidence of a similar discriminative power for CMR and FFR, the assumption of FFR being the gold standard, and thus, classifying CMR results differing from FFR as incorrect, might induce a bias towards an underestimation of the cost-effectiveness of the CMR + CXA strategy.

Limitations

In the four countries, the unit costs for the cardiac examinations fed into the model may vary between different geographical regions and therefore, the results are representative for the entire health care systems under study, but not for smaller geographical regions. In the current model, no treatment costs were included. Correct absence of disease was not directly included in the criterion of effectiveness but the effect was captured indirectly through the costs of complications induced by false negative results. The model does not take into account intangible costs associated with cardiac death. This is because of the third-party-payer-perspective study design. For the US context, we decided to use costs for the material and a reimbursement of the physician to represent FFR costs similar to the approach used by Fearon et al. [7] as the current US reimbursement system does not consider costs for infrastructure nor material. The sensitivity analyses showed a rather moderate effect of prices for FFR on the cost-effectiveness shifting the crossing point by ±6, ±8, ±8, and ±11 percent points for the Swiss, the German, the UK, and the US system, respectively.

Finally, the modeling approach used here implies that some simplifications are built in and the decision process to revascularize or not is reduced to the presence or absence of hemodynamically significant stenoses. It does therefore not consider the clinical background of the patient, which is always important to guide treatment. Accordingly, the presented results might be helpful for trials planning whereas the use of the presented model with real CMR and FFR data acquired in ongoing trials [11] would most likely yield more relevant results.

Conclusions

With a focus on the latest imaging techniques to detect ischemia, this study shows to what extent the cost-effectiveness of two strategies to diagnose hemodynamically significant coronary lesions, i.e. significant CAD, depends on the prevalence of the disease. The CMR + CXA strategy is more cost-effective than CXA + FFR below a CAD prevalence of 62%, 65%, 83%, and 82% for the Swiss, the German, the UK, and the US health care systems, respectively. These findings may help the decision-making with regard to resource utilization.

Abbreviations
CAD: Coronary artery disease; CMR: Cardiovascular magnetic resonance; CXA: Invasive x-ray coronary angiography; FFR: Fractional flow reserve; PCI: Percutaneous coronary interventions.

Competing interests
The authors declare that they have no competing interests.

Authors' contributions
KM is responsible for the conception and design of the cost-effectiveness analysis; she performed the cost-effectiveness analysis, participated to the data collection and drafted the manuscript. DF participated to data collection and was involved in the calculations of the cost-effectiveness analysis. CP provided advices on the cost-effectiveness analysis. GP provided precisions on how the German health care system works and actively participated in the acquisition of required data in this context. SP provided information on how the UK health care system works and participated in the data acquisition in this context. AW provided explanations on how the US health care system

works and participated in the data acquisition in this context. JBW provided explanations on how the Swiss health care system works. JS is responsible for the design of the study, participated to data collection and was involved in the interpretation of the results and drafting the manuscript; he critically revised its intellectual content. In addition, all authors provided helpful comments and relevant suggestions to improve the manuscript and its intellectual content; all authors read and approved the final manuscript.

Acknowledgements
This work forms part of the research areas of SEP contributing to the translational research portfolio of Barts Cardiovascular Biomedical Research Unit which is supported and funded by the National Institute for Health Research. This study was support by a grant of the Swiss Heart Foundation.

Author details
[1]Institute of Health Economics and Management (IEMS), University of Lausanne, Route de Chavannes 31, VIDY, 1015 Lausanne, Switzerland. [2]Technology Assessment Unit (UET), University Hospital (CHUV), Lausanne, Switzerland. [3]Klinik Agatharied, Akademisches Lehrkrankenhaus der LMU Munich, Hausham, Germany. [4]National Institute for Health Research Cardiovascular Biomedical Research Unit at Barts, Queen Mary University of London, London, UK. [5]Comprehensive Cardiology of Stamford and Greenwich, Stamford, CT 06902, USA. [6]Cardiac MR Center, University Hospital (CHUV), Lausanne, Switzerland.

References
1. Allender S, Scarborough P, O'Flaherty M, Capewell S. **Patterns of coronary heart disease mortality over the 20th century in England and Wales: Possible plateaus in the rate of decline.** BMC Public Health. 2008; 8:148.
2. Roger VL, Go AS, Lloyd-Jones DM, Benjamin EJ, Berry JD, Borden WB, Bravata DM, Dai S, Ford ES, Fox CS, Fullerton HJ, Gillespie C, Hailpern SM, Heit JA, Howard VJ, Kissela BM, Kittner SJ, Lackland DT, Lichtman JH, Lisabeth LD, Makuc DM, Marcus GM, Marelli A, Matchar DB, Moy CS, Mozaffarian D, Mussolino ME, Nichol G, Paynter NP, Soliman EZ, et al. **Heart disease and stroke statistics–2012 update: a report from the American Heart Association.** Circulation. 2012; 125:e2–220.
3. Bech GJ, De Bruyne B, Bonnier HJ, Bartunek J, Wijns W, Peels K, Heyndrickx GR, Koolen JJ, Pijls NH. **Long-term follow-up after deferral of percutaneous transluminal coronary angioplasty of intermediate stenosis on the basis of coronary pressure measurement.** J Am Coll Cardiol. 1998; 31:841–7.
4. Rieber J, Schiele TM, Koenig A, Erhard I, Segmiller T, Stempfle HU, Theisen K, Jung P, Siebert U, Klauss V. **Long-term safety of therapy stratification in patients with intermediate coronary lesions based on intracoronary pressure measurements.** Am J Cardiol. 2002; 90:1160–4.
5. Pijls NH, van Schaardenburgh P, Manoharan G, Boersma E, Bech JW, van't Veer M, Bär F, Hoorntje J, Koolen J, Wijns W, de Bruyne B. **Percutaneous coronary intervention of functionally nonsignificant stenosis: 5-year follow-up of the DEFER Study.** J Am Coll Cardiol. 2007; 49:2105–11.
6. Tonino PA, De Bruyne B, Pijls NH, Siebert U, Ikeno F, van' t Veer M, Klauss V, Manoharan G, Engstrøm T, Oldroyd KG, Ver Lee PN, MacCarthy PA, Fearon WF, FAME Study Investigators. **Fractional flow reserve versus angiography for guiding percutaneous coronary intervention.** N Engl J Med. 2009; 360:213–24.
7. Fearon WF, Bornschein B, Tonino PA, Gothe RM, Bruyne BD, Pijls NH, Siebert U, Fractional Flow Reserve Versus Angiography for Multivessel Evaluation (FAME) Study Investigators. **Economic evaluation of fractional flow reserve-guided percutaneous coronary intervention in patients with multivessel disease.** Circulation. 2010; 122:2545–50.
8. Brooks MM, Chaitman BR, Nesto RW, Hardison RM, Feit F, Gersh BJ, Krone RJ, Sako EY, Rogers WJ, Garber AJ, King SB 3rd, Davidson CJ, Ikeno F, Frye RL, BARI 2D Study Group. **Clinical and Angiographic Risk Stratification and Differential Impact on Treatment Outcomes in the Bypass Angioplasty Revascularization Investigation 2 Diabetes (BARI 2D) Trial.** Circulation. 2012; 126:2115–24.
9. Task Force on Myocardial Revascularization of the European Society of Cardiology (ESC) and the European Association for Cardio-Thoracic Surgery (EACTS), European Association for Percutaneous Cardiovascular Interventions (EAPCI), Wijns W, Kolh P, Danchin N, Di Mario C, Falk V,

Folliguet T, Garg S, Huber K, James S, Knuuti J, Lopez-Sendon J, Marco J, Menicanti L, Ostojic M, Piepoli MF, Pirlet C, Pomar JL, Reifart N, Ribichini FL, Schalij MJ, Sergeant P, Serruys PW, Silber S, Sousa Uva M, Taggart D. **Guidelines on myocardial revascularization: The Task Force on Myocardial Revascularization of the European Society of Cardiology (ESC) and the European Association for Cardio-Thoracic Surgery (EACTS).** *Eur Heart J.* 2010; 31:2501–55.

10. Task Force Members, Montalescot G, Sechtem U, Achenbach S, Andreotti F, Arden C, Budaj A, Bugiardini R, Crea F, Cuisset T, Di Mario C, Ferreira JR, Gersh BJ, Gitt AK, Hulot JS, Marx N, Opie LH, Pfisterer M, Prescott E, Ruschitzka F, Sabaté M, Senior R, Taggart DP, van der Wall EE, Vrints CJ, ESC Committee for Practice Guidelines, Zamorano JL, Achenbach S, Baumgartner H, Bax JJ, et al. **2013 ESC guidelines on the management of stable coronary artery disease: The Task Force on the management of stable coronary artery disease of the European Society of Cardiology.** *Eur Heart J.* 2013; 34:2949–3003.

11. Hussain S, Paul M, Plein S, McCann GP, Shah AM, Marber MS, Chiribiri A, Morton G, Redwood S, MacCarthy P, Schuster A, Ishida M, Westwood MA, Perera D, Nagel E. **Design and rationale of the MR-INFORM study: stress perfusion cardiovascular magnetic resonance imaging to guide the management of patients with stable coronary artery disease.** *J Cardiovasc Magn Reson.* 2012; 14:65.

12. Li J, Elrashidi MY, Flammer AJ, Lennon RJ, Bell MR, Holmes DR, Bresnahan JF, Rihal CS, Lerman LO, Lerman A. **Long-term outcomes of fractional flow reserve-guided vs. angiography-guided percutaneous coronary intervention in contemporary practice.** *Eur Heart J.* 2013; 34:1375–83.

13. De Bruyne B, Pijls NH, Kalesan B, Barbato E, Tonino PA, Piroth Z, Jagic N, Möbius-Winkler S, Rioufol G, Witt N, Kala P, MacCarthy P, Engström T, Oldroyd KG, Mavromatis K, Manoharan G, Verlee P, Frobert O, Curzen N, Johnson JB, Jüni P, Fearon WF, FAME 2 Trial Investigators. **Fractional Flow Reserve–Guided PCI versus Medical Therapy in Stable Coronary Disease.** *N Engl J Med.* 2012; 367:991–1001.

14. Bech GJ, De Bruyne B, Pijls NH, de Muinck ED, Hoorntje JC, Escaned J, Stella PR, Boersma E, Bartunek J, Koolen JJ, Wijns W. **Fractional flow reserve to determine the appropriateness of angioplasty in moderate coronary stenosis: a randomized trial.** *Circulation.* 2001; 103:2928–34.

15. Fearon WF, Tonino PA, de Bruyne B, Siebert U, Pijls NH, Investigators FS. **Rationale and design of the Fractional Flow Reserve versus Angiography for Multivessel Evaluation (FAME) study.** *Am Heart J.* 2007; 154:632–6.

16. Costa MA, Shoemaker S, Futamatsu H, Klassen C, Angiolillo DJ, Nguyen M, Siuciak A, Gilmore P, Zenni MM, Guzman L, Bass TA, Wilke N. **Quantitative magnetic resonance perfusion imaging detects anatomic and physiologic coronary artery disease as measured by coronary angiography and fractional flow reserve.** *J Am Coll Cardiol.* 2007; 50:514–22.

17. Horstkotte D, Wiemer M, van Buuren F. **Performance figures of invasive cardiology in Germany 2006 and 2007 focussing on coronary artery disease.** *Clin Res Cardiol.* 2011; 100:187–90.

18. Patel MR, Peterson ED, Dai D, Brennan JM, Redberg RF, Anderson HV, Brindis RG, Douglas PS. **Low diagnostic yield of elective coronary angiography.** *N Engl J Med.* 2010; 362:886–95.

19. Schwitter J, Wacker CM, Wilke N, Al-Saadi N, Sauer E, Huettle K, Schönberg SO, Luchner A, Strohm O, Ahlstrom H, Dill T, Hoebel N, Simor T, MR-IMPACT Investigators. **MR-IMPACT II: Magnetic Resonance Imaging for Myocardial Perfusion Assessment in Coronary artery disease Trial: perfusion-cardiac magnetic resonance vs. single-photon emission computed tomography for the detection of coronary artery disease: a comparative multicentre, multivendor trial.** *Eur Heart J.* 2012; 34:775–81.

20. Schwitter J, Wacker CM, van Rossum AC, Lombardi M, Al-Saadi N, Ahlstrom H, Dill T, Larsson HB, Flamm SD, Marquardt M, Johansson L. **MR-IMPACT: Magnetic Resonance Imaging for Myocardial Perfusion Assessment in Coronary Artery Disease Trial: Comparison of perfusion CMR with Single Photon Emission Computed Tomography for the Detection of Coronary Artery Disease in a Multicenter, Multivendor, Randomized Trial.** *Eur Heart J.* 2008; 29:480–9.

21. Plein S, Schwitter J, Suerder D, Greenwood JP, Boesiger P, Kozerke S. **k-Space and time sensitivity encoding-accelerated myocardial perfusion MR imaging at 3.0 T: comparison with 1.5 T.** *Radiology.* 2008; 249:493–500.

22. Greenwood JP, Maredia N, Younger JF, Brown JM, Nixon J, Everett CC, Bijsterveld P, Ridgway JP, Radjenovic A, Dickinson CJ, Ball SG, Plein S. **Cardiovascular magnetic resonance and single-photon emission computed tomography for diagnosis of coronary heart disease (CE-MARC): a prospective trial.** *Lancet.* 2012; 379:453–60.

23. Coelho-Filho O, Seabra L, Mongeon F, Abdullah S, Francis S, Blankstein R. **Stress Myocardial perfusion Imaging by CMR provides strong prognostic values to cardiac events regardless of patient's sex.** *JACC Cardiovasc Imaging.* 2011; 4:850–61.

24. Bruder O, Wagner A, Lombardi M, Schwitter J, van Rossum A, Pilz G, Nothnagel D, Steen H, Petersen S, Nagel E, Prasad S, Schumm J, Greulich S, Cagnolo A, Monney P, Deluigi CC, Dill T, Frank H, Sabin G, Schneider S, Mahrholdt H. **European Cardiovascular Magnetic Resonance (EuroCMR) registry–multinational results from 57 centers in 15 countries.** *J Cardiovasc Magn Reson.* 2013; 15:9.

25. Jahnke C, Nagel E, Gebker R, Kokocinski T, Kelle S, Manka R, Fleck E, Paetsch I. **Prognostic value of cardiac magnetic resonance stress tests: Adenosine stress perfusion and dobutamine stress wall motion imaging.** *Circulation.* 2007; 115:1769–76.

26. Forrester J, Diamond G, Vas R, Charuzi Y, Silverberg R, Pichler M, Berman D. **Early detection of coronary artery disease.** *Adv Cardiol.* 1979; 26:1–14.

27. Patterson RE, Eisner RL, Horowitz SF. **Comparison of cost-effectiveness and utility of exercise ECG, single photon emission computed tomography, positron emission tomography, and coronary angiography for diagnosis of coronary artery disease.** *Circulation.* 1995; 91:54–65.

28. Dorenkamp M, Bonaventura K, Sohns C, Becker CR, Leber AW. **Direct costs and cost-effectiveness of dual-source computed tomography and invasive coronary angiography in patients with an intermediate pretest likelihood for coronary artery disease.** *Heart.* 2011; 98:460–7.

29. Dewey M, Hamm B. **Cost effectiveness of coronary angiography and calcium scoring using CT and stress MRI for diagnosis of coronary artery disease.** *Eur Radiol.* 2006; 17:1301–9.

30. Boldt J, Leber AW, Bonaventura K, Sohns C, Stula M, Huppertz A, Haverkamp W, Dorenkamp M. **Cost-effectiveness of cardiovascular magnetic resonance and single-photon emission computed tomography for diagnosis of coronary artery disease in Germany.** *J Cardiovasc Magn Reson.* 2013; 15:30.

31. Rieber J, Huber A, Erhard I, Mueller S, Schweyer M, Koenig A, Schiele TM, Theisen K, Siebert U, Schoenberg SO, Reiser M, Klauss V. **Cardiac magnetic resonance perfusion imaging for the functional assessment of coronary artery disease: a comparison with coronary angiography and fractional flow reserve.** *Eur Heart J.* 2006; 27:1465–71.

32. Bruder O, Schneider S, Nothnagel D, Dill T, Hombach V, Schulz-Menger J, Nagel E, Lombardi M, van Rossum AC, Wagner A, Schwitter J, Senges J, Sabin GV, Sechtem U, Mahrholdt H. **EuroCMR (European Cardiovascular Magnetic Resonance) Registry: Results of the German Pilot Phase.** *J Am Coll Cardiol.* 2009; 54:1457–66.

33. Bruder O, Schneider S, Nothnagel D, Pilz G, Lombardi M, Sinha A, Wagner A, Dill T, Frank H, van Rossum A, Schwitter J, Nagel E, Senges J, Sabin G, Sechtem U, Mahrholdt H. **Acute Adverse Reactions to Gadolinium-Based Contrast Agents in CMR: Multicenter Experience With 17,767 Patients From the EuroCMR Registry.** *J Am Coll Cardiol - Cardiovasc Imaging.* 2011; 4:1171–6.

34. Weinstein MC, Siegel JE, Gold MR, Kamlet MS, Russell LB. **Recommendations of the Panel on Cost-effectiveness in Health and Medicine.** *JAMA.* 1996; 276:1253–8.

35. Francis S, Daly C, Heydari B, Abbasi S, Shah R, Kwong R. **Cost-effectiveness analysis for imaging techniques with a focus on cardiovascular magnetic resonance.** *J Cardiovasc Magn Reson.* 2013; 15:52.

36. *Gov.uk [internet] Department of Health, England, NHS reference costs: financial year 2011 to 2012. [Consulted 2013].* Available from https://www.gov.uk/government/publications/nhs-reference-costs-financial-year-2011-to-2012.

37. Maeder M, et al. *Swiss society of cardiology, Cardiovascular Medicine acts.* Basel; 2011. 8–10 June 2011 (abstract).

38. Moschetti K, Muzzarelli S, Pinget C, Wagner A, Pilz G, Wasserfallen JB, Schulz-Menger J, Nothnagel D, Dill T, Frank H, Lombardi M, Bruder O, Mahrholdt H, Schwitter J. **Cost evaluation of cardiovascular magnetic resonance versus coronary angiography for the diagnostic work-up of coronary artery disease: application of the European Cardiovascular Magnetic Resonance registry data to the German, United Kingdom, Swiss, and United States health care systems.** *J Cardiovasc Magn Reson.* 2012; 14:35.

39. Walker S, Girardin F, McKenna C, Ball SG, Nixon J, Plein S, Greenwood JP, Sculpher M. **Cost-effectiveness of cardiovascular magnetic resonance in the diagnosis of coronary heart disease: an economic evaluation using data from the CE-MARC study.** *Heart.* 2013; 99(12):873–81.

40. Cullen KA, Hall MJ, Golosinskiy A, Division of Health Care Statistics. *Ambulatory Surgery in the United States.* National Health Statistics Reports; 2006. 2009;Number 11.

41. Buie VC, Owings M, DeFrances C, Golosinskiy A. **National Hospital Discharge Survey: 2006 summary. U.S. DEPARTMENT OF HEALTH AND HUMAN SERVICES National Center for Health Statistics.** *Vital Health Stat.* 2010; **13:**168.

42. Bruckenberger E, Winkler P. *Herzbericht 2008 mit Transplantationschirurgie;* 2009.

43. Lockie T, Ishida M, Perera D, Chiribiri A, De Silva K, Kozerke S, Marber M, Nagel E, Rezavi R, Redwood S, Plein S. **High-resolution magnetic resonance myocardial perfusion imaging at 3.0-Tesla to detect hemodynamically significant coronary stenoses as determined by fractional flow reserve.** *J Am Coll Cardiol.* 2011; **57:**70–5.

44. Watkins S, McGeoch R, Lyne J, Steedman T, Good R, McLaughlin MJ, Cunningham T, Bezlyak V, Ford I, Dargie HJ, Oldroyd KG. **Validation of Magnetic Resonance Myocardial Perfusion Imaging With Fractional Flow Reserve for the Detection of Significant Coronary Heart Disease.** *Circulation.* 2009; **120:**2207–13.

Perfusion cardiovascular magnetic resonance and fractional flow reserve in patients with angiographic multi-vessel coronary artery disease

Shazia T. Hussain[1,9*], Amedeo Chiribiri[2], Geraint Morton[3], Nuno Bettencourt[4], Andreas Schuster[5], Matthias Paul[6], Divaka Perera[7] and Eike Nagel[8]

Abstract

Background: Perfusion cardiovascular magnetic resonance (CMR) and fractional flow reserve (FFR) are emerging as the most accurate tools for the assessment of myocardial ischemia noninvasively or in the catheter laboratory. However, there is limited data comparing CMR and FFR in patients with multi-vessel disease. This study aims to evaluate the correlation between myocardial ischemia detected by CMR with FFR in patients with multivessel coronary disease at angiography.

Methods and results: Forty-one patients (123 vascular territories) with angiographic 2- or 3-vessel coronary artery disease (visual stenosis >50 %) underwent high-resolution adenosine stress perfusion CMR at 1.5 T and FFR measurement. An FFR value of <0.75 was considered significant.

On a per patient basis, CMR and FFR detected identical ischemic territories in 19 patients (46 %) (mean number of territories 0.7+/−0.7 in both ($p = 1.0$)). On a per vessel basis, 89 out of 123 territories demonstrated concordance between the CMR and FFR results (72 %). In 34 % of the study population, CMR resulted in fewer ischemic territories than FFR; in 12 % CMR resulted in more ischemic territories than FFR. There was good concordance between the two methods to detect myocardial ischemia on a per-patient (k =0.658 95 % CI 0.383-0.933) level and moderate concordance on a per-vessel (k = 0.453 95 % CI 0.294–0.612) basis.

Conclusions: There is good concordance between perfusion CMR and FFR for the identification of myocardial ischemia in patients with multi-vessel disease. However, some discrepancy remains and at this stage it is unclear whether CMR underestimates or FFR overestimates the number of ischemic segments in multi-vessel disease.

Keywords: Ischemia, Fractional flow reserve, Coronary artery disease, Perfusion CMR

Background

Revascularization of patients with stable coronary artery disease (CAD) should be guided by functional information rather than anatomy [1, 2]. A large body of evidence for the non-invasive assessment of ischemia is based on single photon emission computed tomography (SPECT), however, especially in the last decade, cardiovascular magnetic resonance (CMR) has shown advantages such

as higher spatial resolution [3, 4] and potentially better diagnostic accuracy [5].

Guiding revascularization by fractional flow reserve (FFR) has demonstrated improved outcome in comparison to anatomy-guided strategies [6]. The accuracy of CMR and FFR for the detection of CAD has been well demonstrated and comparative studies have shown excellent diagnostic accuracy of perfusion CMR to detect functionally significant CAD identified by FFR [3, 7]. However, there are limited data on their comparability in defining ischemic segments in patients with multi-vessel disease. Detection of 3VD with non-invasive

* Correspondence: shaziathussain@icloud.com
[1]Papworth Hospital NHS trust, Papworth Everard, Papworth Everard, Cambridgeshire, UK
[9]Cardiology Department, Papworth Hospital, Papworth Everard CB23 3RE, UK
Full list of author information is available at the end of the article

imaging can be challenging due to the effects of balanced ischemia leading to false-negative results in up to 20 % of cases [8]. A comparative accuracy study done by Chung et al. [9] compared SPECT and perfusion CMR in patients with angiographically proven three vessel disease and showed that CMR detected perfusion defects in all three vascular territories in 57 % of patients vs only 11 % with SPECT. Data comparing SPECT and FFR have also shown fewer ischemic territories with SPECT than FFR in this group [10]. The low spatial resolution of SPECT may also lead to underestimation of perfusion defects [11].

It is unknown, whether the use of a high-resolution perfusion technique such as CMR leads to improved concordance for the identification of ischemic segments in multi-vessel disease in comparison with FFR. The aim of this study was to compare the extent of myocardial ischemia based on CMR and FFR in patients with angiographically defined multi-vessel disease.

Methods

The study was approved by the Kings College London (KCL) research ethics committee and all patients gave written informed consent to participate. Potential participants were identified after elective diagnostic coronary angiography and informed consent was obtained. A total of 41 patients with inclusion criteria of angina and stable 2- or 3-vessel disease designated on a visual basis by angiography (diameter stenosis >50 %) were recruited. All patients underwent FFR assessment during the subsequent PCI procedure and CMR (performed as part of the research protocol) which occurred prior (within 4 weeks) to the PCI procedure.

Exclusion criteria were contra-indications to CMR (i.e., claustrophobia, metallic implant, pacemaker), contra-indications to adenosine therapy, previous coronary artery bypass graft (CABG), left main stem disease, recent myocardial infarction (MI) within 6 months, unstable angina and left ventricular (LV) ejection fraction <30 %.

CMR image acquisition

Data were acquired with a 1.5 T scanner (Achieva, Philips, Best, The Netherlands) using 32-channel coils. Examinations included high-resolution perfusion, cine and scar imaging. Perfusion imaging consisted of 3 short axis slices acquired every heartbeat covering 16 of the standard myocardial segments (apex excluded) [12] first during adenosine stress followed by a short axis cine imaging stack and then rest perfusion imaging. Imaging parameters for perfusion imaging: kt BLAST acceleration factor 5 SSFP sequence, shortest TE (range 1.35–1.54 ms), shortest TR (range 2.64–3.12 ms), 50° flip angle; 90° prepulse, 100 ms prepulse delay and typical

acquired resolution 1.7 × 1.9 × 10 mm. 0.075 mmol of weight adjusted contrast agent (Gadobutrol/Gadovist, Bayer Healthcare, Germany) was injected at 4 ml/s by a power injector, followed by a 20 ml flush for stress imaging with adenosine infused according to a standard adenosine protocol (140 μg/kg/min for 3 min, if no response after 2 min increase to 170 μg/kg/min). There was a 10 min delay between stress and rest imaging. The cine images were completed with a set of long axis views. Late Gadolinium enhancement (LGE) images were acquired after 10 min (Gadovist 0.2 mmol/kg cumulative dose) using an inversion recovery sequence.

CMR image analysis

Perfusion CMR images were analyzed by two experienced observers blinded to the angiographic data and clinical history (AC and SH). They reported all scans with consensus; any disagreement was arbitrated by a third reader (EN). The CMR images were also graded for quality on a grading system of 1 (poor), 2(moderate) and 3 (good).

A perfusion defect was defined as reduced contrast uptake at peak stress persisting for 5 consecutive heart beats but not present at rest. Corresponding late gadolinium enhanced images were reviewed side by side with the perfusion data and enhanced myocardium was disregarded for ischemia.

Designation of vascular territories was done according to AHA 16 segment classification [13] Segments 1, 2, 7, 8, 13, and 14, were assigned to the left anterior descending coronary artery (LAD). Segments 3, 4, 9, 10, and 15 were assigned to the right coronary artery (RCA). Segments 5, 6, 11, 12, and 16 were assigned to the left circumflex artery (CX). This analysis was performed without knowledge of angiographic variation as per clinical practice.

Coronary angiography and FFR measurement

After obtaining arterial access, a standard Judkin's technique was used to obtain angiographic views. Intracoronary pressure measurements were obtained in all vessels that showed a ≥50 % diameter stenosis, assessed angiographically, using a 0.014-inch intracoronary pressure wire (Volcano Therapeutics, San Diego, CA, USA or Pressure-Wire Certus, St Jude Medical Systems AB, Uppsala, Sweden). FFR was calculated during hyperemia (intravenous adenosine infused at 140 micrograms kg/min for at least 90 s) as P_d/P_a, where P_d and P_a are distal coronary and aortic pressure respectively. In cases of serial stenoses or when there was diffuse disease, the pressure sensor was positioned beyond the most distal diseased segment and if the FFR indicated hemodynamically significant disease, this was ascribed to the most proximal lesion for the purpose of this analysis. A FFR of <0.75 was

Table 1 Pt clinical characteristics and angiographic details

Parameter	Number or mean (+/− SD)
Age (years)	62 (9)
Sex (male)	30
Body Mass Index	27.8 (4.1)
CAD risk factors (%)	
Diabetes	20.6
Hypertension	60.0
Smoking	14.3
Hypercholesterolaemia	93.3
Previous PCI	18.5
Previous myocardial infarction	4.0
Drug therapy (%)	
Aspirin	81.5
Statin	80.0
B blocker	61.3
ACE I	29.6
Angiographic details	
Vessels with FFR >0.75	72
Vessels with FFR ≤0.75	51

Abbreviations: *ACEI* angiotensin converting enzyme, *FFR* fractional flow reserve, *PCI* percutaneous intervention

considered significant. Coronary occlusions or lesions of ≥99 % were defined as FFR positive. Arteries with angiographic plaque < 50 % diameter stenosis were defined as FFR negative.

Statistical analysis

Data analysis was performed with SPSS version 20 (SPSS Inc., Chicago Illinois). Continuous variables were presented as mean ± standard deviation (SD). The k statistic

values were derived to investigate per-patient and per-vessel concordance between FFR and CMR derived evidence for ischemia (a k statistic of +1 indicating perfect agreement, 0 indicating agreement as expected by chance, and −1 indicating complete disagreement). In groups where kappa statistics could not be performed (i.e., where the value in one group was constant) concordance was assessed by percentage agreement.

A subgroup analysis according to different FFR thresholds was also performed. Where possible the kappa statistic was used, otherwise percentage agreement was used.

Results

All 41 patients (29 males, average age 62 ± 9 years) and 123 territories were included in the analysis Table 1 summarizes the clinical characteristics of the patients and the angiographic features. There was an adequate stress response during the CMR scan with a mean heart rate increase from 63 to 80 and an increase in rate pressure product from 8243 to 9889. 27 were good quality scans, 12 were moderate and 2 scans were of poor diagnostic quality Two patients had subendocardial scar, none had transmural scarring. Within the 123 arteries, there were 10 occluded vessels.

Comparison of CMR and FFR

If an angiographic cut-off of 50 % stenosis was used to define patients with multivessel disease, 34 patients had 2VD and 7 pts had 3VD (See Fig. 1).

If an angiographic cut-off of 70 % stenosis was used 7 patients had 0 vessel disease (17 %), 9 patients 1- vessel disease (22 %), 23 patients 2- vessel disease (56 %) and 2 patient 3- vessel disease (4 %).

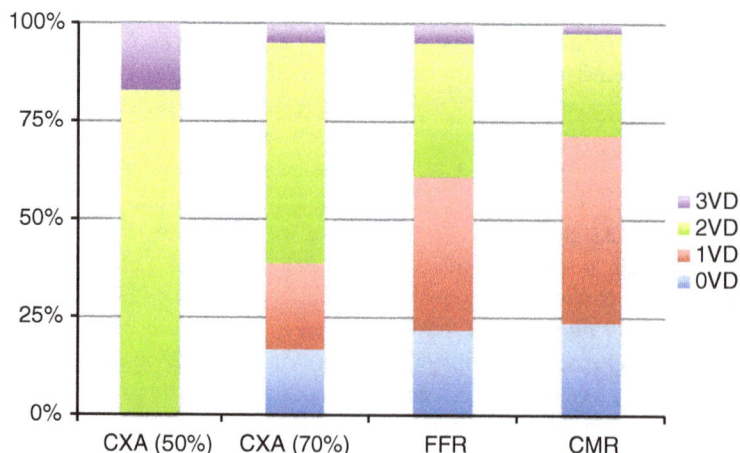

Fig. 1 Respective proportion of number of vascular abnormalities as described by Coronary angiography (based on a angiographic cut off of 50 % and 70 % stenosis), CMR and FFR (CXA = coronary x-ray angiography, CMR = cardiovascular magnetic resonance, FFR = fractional flow reserve)

CMR demonstrated no perfusion defect in 10 patients (24 %), ischemia in one territory in 20 (49 %) patients, two territories in 11 patients (27 %) and 3 territories in one patient (2 %). All cases were read with consensus between two readers with only two cases requiring a third observer.

FFR results were negative in all vessels in 9 patients (22 %), positive in 1 vessel in 16 patients (39 %), in 2 vessels in 13 patients (32 %) and 3 vessels in 3 patients (7 %).

The mean number of territories identified per patient was 1.0 ± 0.8 by CMR and 1.2 ± 0.9 by FFR.

Concordance between FFR and CMR

In 22 patients (54 %), there was complete agreement as to the number of territories of ischemia: mean number of territories 0.7 ± 0.7 for both ($p = 1.0$). Of these there was concordance in territories identified in 93 % of patients.

In 6 patients (15 %), CMR showed more ischemic territories than FFR, in 13 patients (32 %), CMR showed fewer ischemic territories than FFR (See Table 2).

The classification of 91 out of 123 territories (74 %) was identical with CMR and FFR; of the discordant territories, 21 (17 %) were CMR negative and FFR positive and 11 (9 %) CMR positive and FFR negative (See Figs. 2 and 3).

Overall, there was good concordance between the two methods on a per patient basis (k = 0.658) and a fair concordance on a per vessel basis (k = 0.433) (See Table 3).

Concordance between CMR and FFR for various FFR thresholds

Lowering the FFR threshold for FFR improves the percentage agreement for a positive FFR from 56 to 64 % (See Table 4) for result.

Discussion

Our data shows good concordance between CMR and FFR for the identification of myocardial ischemia in patients with angiographic multi-vessel disease. On a per vessel basis, 91 out of 123 territories demonstrated

Table 2 Concordance between CMR and FFR on a per patient basis according to number of significant FFR values and CMR perfusion defects

		FFR result			
		0	1	2	3
CMR result	0	7	2	0	1
	1	1	11	8	0
	2	1	3	4	2
	3	0	0	1	0

Abbreviations: *CMR* cardiovascular magnetic resonance, *FFR* fractional flow reserve

concordance between the CMR and FFR results (74 %). On a per patient basis there was complete concordance of number and localization of territories in 46 % of patients. However, for the presence of ischemia alone, there is 88 % concordance on a per patient basis.

Despite the high resolution of perfusion CMR, in one third of patients, CMR demonstrated a lower number of ischemic territories than FFR. Agreement was best at the extremes of FFR but less strong for intermediate values.

The "true" gold standard functional test

Whilst trying to understand the causes of discrepancy between the two tests, it is important to understand that neither of the tests is a true gold standard for ischemia assessment. FFR is recognized to be highly reproducible measure of ischemia [14] but also has a number of limitations. Originally, FFR was validated against a number of non-invasive imaging modalities, with a Bayesian statistical analysis. This involved a combination of all tests as the reference standard and demonstrated a sensitivity of FFR in the identification of reversible ischemia of 88 % with a specificity of 100 % in patients with single-vessel disease [15]. A meta- analysis of FFR vs QCA and non-invasive imaging by Christou et al. demonstrated less favorable results with a sensitivity and specificity of 76 % and 76 % of FFR compared with non-invasive imaging [16]. As such, discrepant results cannot be assigned to one technique or the other, but should be considered as differences.

Discrepancy between CMR and FFR results

In our study, we demonstrate underestimation by CMR or overestimation by FFR in 33 % of cases. There are four main reasons why two methods measuring the significance of a coronary stenosis may differ:

1.) They measure a different pathophysiology and as such have different definitions of a significant coronary stenosis.
2.) They use different cut-off values to determine "significance".
3.) A significant stenosis is assigned to a different coronary artery/segment.
4.) One of the two tests or both do not measure what they claim to measure.

In the current study each of the four elements contributes to the observed differences.

Pathophysiology

There are physiological differences in the measures of ischemia by the two tests that may contribute to discrepancies. Stress perfusion CMR indicates altered coronary

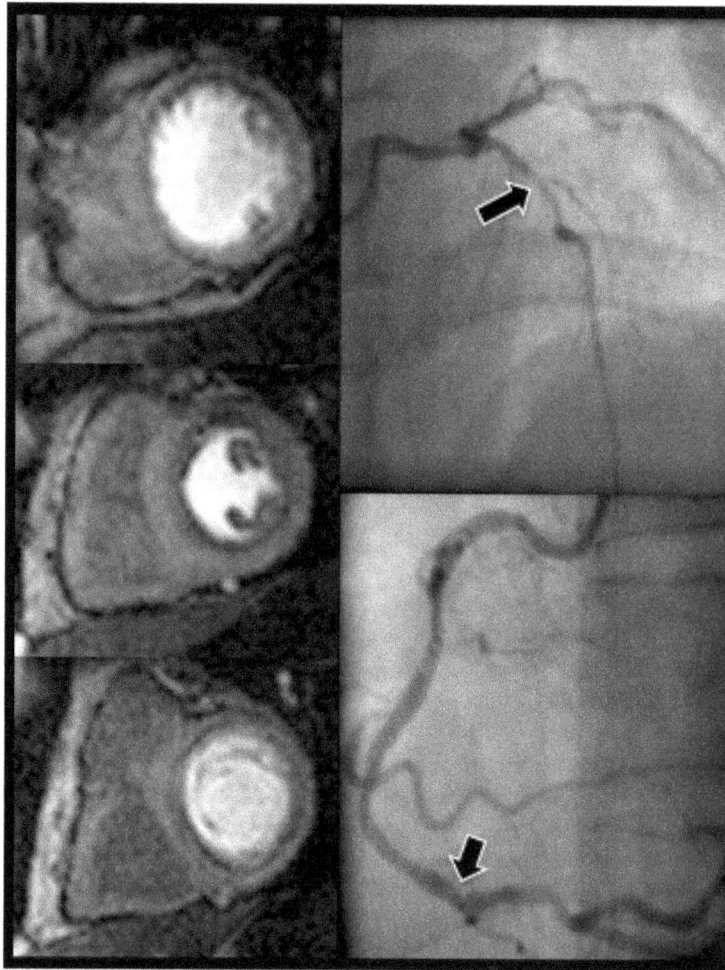

Fig. 2 Case example of concordance between FFR value and CMR. Angiographic images and corresponding perfusion images of a patient with 2-vessel disease. The LAD has a proximal stenosis (FFR value 0.63) (see *arrow*) resulting in a perfusion defect in the anterior wall visible in the apical, mid and basal ventricular slice. The RCA has a distal stenosis (FFR value 0.62) (see *arrow*) resulting in a perfusion defect in the inferior wall visible in the basal and mid slice. (Abbreviations: CMR = cardiovascular magnetic resonance, FFR = fractional flow reserve, LAD = left anterior descending artery, RCA = right coronary artery)

flow reserve (CFR) assessed by contrast delivery through the entire vasculature of the heart and FFR measures the impact of a coronary stenosis on myocardial perfusion in the territory subtended by that vessel and relies on several assumptions regarding minimal microvascular resistance, which may not be true in all cases.

The influence of the microvasculature is important both as a cause of discrepancy, and also in terms of prognosis. An assessment of this is neglected by FFR, which assumes minimal microvascular resistance, but is incorporated within stress perfusion which assesses the whole vascular compartment. In a recent study [17], patients with intermediate stenoses were assessed by both coronary flow velocity reserve and FFR and patients with a normal FFR but an abnormal coronary flow velocity reserve had a significantly higher major adverse cardiac event rate throughout 10 years of follow-up, regardless of the FFR cut-off applied. Since CMR measures perfusion on a myocardial level, it is plausible that such a discrepancy manifests as a CMR perfusion defect in the presence of a negative FFR.

Cut-off values

The sensitivity and specificity of a test can be altered by changing the cut-off value used. In the original validation studies the cut-off value for FFR was set at 0.75 [15], although subsequent studies have used a cut-off of 0.80 [18]. The different cut-off values may explain some of the variation of concordance between FFR and noninvasive imaging in the literature. A study by Melikian et al.[10] used 0.8 as the cut-off value and found poor concordance between SPECT and FFR in patients with multi-vessel disease (k = 0.14 on a per patient and k = 0.28 on a per vessel basis). A study by Ragosta et al. [19]

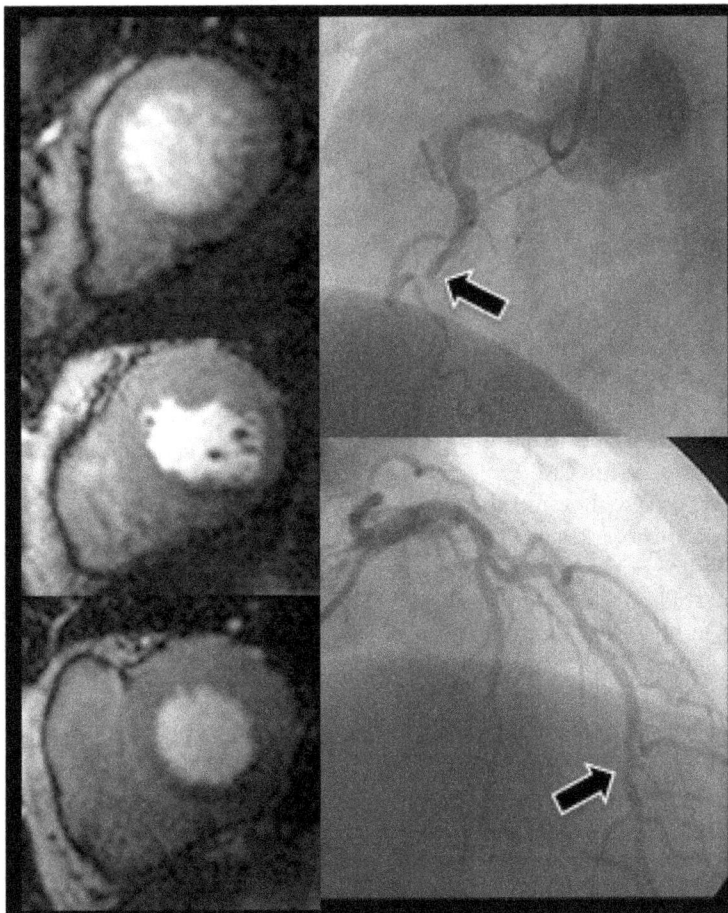

Fig. 3 Case Example of discordance between the FFR value and CMR. Angiographic images and corresponding perfusion images of a patient with 2-vessel disease. The LAD has a distal stenosis (FFR value 0.7) (arrow) with no associated perfusion defect. The RCA has a proximally occluded artery (arrow) resulting in a perfusion defect in the inferior wall visible in all three slices. The combination of a distal lesion and a mildly positive FFR value in the LAD results in no demonstrable ischemia in the anterior wall. (Abbreviations: CMR = cardiovascular magnetic resonance, FFR = fractional flow reserve, LAD = left anterior descending artery, RCA = right coronary artery)

used <0.75 as the cut-off value and found better concordance (69 %). In the current study, we demonstrate that reducing the FFR cut-off value results in improved agreement for positive results, while increasing the cut-off value results in improved agreement for negative results. The resulting accuracy is highly dependent on prevalence but the greatest disparity between FFR and CMR occurred between values of 0.7–0.8. A recent meta-analysis by Johnson et al.[20] assessing outcomes in over 9000 lesions evaluated by FFR found the optimal FFR threshold for a composite endpoint of death, MI, and revascularization at 0.67. Interestingly, the FAME 2 data [21] also showed larger benefit for PCI when FFR was <0.65 with a smaller benefit when FFR was >0.65. Whether a lower or higher threshold value is more important for clinical guidance remains unknown for the time being. There is, however, a general tendency towards less revascularization in mild ischemia making a trend towards stricter cut-off values likely.

Similarly, varying the CMR thresholds will result in a variation of concordance with FFR. Our hypothesis was that the higher spatial resolution of perfusion CMR compared to SPECT would result in a higher concordance with FFR due to a better visualization of small perfusion defects. Interestingly, in the majority of discrepant cases in our study, the stenosis with the lowest FFR was

Table 3 Per vessel and per patient concordance between CMR and FFR

CMR	FFR result			
	Per vessel		Per patient	
	>0.75	≤0.75	>0.75	≤0.75
Negative	60	21	7	3
Positive	11	31	2	29

Concordance for the detection of ischemia between CMR perfusion imaging and fractional flow reserve on a per vessel and a per patient basis
Abbreviations: *CMR* cardiovascular magnetic resonance, *FFR* fractional flow reserve

Table 4 Percentage agreement for different FFR thresholds

FFR threshold		% agreement
0.70	≤0.70	64
	>0.70	80
0.75	≤0.75	60
	>0.75	83
0.80	≤0.80	56
	>0.80	90

Abbreviations: *FFR* fractional flow reserve

identified with both techniques, while less severe FFR results were not seen with perfusion CMR. With SPECT it was suggested [19], that the stenosis with the greatest ischemia is the most evident, leading to visual neglect of subtler perfusion abnormalities. With CMR this is less likely, since perfusion defects usually show as subendocardial defects with normal epicardial perfusion. This allows assessing each coronary artery territory independent of other territories. A recent study by Motwani et al. [22] demonstrated an increase in abnormal territories identified with higher spatial resolution (29 % by standard resolution and 57 % by high resolution imaging ($p = 0.04$)) due to a better visualization of subendocardial defects. However, this may also have been influenced by a higher contrast agent dose used in the high resolution scan. Our study demonstrated concordance on a per vessel level of 74 % which is an improvement on previous studies and may reflect the advantages of higher resolution scanning.

Variable assignment of perfusion territories

Any study that compares a non-invasive with an invasive technique will be limited by the inability to define exact coronary territories by the 17 segment AHA model. Overlap of segments between the coronary arteries may lead to mis-assignment thus affecting concordance. Additionally, in 2- vessel disease, depending on the functional severity of one stenosis compared with the other, it may be difficult to separate out two small areas of ischemia from one larger more confluent area, again affecting concordance.

The majority of validation studies for both CMR and FFR have been done in a single vessel population, and our data suggests that it is difficult to extrapolate those results to apply to a more complex multivessel population. There are many physiological variables that can affect FFR measurement i.e., presence of scar, collaterals, FFR in small diameter vessels, microvascular dysfunction etc. and these are more likely to be present in patients that have extensive CAD such as our patient population. While in general FFR is normalized for the perfusion area subtended by the interrogated vessel, even a highly positive FFR in a small vessel may only lead to a small amount of myocardial ischemia not detectable by CMR.

Study limitations

The main limitation of this study is the use of qualitative visual analysis. Quantitative or semi-quantitative perfusion analyses may further improve concordance and accuracy as recently shown in a study comparing visual and semi-quantitative perfusion CMR versus invasive angiography in patients with known or suspected CAD [23]. We have used visual analysis for the identification of perfusion defects as this is more applicable to clinical practice and our goal was the determination of similarities and differences between two clinically used tests.

Conclusion

This study shows that CMR has good concordance with FFR on a per patient level for the demonstration of ischemia, making it an excellent non-invasive alternative to identify patients suitable for invasive angiography

However, some discrepancies remain in the identification of multiple perfusion defects in patients with multivessel disease. There is a general tendency for CMR to shows fewer diseased vessels than FFR. At this stage it is unclear whether CMR underestimates or FFR overestimates the number of ischemic segments in multi-vessel disease, and thus the utility in using CMR to guide revascularization in these patients remains unresolved.

Abbreviations
AHA, American Heart Association; CABG, coronary artery bypass grafting; CAD, coronary artery disease; CCS, Canadian Class Symptoms; CMR, cardiovascular magnetic resonance; CX, circumflex artery; FFR, fractional flow reserve; HR, heart rate; LAD, left anterior descending artery; LGE, late gadolinium enhancement; LV, left ventricle; MI, Myocardial infarction; PCI, percutaneous intervention; QCA, quantitative coronary angiography; RCA, right coronary artery; RPP, rate pressure product; SBP, systolic blood pressure; SD, standard deviation; SPECT, single photon emission computed tomography

Acknowledgements
The authors acknowledge financial support from the Department of Health via the National Institute for Health Research (NIHR) comprehensive Biomedical Research Centre award to Guy's & St Thomas' NHS Foundation Trust in partnership with King's College London and King's College Hospital NHS Foundation Trust.
Ethical approval for this study was gained from the KCL research and ethics committee (REC).

Authors' contribution
SH conceived the study, and participated in its design and coordination and wrote the manuscript. AC and MP participated in the design of the study and patient recruitment. NB helped with patient recruitment. GM participated in the design of the study, performed the statistical analysis and helped to revise the manuscript. AS helped with statistical analysis, result analysis and final manuscript. DP helped revise the final manuscript. EN conceived of the study, and participated in its design and coordination and helped to draft the manuscript. All authors read and approved the final manuscript.

Competing interests
Prof Nagel received significant grant support from Bayer Schering Pharma and Philips Healthcare. Dr Chiribiri receives minor grant support from Philips Healthcare. The other authors declare that they have no competing interests.

Author details

[1]Papworth Hospital NHS trust, Papworth Everard, Papworth Everard, Cambridgeshire, UK. [2]King's College London BHF Centre of Excellence, NIHR Biomedical Research Centre and Welcome Trust and EPSRC Medical Engineering Centre at Guy's and St. Thomas' NHS Foundation Trust, Division of Imaging Sciences, The Rayne Institute, London, UK. [3]Portsmouth Hospitals NHS trust, Portsmouth, UK. [4]Centro Hospitalar de Vila Nova de Gaia/Espinho, EPE, Vila Nova de Gaia, Portugal. [5]Department of Cardiology and Pulmonology and German Centre for Cardiovascular Research, Göttingen, Germany. [6]Luzerner Kantonsspital, 6000 Luzern 16, Switzerland. [7]King's College London BHF Centre of Excellence, NIHR Biomedical Research Centre at Guy's and St. Thomas' NHS Foundation Trust, Cardiovascular Division, The Rayne Institute, London, UK. [8]DZHK Centre for Cardiovascular Imaging, University Hospital Frankfurt/Main, Frankfurt/Main, Germany. [9]Cardiology Department, Papworth Hospital, Papworth Everard CB23 3RE, UK.

References

1. Hachamovitch R, Hayes SW, Friedman JD, Cohen I, Berman DS. Comparison of the short-term survival benefit associated with revascularization compared with medical therapy in patients with no prior coronary artery disease undergoing stress myocardial perfusion single photon emission computed tomography. Circulation. 2003;107:2900–7.
2. Shaw LJ, Berman DS, Maron DJ, et al. Optimal Medical Therapy With or Without Percutaneous Coronary Intervention to Reduce Ischemic Burden: Results From the Clinical Outcomes Utilizing Revascularization and Aggressive Drug Evaluation (COURAGE) Trial Nuclear Substudy. Circulation. 2008;117:1283–91.
3. Lockie T, Ishida M, Perera D, et al. High-resolution magnetic resonance myocardial perfusion imaging at 3.0-Tesla to detect hemodynamically significant coronary stenoses as determined by fractional flow reserve. J Am Coll Cardiol. 2011;57:70–5.
4. Plein S, Kozerke S, Suerder D, et al. High spatial resolution myocardial perfusion cardiac magnetic resonance for the detection of coronary artery disease. Eur Heart J. 2008;29:2148–55.
5. Greenwood JP, Maredia N, Younger JF, et al. Cardiovascular magnetic resonance and single-photon emission computed tomography for diagnosis of coronary heart disease (CE-MARC): a prospective trial. Lancet. 2012;379:453–60.
6. Tonino PA, De Bruyne B, Pijls NH, et al. Fractional flow reserve versus angiography for guiding percutaneous coronary intervention. N Engl J Med. 2009;360:213–24.
7. Watkins S, McGeoch R, Lyne J, et al. Validation of magnetic resonance myocardial perfusion imaging with fractional flow reserve for the detection of significant coronary heart disease. Circulation. 2009;120:2207–13.
8. Christian TF, Miller TD, Bailey KR, Gibbons RJ. Noninvasive identification of severe coronary artery disease using exercise tomographic thallium-201 imaging. Am J Cardiol. 1992;70:14–20.
9. Chung SY, Lee KY, Chun EJ, et al. Comparison of stress perfusion MRI and SPECT for detection of myocardial ischemia in patients with angiographically proven three-vessel coronary artery disease. AJR Am J Roentgenol. 2010;195:356–62.
10. Melikian N, De Bondt P, Tonino P, et al. Fractional flow reserve and myocardial perfusion imaging in patients with angiographic multivessel coronary artery disease. JACC Cardiovasc Interv. 2010;3:307–14.
11. Beller GA. Underestimation of coronary artery disease with SPECT perfusion imaging. J Nucl Cardiol. 2008;15:151–3.
12. Nagel E, Klein C, Paetsch I, et al. Magnetic resonance perfusion measurements for the noninvasive detection of coronary artery disease. Circulation. 2003;108:432–7.
13. Cerqueira MD, Weissman NJ, Dilsizian V, et al. Standardized myocardial segmentation and nomenclature for tomographic imaging of the heart. A statement for healthcare professionals from the Cardiac Imaging Committee of the Council on Clinical Cardiology of the American Heart Association. Int J Cardiovasc Imaging. 2002;18:539–42.
14. Bech GJ, De Bruyne B, Pijls NH, et al. Fractional flow reserve to determine the appropriateness of angioplasty in moderate coronary stenosis: a randomized trial. Circulation. 2001;103:2928–34.
15. Pijls NH, De Bruyne B, Peels K, et al. Measurement of fractional flow reserve to assess the functional severity of coronary-artery stenoses. N Engl J Med. 1996;334:1703–8.
16. Christou MA, Siontis GC, Katritsis DG, Ioannidis JP. Meta-analysis of fractional flow reserve versus quantitative coronary angiography and noninvasive imaging for evaluation of myocardial ischemia. Am J Cardiol. 2007;99:450–6.
17. van de Hoef TP, van Lavieren MA, Damman P, et al. Physiological basis and long-term clinical outcome of discordance between fractional flow reserve and coronary flow velocity reserve in coronary stenoses of intermediate severity. Circ Cardiovasc Interv. 2014;7:301–11.
18. Pijls NH, Fearon WF, Tonino PA, et al. Fractional flow reserve versus angiography for guiding percutaneous coronary intervention in patients with multivessel coronary artery disease: 2-year follow-up of the FAME (Fractional Flow Reserve Versus Angiography for Multivessel Evaluation) study. J Am Coll Cardiol. 2010;56:177–84.
19. Ragosta M, Bishop AH, Lipson LC, et al. Comparison between angiography and fractional flow reserve versus single-photon emission computed tomographic myocardial perfusion imaging for determining lesion significance in patients with multivessel coronary disease. Am J Cardiol. 2007;99:896–902.
20. Johnson NP, Toth GG, Lai D, et al. Prognostic value of fractional flow reserve: linking physiologic severity to clinical outcomes. J Am Coll Cardiol. 2014;64:1641–54.
21. De Bruyne B, Pijls NH, Kalesan B, et al. Fractional flow reserve-guided PCI versus medical therapy in stable coronary disease. N Engl J Med. 2012;367: 991–1001.
22. Motwani M, Maredia N, Fairbairn TA, Kozerke S, Greenwood JP, Plein S. Assessment of ischaemic burden in angiographic three-vessel coronary artery disease with high-resolution myocardial perfusion cardiovascular magnetic resonance imaging. European heart journal cardiovascular Imaging. 2014;15:701–8.
23. Patel AR, Antkowiak PF, Nandalur KR, et al. Assessment of Advanced Coronary Artery Disease: Advantages of Quantitative Cardiac Magnetic Resonance Perfusion Analysis. J Am Coll Cardiol. 2010;56:561–9.

A clinical combined gadobutrol bolus and slow infusion protocol enabling angiography, inversion recovery whole heart, and late gadolinium enhancement imaging in a single study

Animesh Tandon[1,2,3*] [ID], Lorraine James[1,3], Markus Henningsson[4], René M. Botnar[4,5], Amanda Potersnak[3], Gerald F. Greil[1,2,3] and Tarique Hussain[1,2,3]

Abstract

Background: The use of gadolinium contrast agents in cardiovascular magnetic resonance is well-established and serves to improve both vascular imaging as well as enable late gadolinium enhancement (LGE) imaging for tissue characterization. Currently, gadofosveset trisodium, an intravascular contrast agent, combined with a three-dimensional inversion recovery balanced steady state free precession (3D IR bSSFP) sequence, is commonly used in pediatric cardiac imaging and yields excellent vascular imaging, but cannot be used for late gadolinium enhancement. Gadofosveset use remains limited in clinical practice, and manufacture was recently halted, thus an alternative is needed to allow 3D IR bSSFP and LGE in the same study.

Methods: Here we propose a protocol to give a bolus of 0.1 mL/kg = 0.1 mmol/kg gadobutrol (GADAVIST/ GADOVIST) for time-resolved magnetic resonance angiography (MRA). Subsequently, 0.1 mmol/kg is diluted up to 5 or 7.5 mL with saline and then loaded into intravenous tubing connected to the patient. A 0.5 mL short bolus is infused, then a slow infusion is given at 0.02 or 0.03 mL/s. Image navigated (iNAV) 3D IR bSSFP imaging is initiated 45–60 s after the initiation of the infusion, with a total image acquisition time of ~5 min. If necessary, LGE imaging using phase sensitive inversion recovery reconstruction (PSIR) is performed at 10 min after the infusion is initiated.

Results: We have successfully performed the above protocol with good image quality on 10 patients with both time-resolved MRA and 3D IR bSSFP iNAV imaging. Our initial attempts to use pencil beam respiratory navigation failed due to signal labeling in the liver by the navigator. We have also performed 2D PSIR LGE successfully, with both LGE positive and LGE negative results.

Conclusion: A bolus of gadobutrol, followed later by a slow infusion, allows time-resolved MRA, 3D IR bSSFP using the iNAV navigation technique, and LGE imaging, all in a single study with a single contrast agent.

Keywords: Congenital heart disease, Gadobutrol, Time-resolved magnetic resonance angiography, Steady state magnetic resonance angiography, Late gadolinium enhancement

* Correspondence: Animesh.Tandon@UTSouthwestern.edu
[1]Department of Pediatrics, University of Texas Southwestern Medical Center, 5323 Harry Hines Blvd, Dallas 75390, Texas, USA
[2]Department of Radiology, University of Texas Southwestern Medical Center, 5323 Harry Hines Blvd, Dallas 75390, Texas, USA
Full list of author information is available at the end of the article

Background

Delineation of vascular structures is an especially important part of cardiovascular magnetic resonance (CMR) in congenital heart disease (CHD), due to the frequency of vascular lesions. Current techniques for vascular imaging in CHD are in three major groups:

- Non-contrast three-dimensional (3D), ECG and respiratory navigated, T2-prepared, fat saturated imaging with a balanced steady-state free precession readout (3D T2-prep bSSFP).
- Contrast-enhanced non-gated conventional or time-resolved magnetic resonance angiography (MRA).
- And intravascular contrast-enhanced, 3D, ECG and respiratory navigated, fat saturated imaging with an inversion recovery pulse and balanced steady-state free precession readout (3D IR bSSFP) [1, 2].

This latter technique has been shown to be superior to non-contrast 3D T2-prep bSSFP with both intravascular and extravascular contrast agents [2], and to IR gradient recovery echo sequences [3]. The use of image navigation (iNAV) as opposed to pencil beam navigation further improves the image quality [4]. Thus, the standard of care for imaging at our center was gadofosveset trisodium (ABLAVAR, Lantheus Medical Imaging, N. Billerica, MA)-enhanced 3D IR bSSFP imaging. However, due to gadofosveset trisodium's albumin binding, the kinetics are such that they preclude late gadolinium enhancement (LGE) imaging in the same study.

Gadofosveset is approved for use, but there is currently a disruption in manufacturing (August 1, 2016 (manufacturer communication)). Furthermore, clinical use of this contrast agent was not ubiquitous. Gadobenate dimeglumine (MultiHance, Bracco Diagnostic, Milano, Italy) has been shown to produce similar images as gadofosveset [5] given its partial albumin binding characteristics, but given its linear nature, there are theoretical concerns regarding a higher risk of central nervous system deposition [6] and nephrogenic systemic fibrosis (NSF) than with macrocyclic gadolinium compounds [7]. Gadobutrol (GADAVIST (Bayer Healthcare Pharmaceuticals, Whippany, NJ) or GADOVIST (Bayer Schering Pharma, Berlin, Germany)) is a macrocyclic, ionic gadolinium-containing contrast agent with no known cases of NSF and no protein-binding characteristics [7], and is FDA-approved in adult and pediatric patients (including term neonates) to detect and visualize areas with disrupted blood brain barrier and/or abnormal vascularity of the central nervous system, and for use in magnetic resonance angiography (MRA) in adult and pediatric patients (including term neonates) to evaluate known or suspected supra-aortic or renal artery disease [8]. Gadobutrol has shown equal efficacy for LGE imaging as compared to Gd-DTPA [9].

To address the current disruption of gadofosveset manufacture, we devised a method of dosing gadobutrol in order to achieve high-quality 3D IR bSSFP images while also allowing LGE imaging. Our team was inspired by Dabir et al. (2012) [10], who performed multi-dynamic first-pass MRA followed by single-phase T1-weighted 3D inversion recovery imaging with ECG triggering and respiratory navigator gating. However, they used a 3 Tesla MR scanner and a SENSE acceleration factor of 4, while our protocol used a lower SENSE acceleration factor of 2 at 1.5 Tesla. The novelty of the current study was the use of image navigated respiratory motion correction that further accelerated 3D IR bSSFP image acquisition, since a user-defined scan efficiency can be chosen prior to the scan [11]. In addition, the injector set up of this protocol allows a slow infusion protocol using a commonly available injector, without the need for a separate infusion pump; the use of the injector pump set-up was inspired by Ishida et al. (2011) [12]. The practicality of this protocol makes it easily applied in everyday practice.

Methods

Study population

Consecutive patients underdoing contrast-enhanced CMR with a clinical indication for 3D whole-heart imaging at our institution had the protocol performed. We have IRB approval for retrospective use of clinically-obtained data, and there is a waiver of consent.

Equipment setup

The CMR studies were performed on an Ingenia 1.5 Tesla scanner (Philips, Best, The Netherlands) with the 32-channel phased array digital receiver coil for signal reception. The contrast power injector was a Medrad Spectris Solaris EP (Bayer, Whippany, NJ). The intravenous (IV) tubing used was Medex 450FL 20 in., APV = 2.4 mL (Smiths Medical ASD Inc., Dublin, OH).

An IV line is placed before the examination for contrast administration. Extension tubing is connected between the end of the injector line and the IV line connected to the patient (Figs. 1 and 2 explain the overall contrast and injector use; Fig. 1a defines extension tubing set-up); either 2 pieces (if patient was under 50 kg) or 3 pieces (if patient was over 50 kg). This provides ~5 or 7.5 mL of IV tubing volume between the injector and the patient. A three-way stopcock is attached between the injector and extension tubing. Both pumps of the power injector are loaded with saline.

CMR protocol

Initial and gadobutrol bolus time-resolved MRA

Standard bSSFP cine imaging is performed at the beginning of the study (Fig. 3), followed by phase contrast

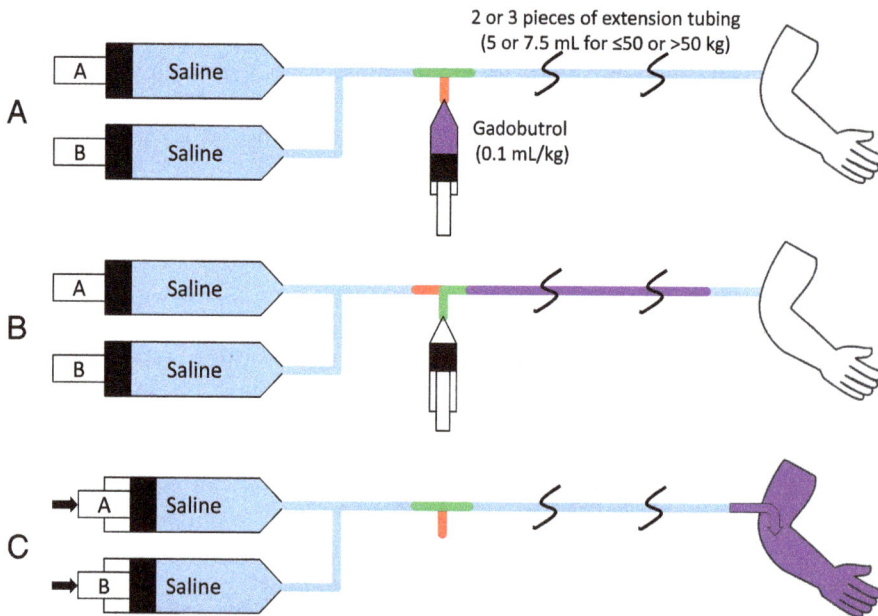

Fig. 1 Gadobutrol bolus infusion setup. **a** Intravenous (IV) extension tubing is connected between the end of the injector line and the IV connected to the patient; either 2 pieces (if patient is ≤50 kg) or 3 pieces (if patient is >50 kg). This provides 5 or 7.5 mL of IV tubing volume between the injector and the patient, respectively. A three-way stopcock is attached between the injector and extension tubing. Both pumps of the power injector are loaded with saline. **b** When the patient is ready for time-resolved MRA, the technician turns the stopcock off to the injector, and 0.1 mL/kg undiluted gadobutrol is infused into the extension tubing. The power injector is set for pump A to inject 10 mL at 2 mL/s, and pump B is set to inject 20 mL/s at 2 mL/s. The stopcock is then turned back to allow flow from injector to patient. **c** Injection is then started at the appropriate time, and thus the contrast in the tubing is injected into the patient

imaging. At the time of time-resolved MRA, undiluted gadobutrol is loaded into the tubing through the stopcock (Fig. 1b). At the appropriate time, the injection is started for time-resolved MRA. The gadobutrol in the extension tubing is thus injected into the patient. After time-resolved MRA, contrast-neutral imaging such as further phase contrast or bSSFP imaging is performed (Fig. 3).

Gadobutrol slow infusion

When the patient is ready for 3D IR bSSFP iNAV imaging, the patient is prepared for gadobutrol slow infusion, as shown in Fig. 2a. In short, diluted gadobutrol is loaded into the IV extension tubing through the stopcock. The 3D IR bSSFP iNAV sequence is set up to image for approximately 2 to 2.5 min with gating efficiency = 50 % (total imaging time 4 to 5 min). Field of view and voxel size are usually manipulated to get the correct imaging time; representative sequence parameters include repetition time/echo time (TR/TE) = 3.7/1.86 ms, flip angle = 70°, field-of-view (FOV) = 320 × 320 × 120 mm, voxel size = 1.5 × 1.5 × 1.5 mm, k space profile order was centric (low-high), SENSE factor = 2, inversion time = 220 ms (if run in systole) or 240 ms (if run in diastole) [4]. This sequence may be run in systole or diastole,

depending on clinical indication, heart rate, and duration of the quiescent phases in the cardiac cycle [13].

When the 3D IR bSSFP iNAV is ready to run, the continuous infusion is started, and then after a 45–60 s delay, the imaging is started, as detailed in Figs. 2b, c, and 3. The pump rates suggested give about 225–234 s of injection of the contrast itself, followed by flush. The imaging sequence time extends beyond the time the contrast is infusing, but the initial delay between starting the injection and starting the imaging seems to allow the gadobutrol to build to a sufficient blood level.

Late gadolinium enhancement imaging

After the 3D IR bSSFP imaging is complete, further post-contrast imaging can be performed. At 10 to 15 min after the start of the infusion, 2D phase-sensitive inversion recovery (PSIR) LGE imaging can be performed, if necessary; representative sequence parameters include repetition time/echo time (TR/TE) = 5.5/6 ms, flip angle = 25°, echo train length = 22, in-plane resolution = 1.9 × 1.9 mm, slice thickness = 8 mm.

Results

We successfully completed both time-resolved MRA and 3D IR bSSFP iNAV imaging with the above technique for 10 patients (Fig. 4) with a variety of diagnoses including: pulmonary stenosis and sinus venosus atrial septal

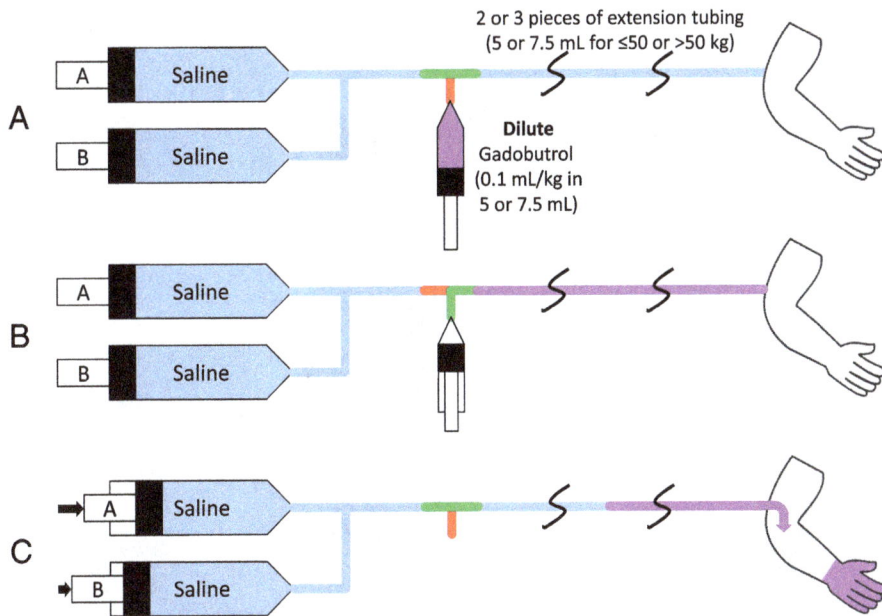

Fig. 2 Gadobutrol slow infusion setup. **a** Gadobutrol 0.1 mL/kg is diluted with saline to 5 (≤50 kg patient) or 7.5 mL (>50 kg patient). **b** When ready for 3D IR bSSFP iNAV imaging, the dilute gadobutrol is loaded into the extension tubing. The 3D IR bSSFP iNAV sequence is set up to image for approximately 4 to 5 total minutes. **c** Injector pump A is set to inject 0.5 mL at 2 mL/s, to overcome dead space/saline in the extension tubing. Injector pump B is set to inject 20 mL at 0.02 mL/s (≤50 kg patient) or 0.03 mL/s (>50 kg patient). The injection is started, and after a delay of 45–60 s, 3D IR bSSFP iNAV imaging is started

defect (ASD) status post surgical intervention (Fig. 4a, b); hypoplastic right pulmonary artery (RPA) with severe distal RPA stenosis, secundum ASD, coronary sinus septal defect (Fig. 4c, d); and bicuspid aortic valve with dilated aortic root (Fig. 4e, f). The patient age ranged from 4.7 to 29.4 years (median 11.7 years); weight ranged from 15.1 to 92.4 kg (median 29.6 kg); body surface area was 0.64 to 2.02 m^2 (median 1.10 m^2); heart rate was 60–101 beats per minute (median 79); and all patients had normal creatinine for their age (0.3–1.0 mg/dL). Our initial three

attempts used the pencil beam respiratory navigator with the 3D IR bSSFP sequence; however, all of these proved to be unusable. This is likely due to artifact generated by the navigator restore pulse labeling blood as has been described previously [14]. This likely caused a compression of the dynamic range and thus the overall image quality was degraded (Fig. 5). We have also run 2D PSIR LGE sequences as described above, with both positive and negative results (Fig. 6). Image quality for LGE was excellent in these cases.

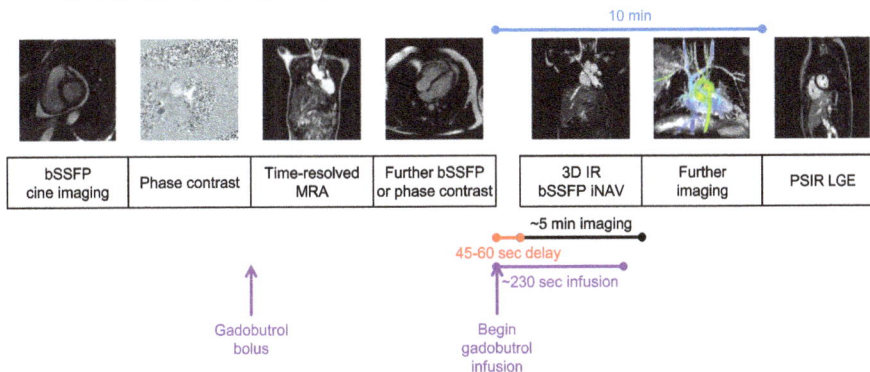

Fig. 3 Example study timeline. This diagram graphically depicts the timeline of an example study using the gadobutrol bolus and slow infusion protocol

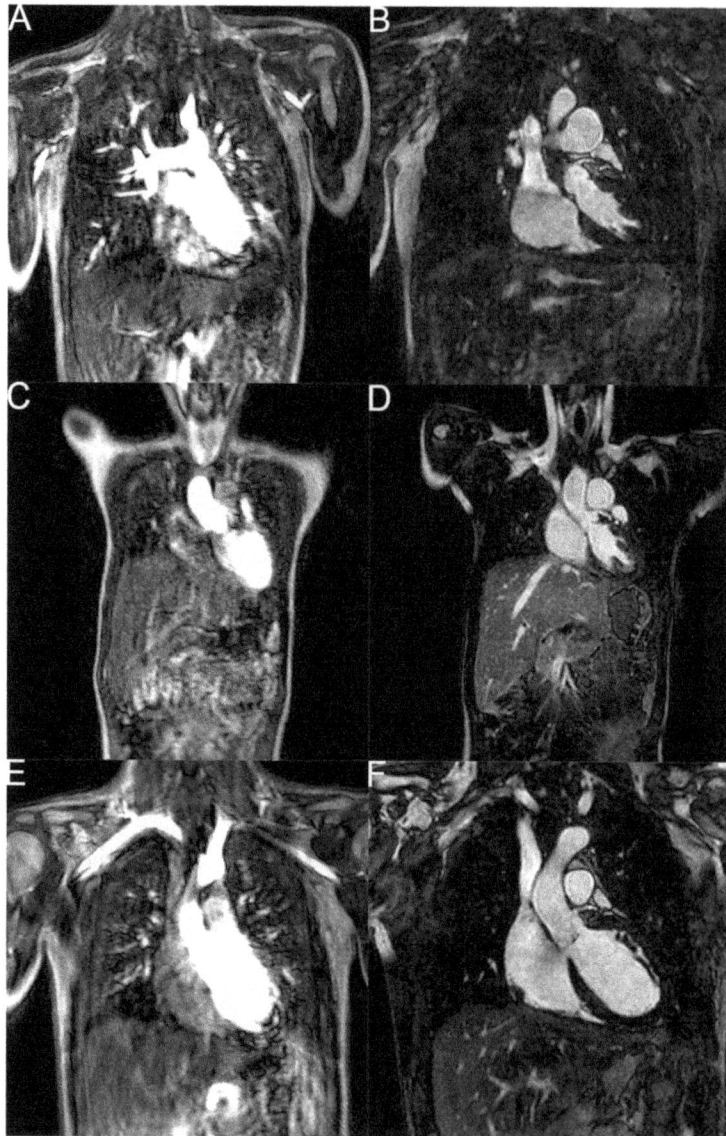

Fig. 4 Time-resolved MRA and 3D IR bSSFP iNAV example images. MRA and 3D IR bSSFP iNAV images, respectively, from (**a**, **b**) patient with pulmonary stenosis and sinus venosus atrial septal defect (ASD) status post surgical intervention; (**c**, **d**) patient with hypoplastic right pulmonary artery (RPA) with severe distal RPA stenosis, secundum ASD, coronary sinus septal defect; (**e**, **f**) patient with bicuspid aortic valve with dilated aortic root

Conclusion

Given the importance of time-resolved MRA, steady state 3D IR bSSFP, and LGE in fully evaluating patients with congenital heart disease, our protocol represents a step forward in being able to acquire all of these datasets in a single exam with a single contrast agent. The individual features of this protocol are not novel. The slow infusion, image navigator, bolus technique and late gadolinium enhancement techniques have been described [10–12]. The purpose of the protocol is to provide practical guidance on how to combine these techniques to enable acquisition of these datasets using existing injector equipment at 1.5 Tesla magnet field strength. Our choice of inversion time was influenced by our previous clinical experience, and by previous work suggesting 280 ms for gadobutrol by Dabir et al. (2012) [10]. However, unlike that study, our contrast agent could not be completely injected as a slow infusion, because a bolus injection is required for first-pass MRA. This, in turn, results in a broader variation of contrast agent concentration in the blood and so benefits from a shorter inversion time. In addition, our goal was not to completely null the myocardium, as might be desired for coronary imaging, but to have some myocardial

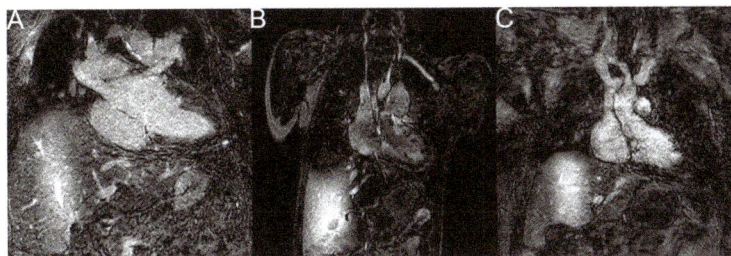

Fig. 5 Example images of 3D IR bSSFP imaging using pencil beam navigation. As can be seen in all three panels, these proved to be unusable because the navigator labeled the blood in the liver and thus the overall image quality was degraded. This is perhaps due to the high signal in the liver causing an overall compression of the dynamic range. **a** Image from a patient with d-transposition of the great arteries, ventricular septal defect (VSD), and pulmonary stenosis status post aortic root translocation and VSD closure. **b** Image from a patient with a large secundum atrial septal defect. **c** Image from a patient with trisomy 21 and common AV canal status post surgical repair

visualization to allow better identification of the anatomy in patients with congenital heart disease. We additionally confirmed our initial choice of 240 ms by running a Look-Locker immediately after the infusion. We used 220 ms for systole due to the practical need for a shorter inversion time at higher heart rates to allow systolic imaging. This protocol should be further evaluated in prospective studies to ensure that the image quality of all three image types are comparable to current standards, and to further optimize imaging parameters such as inversion time, image acquisition length compared to infusion duration, and other factors, but our subjective experience is that it delivers comparable images to gadofosveset trisodium-based 3D IR bSSFP while allowing the added advantage of LGE imaging. One potential alternative for centers that do not have access to image-based navigation techniques may be to use pencil beam navigation with a higher flip angle and the navigator restore pulse turned off. However, given that this reduces the effectiveness of navigation on the Philips platform, we did not evaluate this option. In addition, pencil-beam navigation with 3D IR GRE sequences on Siemens uses a different implementation of pulse sequences that does not require the navigator restore pulse. We would surmise, therefore, that these scanners can continue to use the conventional pencil-beam navigator without incurring the labeling artifact described above. Our correspondence with pediatric centers employing Siemens hardware supports this assumption (T. Slesnick, personal communication). Given the current disruption in gadofosveset trisodium production, the importance of this alternative protocol will be evident to CMR practitioners who care for patients with congenital heart disease.

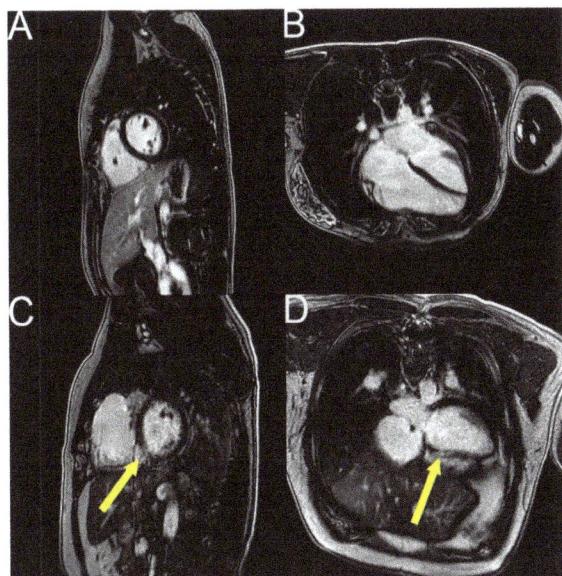

Fig. 6 Example phase sensitive inversion recovery late gadolinium enhancement images. **a, b** LGE negative short axis (**a**) and 4 chamber (**b**) images from previously mentioned patient with pulmonary stenosis and sinus venosus atrial septal defect (ASD) status post surgical intervention. **c, d** A small area of full-thickness LGE (yellow arrows) in the mid inferoseptal segment correlating to the RCA distribution is shown in short axis (**a**) and 4 chamber (**b**) images from a patient with d-transposition of the great arteries, ventricular septal defect (VSD), and pulmonary stenosis status post aortic root translocation and VSD closure, and known previous right coronary kinking status post reimplantation

Abbreviations
3D IR bSSFP: Three-dimensional inversion recovery balanced steady state free precession; ASD: Atrial septal defect; iNAV: Image navigation; IV: Intravenous; LGE: Late gadolinium enhancement; MRA: Magnetic resonance angiography; NSF: Nephrogenic systemic fibrosis; PSIR: Phase-sensitive inversion recovery; RPA: Right pulmonary artery

Acknowledgements
We would like to acknowledge the help of Dr. Tim Slesnick, Emory University/Children's Healthcare of Atlanta.

Funding
The authors acknowledge partial support from a British Heart Foundation (BHF) programme grant (RG/12/1/29262).

Authors' contributions

AT, LJ, MH, RMB, AP, GFG, and TH contributed to the development of the protocol. AT, LJ, MH, RMB, AP, GFG, and TH reviewed the manuscript and agree with its publication. All authors read and approved the final manuscript.

Authors' information

Not applicable.

Competing interests

The authors declare that they have no competing interests.

Consent for publication

The UT Southwestern IRB approved the use of images and content from this study and waived the need for consent, STU 032016–009.

Author details

[1]Department of Pediatrics, University of Texas Southwestern Medical Center, 5323 Harry Hines Blvd, Dallas 75390, Texas, USA. [2]Department of Radiology, University of Texas Southwestern Medical Center, 5323 Harry Hines Blvd, Dallas 75390, Texas, USA. [3]Pediatric Cardiology, Children's Medical Center Dallas, 1935 Medical District Dr, Dallas 75235, Texas, USA. [4]Department of Imaging and Biomedical Engineering, King's College London, London, UK. [5]Pontificia Universidad Católica de Chile, Escuela de Ingeniería, Santiago, Chile.

References

1. Fratz S, Chung T, Greil GF, Samyn MM, Taylor AM, Valsangiacomo Buechel ER, Yoo SJ, Powell AJ. Guidelines and protocols for cardiovascular magnetic resonance in children and adults with congenital heart disease: SCMR expert consensus group on congenital heart disease. J Cardiovasc Magn Reson. 2013;15:51.
2. Makowski MR, Wiethoff AJ, Uribe S, Parish V, Botnar RM, Bell A, Kiesewetter C, Beerbaum P, Jansen CH, Razavi R, et al. Congenital heart disease: cardiovascular MR imaging by using an intravascular blood pool contrast agent. Radiology. 2011;260:680–8.
3. Febbo JA, Galizia MS, Murphy IG, Popescu A, Bi X, Turin A, Collins J, Markl M, Edelman RR, Carr JC. Congenital heart disease in adults: Quantitative and qualitative evaluation of IR FLASH and IR SSFP MRA techniques using a blood pool contrast agent in the steady state and comparison to first pass MRA. Eur J Radiol. 2015;84:1921–9.
4. Henningsson M, Hussain T, Vieira MS, Greil GF, Smink J, Ensbergen GV, Beck G, Botnar RM. Whole-heart coronary MR angiography using image-based navigation for the detection of coronary anomalies in adult patients with congenital heart disease. J Magn Reson Imaging. 2016;43:947–55.
5. Camren GP, Wilson GJ, Bamra VR, Nguyen KQ, Hippe DS, Maki JH. A comparison between gadofosveset trisodium and gadobenate dimeglumine for steady state MRA of the thoracic vasculature. Biomed Res Int. 2014;2014:625614.
6. Robert P, Violas X, Grand S, Lehericy S, Idee JM, Ballet S, Corot C. Linear gadolinium-based contrast agents are associated with brain gadolinium retention in healthy rats. Invest Radiol. 2016;51:73–82.
7. Reiter T, Ritter O, Prince MR, Nordbeck P, Wanner C, Nagel E, Bauer WR. Minimizing risk of nephrogenic systemic fibrosis in cardiovascular magnetic resonance. J Cardiovasc Magn Reson. 2012;14:31.
8. Gadavist package insert [http://www.accessdata.fda.gov/drugsatfda_docs/label/2016/201277s011lbl.pdf], Accessed 29 July 2016.
9. Rudolph A, Messroghli D, von Knobelsdorff-Brenkenhoff F, Traber J, Schuler J, Wassmuth R, Schulz-Menger J. Prospective, randomized comparison of gadopentetate and gadobutrol to assess chronic myocardial infarction applying cardiovascular magnetic resonance. BMC Med Imaging. 2015;15:55.
10. Dabir D, Naehle CP, Clauberg R, Gieseke J, Schild HH, Thomas D. High-resolution motion compensated MRA in patients with congenital heart disease using extracellular contrast agent at 3 Tesla. J Cardiovasc Magn Reson. 2012;14:75.
11. Henningsson M, Koken P, Stehning C, Razavi R, Prieto C, Botnar RM. Whole-heart coronary MR angiography with 2D self-navigated image reconstruction. Magn Reson Med. 2012;67:437–45.
12. Ishida M, Schuster A, Morton G, Chiribiri A, Hussain S, Paul M, Merkle N, Steen H, Lossnitzer D, Schnackenburg B, et al. Development of a universal dual-bolus injection scheme for the quantitative assessment of myocardial perfusion cardiovascular magnetic resonance. J Cardiovasc Magn Reson. 2011;13:28.
13. Hussain T, Lossnitzer D, Bellsham-Revell H, Valverde I, Beerbaum P, Razavi R, Bell AJ, Schaeffter T, Botnar RM, Uribe SA, Greil GF. Three-dimensional dual-phase whole-heart MR imaging: clinical implications for congenital heart disease. Radiology. 2012;263:547–54.
14. Moghari MH, Peters DC, Smink J, Goepfert L, Kissinger KV, Goddu B, Hauser TH, Josephson ME, Manning WJ, Nezafat R. Pulmonary vein inflow artifact reduction for free-breathing left atrium late gadolinium enhancement. Magn Reson Med. 2011;66:180–6.

4

Infarct size following complete revascularization in patients presenting with STEMI: a comparison of immediate and staged in-hospital non-infarct related artery PCI subgroups in the CvLPRIT study

Jamal N. Khan[1], Sheraz A. Nazir[1], John P. Greenwood[2], Miles Dalby[3], Nick Curzen[4], Simon Hetherington[5], Damian J. Kelly[6], Daniel Blackman[2], Arne Ring[7], Charles Peebles[4], Joyce Wong[3], Thiagarajah Sasikaran[3], Marcus Flather[8], Howard Swanton[9], Anthony H. Gershlick[1] and Gerry P. McCann[1*]

Abstract

Background: The CvLPRIT study showed a trend for improved clinical outcomes in the complete revascularisation (CR) group in those treated with an immediate, as opposed to staged in-hospital approach in patients with multivessel coronary disease undergoing primary percutaneous intervention (PPCI). We aimed to assess infarct size and left ventricular function in patients undergoing immediate compared with staged CR for multivessel disease at PPCI.

Methods: The Cardiovascular Magnetic Resonance (CMR) substudy of CvLPRIT was a multicentre, prospective, randomized, open label, blinded endpoint trial in PPCI patients with multivessel disease. These data refer to a post-hoc analysis in 93 patients randomized to the CR arm (63 immediate, 30 staged) who completed a pre-discharge CMR scan (median 2 and 4 days respectively) after PPCI. The decision to stage non-IRA revascularization was at the discretion of the treating interventional cardiologist.

Results: Patients treated with a staged approach had more visible thrombus (26/30 vs. 31/62, $p = 0.001$), higher SYNTAX score in the IRA (9.5, 8–16 vs. 8.0, 5.5–11, $p = 0.04$) and a greater incidence of no-reflow (23.3 % vs. 1.6 % $p < 0.001$) than those treated with immediate CR. After adjustment for confounders, staged patients had larger infarct size (19.7 % [11.7–37.6] vs. 11.6 % [6.8–18.2] of LV Mass, $p = 0.012$) and lower ejection fraction (42.2 ± 10 % vs. 47.4 ± 9 %, $p = 0.019$) compared with immediate CR.

Conclusions: Of patients randomized to CR in the CMR substudy of CvLPRIT, those in whom the operator chose to stage revascularization had larger infarct size and lower ejection fraction, which persisted after adjusting for important covariates than those who underwent immediate CR. Prospective randomized trials are needed to assess whether immediate CR results in better clinical outcomes than staged CR.

Keywords: Myocardial infarction, Primary percutaneous coronary intervention, Multivessel disease, Cardiovascular magnetic resonance, Infarct size

---

* Correspondence: gpm12@le.ac.uk
[1]Department of Cardiovascular Sciences, University of Leicester and the NIHR Leicester Cardiovascular Biomedical Research Unit, University Hospitals of Leicester NHS Trust, Glenfield Hospital, Leicester, UK
Full list of author information is available at the end of the article

Background

The management of multivessel coronary artery disease in patients with ST-segment myocardial infarction at primary percutaneous coronary intervention (PPCI) is controversial (1). Registry data have suggested that a staged complete revascularization (CR) strategy results in better clinical outcomes than immediate CR at the time of PCI. However two recent randomised, controlled trials (2, 3) demonstrated reduced medium-term major adverse cardiovascular event (MACE) rates compared with infarct related artery (IRA)-only revascularization. These findings have resulted in the withdrawal of the American College of Cardiology Choosing Wisely advice of not to undertake CR at the time of PPCI (4). In addition we have shown that CR is not associated with an increase in total infarct size assessed by in-patient cardiovascular magnetic resonance (CMR), despite a small increase in type 4a MI compared to an IRA-only revascularization strategy (5).

There remains however no consensus on whether in-hospital complete revascularisation should be staged (staged CR) or undertaken immediately after PPCI (Immediate CR). In the CvLPRIT study (3), there was a trend for reduced clinical events (death/MI/heart failure) in patients who had immediate (3.1 %) rather than staged (11.9 %) CR.

The aim of this post hoc analysis of the CvLPRIT CMR substudy (5) was to assess infarct size and LV function in patients who underwent immediate compared to staged CR, in order to gain insight into the likely mechanisms to explain the differences in clinical outcomes.

Methods

Study design

The study design and main results have been published previously (3, 6). CvLPRIT CMR was a prespecified substudy of a multicenter, prospective, randomized, controlled, open- label, clinical trial with blinded CMR endpoint analysis (PROBE design) conducted in 7 UK centers between May 2011 and May 2014 (5). Inclusion and exclusion criteria were as for the main trial with absolute contraindications to CMR imaging as an additional exclusion.

Patient recruitment and treatment

After verbal assent patients were randomized after coronary angiography but before IRA PCI, to IRA-only or in-hospital complete revascularization. If there were no clinical contraindications, immediate CR was recommended but the non-IRA procedure could be staged, at the operator's discretion, but completed during the index admission. Reasons for staging revascularization were not recorded. Recruitment is shown in Fig. 1. Ninety-eight patients in the substudy were randomised to in-hospital CR, of which 63 were performed immediately and in 30 the procedure was staged. Five patients crossed over into the IRA-only treatment arm.

Angiographic analysis

Pre and post-PPCI epicardial coronary flow was assessed using Thrombolysis In Myocardial Infarction scoring (7). Collateral flow to the IRA pre-PPCI was graded using the Rentrop system (8). Quantitative Coronary Angiography (QCA) was undertaken using *QAngioXA v1.0* software (Medis, Leiden, Netherlands). Myocardium at risk was angiographically quantified using the Alberta Provincial Project for Outcome Assessment in Coronary Heart Disease (APPROACH score) (9, 10).

CMR

The CMR methods have been described in detail previously (5). In brief, CMR was performed pre-discharge and after any staged procedure and at 9 months (follow-up CMR).

Pre-discharge CMR

After localisers and long axis cine images, complete stacks of short axis images covering the entire left ventricle (LV) were acquired with (1) T2w-STIR to determine the area at risk, (2) cine images for LV volumes, mass and ejection fraction and (3) late gadolinium enhanced (LGE) images to determine infarct size and MVO after administration of 0.2 mmol/kg of Magnevist (Bayer, Leverkusen, Germany).

Follow-up CMR

Follow-up CMR was performed at 9 months (±4 weeks) post-PPCI. The protocol for follow-up CMR was similar to the pre-discharge scan, but with T2w-STIR imaging omitted and assessment of reversible ischemia with first-pass perfusion after pharmacological stress with adenosine included.

CMR analysis

Analysis was performed as previously described by physicians blinded to all clinical data including treatment allocation at the University of Leicester core lab (5). Briefly, infarct size was quantified on LGE imaging using the Full-Width Half-Maximum technique (11). On the pre-discharge CMR scan, ischaemic area-at-risk (oedema) was assessed using Otsu's Automated Technique (12) and myocardial salvage index (MSI) was calculated as the percentage of the area at risk that was not infarcted on LGE (5). If infarction was seen in >1 coronary territory in the pre-discharge CMR, this was recorded as being in the IRA territory (associated oedema and/or MVO) or the non-IRA

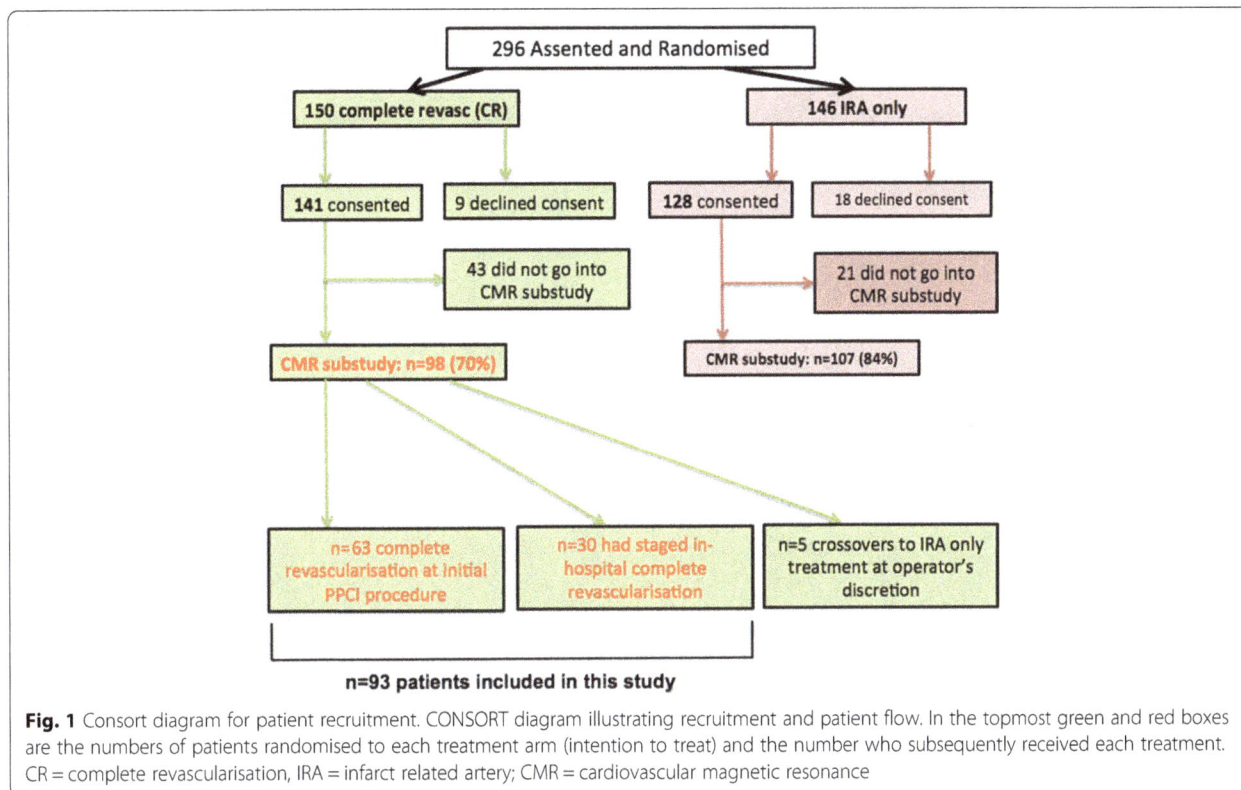

Fig. 1 Consort diagram for patient recruitment. CONSORT diagram illustrating recruitment and patient flow. In the topmost green and red boxes are the numbers of patients randomised to each treatment arm (intention to treat) and the number who subsequently received each treatment. CR = complete revascularisation, IRA = infarct related artery; CMR = cardiovascular magnetic resonance

territory with the consensus of three observers (JNK, GPM, JPG). Non-IRA infarcts were additionally classified as likely to be acute or chronic (presence of wall thinning and no oedema/MVO). Infarct size was recorded for both IRA and non-IRA LGE and total infarct size was the sum of all LGE. On the follow-up CMR, perfusion images were visually assessed for defects and reversible ischaemia burden calculated as a percentage expression of the summed difference score (13).

Clinical outcomes and follow-up

MACE comprised a composite of all-cause mortality, recurrent MI, heart failure and ischemia-driven revascularization. Secondary endpoints included cardiovascular death and individual components of the primary endpoint. Safety endpoints comprised stroke, major bleeding and contrast-induced nephropathy. Data were collected by an independent clinical trials unit (Royal Brompton Hospital, London) and events adjudicated by blinded clinicians.

Statistical analysis

The primary outcome of the CMR substudy was infarct size (expressed as % of LV mass) on pre-discharge CMR, analysed on a log-transformed scale due to right skew. This was adjusted for known baseline predictors of infarct size (anterior MI, time to revascularization, diabetes, TIMI

flow pre-PPCI) and important baseline variables that significantly differed between the two groups (TIMI flow post-PPCI, SYNTAX score, dual antiplatelet therapy choice, glycoprotein inhibitor/bivalirudin use for N-IRA PCI) using generalized mixed models. Normally distributed continuous variables were expressed as mean ± standard deviation and comparison was with student's t-tests. Non-normally distributed data were expressed as median (25th–75th quartiles) and analysed using Mann-Whitney testing. Categorical variables were compared using Chi-squared testing. Clinical outcomes were assessed using time-to-first event survival analysis (log-rank test with right censoring). Kaplan-Meier curves were plotted for the period of randomization to the occurrence of the clinical outcomes and compared using log-rank test, and Cox proportional hazard models were fitted to estimate hazard ratios and 95 % confidence intervals for treatment comparisons.

Results

Baseline characteristics

Baseline characteristics and comorbidities were closely matched in the in-hospital staged and Immediate CR subgroups and were similar to those in the overall CvLPRIT study population (Table 1). Four patients in the immediate CR group versus none in the staged group had a history of non-STEMI and previous PCI.

Table 1 Baseline characteristics of main CvLPRIT trial and immediate versus staged in-hospital complete revascularisation CMR substudy participants

Variable	CvLPRIT cohort (n = 296)	Immediate CR (n = 63)	Staged CR (n = 30)	p
Age (y)	64.9 ± 11.6	63.0 ± 11.6	65.0 ± 10.3	0.42
Male sex (%)	240/296 (81.1)	55 (87.3)	28 (93.3)	0.38
BMI (kg/m²)	27.3 (24.4–30.2)	27.7 ± 4.5	27.6 ± 4.1	0.95
Heart rate (beats per minute)	74.4 ± 17.6	71.9 ± 16.4	73.5 ± 18.0	0.68
Systolic BP (mmHg)	137.6 ± 27.1	132.6 ± 26.8	140.0 ± 27.7	0.23
Anterior infarct (%)	106 (35.6)	21 (33.3)	11 (36.7)	0.75
eGFR (ml/min/1.73)	95.74 ± 34.7	96.1 ± 30.2	101.5 ± 41.0	0.49
Hypertension (%)	105/287 (36.6)	24 (38.1)	10 (33.3)	0.66
Hypercholesterolemia (%)	75/287 (26.1)	16 (25.4)	12 (40.0)	0.15
Diabetes Mellitus (%)	39/287 (13.6)	11 (17.5)	4 (13.3)	0.61
Current smoker (%)	87/285 (30.5)	23 (36.5)	10 (33.3)	0.77
Previous MI (%)	12/287 (4.2)	4 (6.3)	0 (0.0)	0.16
Previous PCI (%)	9/287 (3.1)	4 (6.3)	0 (0.0)	0.16
Anti-anginal medication (B/N)	54/287 (18.8)	8/63 (12.7)	5/29 (17.2)	0.56
Killip Class II-III (%)	24/286 (8.4)	4 (6.3)	2 (6.7)	0.95

Abbreviations: *CR* complete revascularization, *BME* black or minority ethnicity, *BMI* body mass index, *eGFR* estimated glomerular filtration rate, *CK* creatine kinase, *MI* myocardial infarction, *PCI* percutaneous coronary intervention
Anti-anginal medication (B/N) = beta-blocker or nitrate at admission

Angiographic and PCI details

The median time to staged non-IRA PCI was 34.2 h post-PPCI (IQR 24.8–48.9). There was increased visible thrombus, subsequent thrombectomy catheter use, a higher incidence of IRA no-reflow and reduced TIMI grade post-PPCI in staged CR patients (Table 2). There was a small but significant increase in CAD complexity in the staged group (SYNTAX score 18.3 vs. 16, p = 0.021) involving the IRA (p = 0.043). The prevalence of well collateralised IRA territory and LAD IRA were similar in both groups. The angiographically derived AAR on APPROACH score was similar in the groups. Patients with right coronary artery IRA were more likely, and those with circumflex IRA less likely, to have a staged procedure. There was less glycoprotein IIb/IIIa inhibitor and bivalirudin use during the non-IRA PCI in the staged compared to the immediate CR group. When the staged and PPCI procedures were added, there was significantly increased cumulative screening time, contrast dose, number of stents (non-IRA PCI and total number of stents) and total procedure lengths in staged versus immediate CR (Table 2).

CMR data

Pre-discharge CMR

Results are displayed in Table 3. Pre-discharge CMR was undertaken later in staged CR patients than in those undergoing immediate CR (4.1 [2.7–5.4] days post PPCI vs. 2.3 days [1.7–3.2], p < 0.001). LV ejection fraction was significantly lower in staged patients. Median total infarct size was significantly greater in staged patients (19.7 % (11.7–37.6) vs. 11.6 % (6.8–18.2) LVM, p = 0.016) and this was associated with an increase in peak creatine kinase of borderline statistical significance. When corrected for important covariates, infarct size remained greater (p = 0.012). In 22 patients (24 %), area at risk could not be quantified. MSI was lower in staged CR patients and there was a greater extent of MVO (p = 0.032).

The prevalence of non-IRA territory infarcts in staged patients was almost three-fold that of the Immediate CR group (40 % vs. 14 %, p = 0.006), including when only acute non-IRA infarcts were included (30 % vs. 11 %, p = 0.024). Examples are shown in Fig. 2 and the location, size of infarct, expected coronary artery territory and additional non-IRA PCI are shown in Additional file 1: Table S1. Non-IRA territory infarcts varied considerably in size from 0.1 to 11.9 % of LV mass and averaged 3.7 % (immediate) and 2.9 % (staged) of LV mass. Two patients (3 %) in the immediate and three (10 %) in the staged CR group had chronic non-IRA infarcts (evidenced by wall thinning). Excluding these patients from the analysis did not significantly alter the results (Additional file 1: Table S2).

Follow-up CMR

Results are shown in Table 3. Fifty-three patients in the immediate group and 26 in the staged group underwent follow-up CMR. There were no differences in baseline

Table 2 Periprocedural details in the immediate and staged in-hospital complete revascularisation groups

Variable	Immediate CR ($n = 63$)	Staged CR ($n = 30$)	p
Symptom to PCI time (min)	180 (128–307)	203 (152–296)	0.95
Radial access (%)	50 (80.6)	27 (90.0)	0.26
Aspirin	62 (98.4)	30 (100)	0.49
Second antiplatelet agent (n, %)	63 (100)	30 (100)	1.00
GPI during PPCI (n, %)	20 (31.7)	11/29 (37.9)	0.56
Bivalirudin during PPCI (n, %)	32 (53.3)	17/27 (63.0)	0.40
Infarct related artery:			
Left Anterior Descending (n, %)	20 (31.7)	11 (36.7)	0.64
Right Coronary (n, %)	24 (38.1)	19 (63.3)	0.022
Circumflex (n, %)	19 (30.2)	0 (0)	0.001
Visible thrombus (n, %)	31/62 (50.0)	26/30 (86.7)	0.001
Thrombectomy catheter (%)	39/63 (61.9)	26/30 (86.7)	0.015
Vessels with ≥75 % stenosis (n)	1.5 ± 0.6	1.6 ± 0.6	0.82
Stenosis in non-IRA lesions (%)	73.4	72.9	0.85
SYNTAX score (total)	16 (12–21.5)	18.3 (15–26)	0.021
SYNTAX score (IRA)	8 (5.5–11)	9.5 (8–16)	0.043
SYNTAX score (NIRAs)	6 (4–9)	7 (4.8–12)	0.24
Rentrop grade	0 (0–1)	1 (0–1)	0.35
Rentrop grade 2–3 pre PCI (n, %)	7/63 (11.1)	3/30 (10.0)	0.87
APPROACH area at risk (%)	26.0 ± 11.7	29.2 ± 10.8	0.21
TIMI grade pre PCI	0 (0–1)	0 (0–0)	0.47
TIMI grade post PCI	3 (3–3), 2.92 ± 0.4	3 (3–3), 2.77 ± 0.5	0.023
IRA no-reflow (n, %)	1 (1.6)	7 (23.3)	<0.001
GPI at NIRA PCI (n, %)	20 (31.7)	4 (7.7)	0.06
Bivalirudin during NIRA PCI (n, %)	32/60 (53.3)	3/28 (10.7)	<0.001
GPI or Bivalirudin at NIRA PCI (n, %)	50/60 (87.7)	7/28 (25.0)	<0.001
Total Contrast dose (ml)	295 (213–350)	390 (266–555)	0.002
Total Screening time (min)	15.5 (12–21)	21 (17–43.3)	0.001
Total Procedure length (IRA + NIRA, min)	58 (38.5–72.8)	91 (67–154.3)	<0.001
IRA PCI procedure length (min)	53 (35–70.5)	55 (37.5–81.3)	0.08
Total number of stents (n)	2.8 ± 1.1	3.4 ± 1.4	0.034
Number of stents in IRA (n)	1.3 ± 0.6	1.6 ± 0.8	0.09
Number of stents in NIRAs (n)	1.5 ± 0.8	1.8 ± 1.0	0.026

Data presented as n/N (%), mean ± SD or median (IQR)

Abbreviations: *CR* complete revascularization, *IRA* infarct related artery, *PCI* percutaneous coronary intervention, *GPI* glycoprotein IIa/IIIb inhibitor, *QCA* quantitative coronary angiography, *TIMI* thrombolysis in myocardial infarction

characteristics or pre-discharge CMR findings between those who did and did not attend the follow-up CMR (data not shown). Total infarct size remained greater in staged CR patients (13.5 % vs. 5.7 %, $p = 0.004$, corrected $p = 0.044$). Reversible perfusion defects were seen in 20 % of the immediate and 27 % of the staged patients but the overall ischemic burden was small (2.6 ± 6.9 and 5.2 ± 12.1 % respectively) and not significantly different between groups.

Clinical outcomes

Discharge medication was similar between groups (Additional file 1: Table S3). Median follow-up was 365 days (immediate CR 365 days, staged CR 361 days, $p = 0.75$). Length of inpatient stay was longer in staged CR (4.2 ± 3.2 vs. 3.1 ± 1.9, $p = 0.002$) compared to immediate CR. The overall MACE rate was low (6.5 %) at 1 year. The incidence of in-hospital clinical

Table 3 Peak creatine kinase and pre-discharge and follow-up CMR data

Variable	Immediate CR (n = 63)	Staged CR (n = 30)	p
Peak CK (IU/L)	939 (627–1567)	1508 (938–2280)	0.05
Pre-discharge CMR			
Total Infarct Size (% LVM)	11.6 (6.8–18.2) 13.5 ± 11.4	19.7 (11.7–37.6) 22.6 ± 14.5	0.016 (0.012)*
Time from PPCI (days)	2.3 (1.7–3.2)	4.1 (2.7–5.4)	<0.001
Infarct on LGE (%)	60 (95.2)	30 (100)	0.22
Patients with >1 acute infarct	7 (11.1)	9 (30.0)	0.024
IRA Infarct size (% LVM)	11.1 (5.4–17.4) 12.5 ± 10.0	19.1 (8.8–35.2) 20.9 ± 14.6	0.039 (0.05)*
Non-IRA Infarct size (% LVM)	0.9 ± 3.2	1.7 ± 3.6	0.11 (0.65)*
Total acute infarcts (% LVM)	11.6 (6.8–17.6) 13.0 ± 10.3	19.1 (10.2–37.1) 21.7 ± 14.8	0.006 (0.025)*
Area at risk (% LVM)	31.4 ± 12.5	33.1 ± 10.8	0.57
MSI§ (%)	61.7 (37.4–75.5)	35.1 (5.9–66.4)	0.008 (0.034)*
MVO present (n %)	34/63 (54.0)	21/30 (70.0)	0.14
MVO (% LVM)	0.07 (0.00–0.93)	0.44 (0.00–6.1)	0.032 (0.024)*
LVMI (g/m2)	52.5 (47.7–61.0)	51.5 (45.6–63.0)	0.55
LVEDVI (ml/m2)	89.9 (78.4–110.0)	89.7 (82.8–102.9)	0.43
LVEF (%)	47.4 ± 9.4	42.2 ± 10.2	0.019
Follow-up CMR	n = 53	n = 26	
LVMI (g/m2)	45.2 (38.8–52.3)	47.4 (40.9–51.6)	0.71
LVEDVI (ml/m2)	92.5 (80.5–105.5)	93.9 (83.3–113.6)	0.28
LVEF (%)	50.9 ± 9.4	46.7 ± 8.9	0.06
Infarct on LGE (n,%)	51 (96.2)	26 (100)	0.32
Patients with >1 infarct (%)	9 (17.0)	9 (34.6)	0.08
IS (% LVM)	5.7 (2.4–10.4)	13.5 (4.6–23.3)	0.004 (0.044)*

Data presented as n/N (%), mean ± SD or median (IQR)

Abbreviations: CR complete revascularization, IRA infarct related artery, LVMI left ventricular mass index, LVEDVI left ventricular end-diastolic volume index, LVEF left ventricular ejection fraction, LGE late gadolinium enhancement, IS infarct size, MVO microvascular obstruction, MSI myocardial salvage index

§Analyzable oedema imaging available in 76 % of patients in both groups

*Adjusted for known predictors of IS (anterior MI, time to revascularization, diabetes, TIMI flow pre-PPCI) and important baseline variables significantly varying between the two groups (TIMI flow post-PPCI, SYNTAX score, dual antiplatelet therapy choice, glycoprotein inhibitor/bivalirudin use for N-IRA PCI)

events, overall MACE and individual components were similar in the treatment arms (Additional file 1: Table S4), apart from a higher frequency of major bleeds in staged CR (10.0 % vs. 0.0 %, p = 0.011).

Discussion

This post hoc analysis of patients in the CvLPRIT CMR substudy is the first report of infarct size following immediate and staged CR for multivessel disease at PPCI. We have shown that patients in the CvLPRIT study who were randomized to CR, and in whom experienced interventional cardiologists chose to stage non-IRA PCI, had more visible IRA thrombus, slightly but significantly higher SYNTAX score, lower TIMI scores and more no-flow after PPCI. These differences in baseline angiographic and PPCI results were associated with larger infarcts, less myocardial salvage and reduced ejection fraction compared to patients who had immediate CR. It is important to highlight that patients in this analysis were not randomized to immediate or staged CR and there were many differences in baseline characteristics between the groups. Therefore, despite adjusting for known baseline predictors of infarct size and other variables that significantly differed between the two groups, the results are still likely to suffer from unknown biases and we cannot conclude that staging results in larger

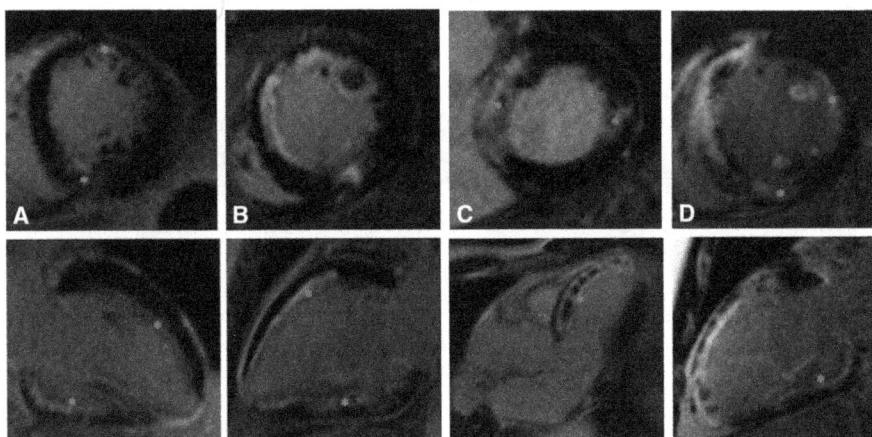

Fig. 2 Examples of patients with >1 'acute' MI on CMR. Late gadolinium enhanced short axis (*top row*) and long axis (*bottom row*). * IRA-related infarct; * NIRA-related infarct(s). **a** (X511 Immediate CR): IRA (RCA) inferior infarct 19.1 % LVM, NIRA (LAD) anterior infarct 3.8 % LVM, total IS 22.9 % LVM. **b** (X695 Immediate CR): IRA (RCA) inferior infarct 7.8 % LVM, NIRA (LAD) anteroseptal infarct 5.0 % LVM, total IS 12.8 % LVM. **c** (X757 Staged CR): IRA (LAD) anteroseptal infarct 20.8 % LVM, NIRA (LCX) lateral infarct 0.6 % LVM, total IS 21.4 % LVM. **d** (X798 Staged CR): 3 acute infarcts, IRA (LAD) anteroseptal infarct 35 % LVM, NIRA-1 (RCA) inferior infarct 0.7 % LVM, NIRA-2 (LCX) lateral infarct 2.0 % LVM, total IS 37.6 % LVM. IRA infarct size and non-IRA PCI in Additional file 1: Table S1

infarcts than immediate CR. These data can therefore be considered hypothesis-generating only, but warrant further investigation in larger studies.

Infarct size, MVO and myocardial salvage

The lower total infarct size and MVO extent, higher MSI and LV ejection fraction observed with immediate CR may be due to a number of possible factors. There could be real differences arising from treatment strategies; the staged group may have been having larger infarcts and thirdly the decision to stage the procedure, at least in some cases, may have been as a direct result of poor technical success e.g. no-reflow of the IRA. We think it is unlikely that staged patients were having larger infarcts at baseline as the time to presentation, proportion having anterior MI, degree of collateralization of the IRA and Killip Class were not significantly different from the immediate CR group and adjusting for these variables did not significantly alter the results. In addition, the ischaemic area at risk was not significantly different in the two groups. This was the case both when quantified on CMR and on the angiographically derived APPROACH score, which would negate any effect of differing CMR timing. A significant effect of ischemic preconditioning is also unlikely given the low prevalence of anti-anginal medication use in both groups (14).

Immediate CR to non-IRA's could theoretically reduce infarct size by increasing collateral flow or by improved blood flow to the watershed region of the infarct (15). The severity of the non-IRA lesions (average stenosis diameter 73 % in both groups) also indicates that these were likely to have been flow-limiting stenoses. In support of a real effect of immediate CR is the increase in MSI compared to staged patients.

However, and most importantly, differences in angiographic and PPCI results most likely explain the reductions in MSI and increased infarct size in the staged v immediate CR groups. The staged group had significantly more visible thrombus in the IRA (87 % v 50 %), subsequent thrombectomy catheter use and significantly more no-reflow (23 % v 2 %) than the immediate CR group. These factors are likely to be the main reason for the increase in infarct size, reduced salvage and decreased ejection fraction. We did not prospectively record the operators' reasons for staging the non-IRA procedures in staged patients but we think it is likely that a suboptimal result from the PPCI and the presence of inferior rather than lateral MI influenced the decision to stage the non-IRA PCI.

Non-IRA MI

A surprising finding in this study was that the frequency of non-IRA MI detected by CMR was considerably higher in the staged versus immediate CR groups. PCI related MI (type 4a) are well recognized, (16, 17) although of uncertain clinical significance. In elective PCI patients up to 29 % (18) will have significant increases in troponin and a similar proportion of patients undergoing complex PCI will have evidence of type 4a MI on CMR, even when pre-treated with clopidogrel for >24 h and a glycoprotein IIb/IIIa inhibitor periprocedurally (18). Excluding those patients with evidence of chronic infarction, acute non-IRA MI was seen in 30 % of the staged and only 11 % of the immediate CR groups. Although these type 4a MI were relatively infrequent and small (3.7 and 2.8 % of LV mass for immediate and staged patients respectively) there was considerable variation in size. Revascularization related injury accounting for 4 % of LV mass has been associated with a three-fold increase in MACE (19). Larger randomized studies are required to confirm whether staging CR results in more frequent non-IRA MI and poorer outcomes than immediate CR.

The explanation for the increase in type 4a MI seen with staged CR is likely to be related to greater number of stents implanted in the non-IRA of the staged patients and possibly the different use of adjunctive medication at the time of the non-IRA PCI. Glycoprotein IIb/IIIa inhibitor (8 %) and bivalirudin (11 %) use was low in the staged procedures compared to the immediate CR group (32 and 53 % respectively), which probably reflects clinicians concerns about bleeding with a second in-patient procedure requiring additional vascular access.

Clinical outcomes

The clinical event rate in both groups was similar (immediate 6.3 % and staged 6.7 %) and lower than seen in the main trial for those randomized to CR (10 %). The lack of other significant differences between the two groups in this post-hoc analysis with small numbers mean no conclusions can be drawn. Immediate CR was associated with a shorter inpatient stay of one night compared with staged CR. This finding and the reduction in lab time with second procedures may suggest that an immediate CR is likely to be more cost effective than a staged strategy (20). However these findings could simply be related to the fact the staged patients had larger MI and although cost-effectiveness will be assessed in the entire CVLPRIT population, any differences between staged and immediate CR would have to be confirmed in randomized trials comparing these strategies. The increased frequency of major bleeds with staged CR is likely secondary to the need for two separate procedures and hence two arterial punctures. However, due to the small numbers, this should be confirmed in a larger study.

This is a post-hoc analysis and patients were not randomised to immediate or staged CR. We did not systematically record the reasons for staging the procedure or use of adjunctive medication, which is a significant limitation. The marked differences in angiographic appearances at baseline, and success following PPCI, are likely to contribute to the observed differences in infarct size between the immediate and staged CR groups. However statistical significance persisted after correction for important baseline covariates. Due to the small numbers of patients in this analysis, propensity matching was not possible. The study was not powered for clinical outcomes. Inevitably, patients who died early or who were very ill following PPCI could not participate in the CMR study which likely explains why the clinical event rates are lower than in the main study. The pre-discharge CMR was undertaken later in staged patients (day 4), which is likely to have resulted in a decrease in infarct size and MVO extent compared with scanning at day 2 (21). Hence, the observed differences in CMR outcomes in immediate and staged CR may have been even greater if both groups were scanned at the same timepoint. However, it was important that the CMR was performed after the staged non-IRA procedures to ensure that we captured associated type 4a MI in our results. Finally, as it was not routinely captured, we could not confirm whether the higher incidence of no-reflow in the staged patients was reflected in less ST-segment elevation resolution post PPCI.

Conclusions

Patients with staged CR in the CvLPRIT CMR substudy had more visible thrombus in the IRA, higher SYNTAX score, more stents inserted, higher incidence of no-flow and subsequently larger infarct size and reduced ejection fraction, that persisted after correction for important confounders, than patients treated with immediate CR. Prospective randomized trials are needed to assess whether immediate CR results in better clinical outcomes than staged CR.

Abbreviations

AAR: Area-at-risk; CMR: Cardiovascular magnetic resonance; CR: Complete revascularisation; CvLPRIT: Complete versus Lesion-only Primary PCI Trial; IRA: Infarct related artery; LGE: Late gadolinium enhanced; LV: Left ventricular; MSI: Myocardial salvage index; PPCI: Primary percutaneous coronary intervention; STEMI: ST-Segment elevation myocardial infarction; TIMI: Thrombolysis in myocardial infarction

Acknowledgments

GPM is funded by a NIHR research fellowship. The views expressed in this publication are those of the author(s) and not necessarily those of the NHS, the National Institute for Health Research or the Department of Health.

Funding

The CvLPRIT-CMR substudy was funded by the Medical Research Council and managed by the National Institute for Health Research (NIHR) Efficacy and Mechanism Evaluation programme (10-27-01). The main CvLPRIT trial was funded by the British Heart Foundation (SP/10/001), supported by NIHR Comprehensive Local Research Networks.

Authors' contributions

JNK, GPM and AHG conceived the idea for this substudy. JNK, GPM, SAN, JPG, JW and CP supervised CMR scans. JNK performed CMR and QCA analyses (under supervision of GPM and AHG respectively). JNK performed the statistical analysis and wrote the paper that was revised by GPM. All authors critically reviewed the manuscript for intellectual content.

Authors' information

Affiliations, qualifications and email addresses of all authors are on the title page.

Competing interests

There are no relevant conflicts of interests for any of the authors.

Consent for publication

There is no identifiable patient data in this manuscript. All authors give consent for publication.

Author details

[1]Department of Cardiovascular Sciences, University of Leicester and the NIHR Leicester Cardiovascular Biomedical Research Unit, University Hospitals of Leicester NHS Trust, Glenfield Hospital, Leicester, UK. [2]Multidisciplinary Cardiovascular Research Centre and The Division of Cardiovascular and Diabetes Research, Leeds Institute of Cardiovascular and Metabolic Medicine, University of Leeds, Leeds, UK. [3]Harefield Hospital, Royal Brompton and Harefield Foundation Trust, NIHR Cardiovascular Biomedical Research Unit, Middlesex, UK. [4]University Hospital Southampton NHS Foundation Trust and University of Southampton, Southampton, UK. [5]Kettering General Hospital, Kettering NN16 8UZ, UK. [6]Royal Derby Hospital, Derby, UK. [7]Leicester Clinical Trials Unit, University of Leicester, UK and Department of Mathematical Statistics and Actuarial Science, University of Leicester, University of the Free State, Bloemfontein, South Africa. [8]Norfolk and Norwich University Hospitals NHS Foundation Trust and Norwich Medical School, University of East Anglia, Norwich, UK. [9]The Heart Hospital, University College London Hospitals, London, UK.

References

1. Sorajja P, Gersh BJ, Cox DA, et al. Impact of multivessel disease on reperfusion success and clinical outcomes in patients undergoing primary percutaneous coronary intervention for acute myocardial infarction. Eur Heart J. 2007;28:1709–16.
2. Wald DS, Morris JK, Wald NJ, et al. Randomized trial of preventive angioplasty in myocardial infarction. N Engl J Med. 2013;369:1115–23.
3. Gershlick AH, Khan JN, Kelly DJ, et al. Randomized trial of complete versus lesion-only revascularization in patients undergoing primary percutaneous coronary intervention for STEMI and multivessel disease: the CvLPRIT trial. J Am Coll Cardiol. 2015;65:963–72.
4. Cardiology TACo. Choosing Wisely. Five Things Physicians and Patients Should Question. The American Board of Internal Medicine. 2014. Website (http://www.acc.org/about-acc/press-releases/2014/09/18/15/28/choosing-wisely-statement?w_nav=S).
5. McCann GP, Khan JN, Greenwood JP et al. The Randomised Complete Versus Lesion-only PRimary PCI Trial: Cardiovascular MRI Substudy (CVLPRIT-CMR) JACC 2015;66:2713–2724.
6. Kelly DJ, McCann GP, Blackman D, et al. Complete Versus culprit-Lesion only PRimary PCI Trial (CVLPRIT): a multicentre trial testing management strategies when multivessel disease is detected at the time of primary PCI: rationale and design. Euro Intervent j Eur PCR collab Working Group Intervent Cardiol Eur Soc Cardiol. 2013;8:1190–8.
7. The Thrombolysis in Myocardial Infarction (TIMI) trial. Phase I findings. TIMI Study Group. The New England journal of medicine 1985;312:932–6.
8. Rentrop KP, Cohen M, Blanke H, Phillips RA. Changes in collateral channel filling immediately after controlled coronary artery occlusion by an angioplasty balloon in human subjects. J Am Coll Cardiol. 1985;5:587–92.
9. Graham MM, Faris PD, Ghali WA, et al. Validation of three myocardial jeopardy scores in a population-based cardiac catheterization cohort. Am Heart J. 2001;142:254–61.
10. Ortiz-Perez JT, Meyers SN, Lee DC, et al. Angiographic estimates of myocardium at risk during acute myocardial infarction: validation study using cardiac magnetic resonance imaging. Eur Heart J. 2007;28:1750–8.
11. Amado LC, Gerber BL, Gupta SN, et al. Accurate and objective infarct sizing by contrast-enhanced magnetic resonance imaging in a canine myocardial infarction model. JACC. 2004;44:2383–9.
12. Sjogren J, Ubachs JF, Engblom H, Carlsson M, Arheden H, Heiberg E. Semi-automatic segmentation of myocardium at risk in T2-weighted cardiovascular magnetic resonance. JCMR. 2012;14:10.
13. Hussain ST, Paul M, Plein S, et al. Design and rationale of the MR-INFORM study: stress perfusion cardiovascular magnetic resonance imaging to guide the management of patients with stable coronary artery disease. JCMR. 2012;14:65.
14. Reiter R, Henry TD, Traverse JH. Preinfarction angina reduces infarct size in ST-elevation myocardial infarction treated with percutaneous coronary intervention. Circ Cardiovasc Interv. 2013;6:52–8.
15. Selvanayagam JB, Cheng aSH, Jerosch-Herold M, et al. Effect of Distal Embolization on Myocardial Perfusion Reserve After Percutaneous Coronary Intervention: A Quantitative Magnetic Resonance Perfusion Study. Circulation. 2007;116:1458–64.
16. Prasad A, Rihal CS, Lennon RJ, Singh M, Jaffe AS, Holmes DR. Significance of periprocedural myonecrosis on outcomes after percutaneous coronary intervention: an analysis of preintervention and postintervention troponin T levels in 5487 patients. Circ Cardiovasc Interv. 2008;1:10–9.
17. Thygesen K, Alpert JS, White HD. Universal definition of myocardial infarction. Eur Heart J. 2007;28:2525–38.
18. Selvanayagam JB, Porto I, Channon K, et al. Troponin elevation after percutaneous coronary intervention directly represents the extent of irreversible myocardial injury: insights from cardiovascular magnetic resonance imaging. Circulation. 2005;111:1027–32.
19. Rahimi K, Banning AP, Cheng AS, et al. Prognostic value of coronary revascularisation-related myocardial injury: a cardiac magnetic resonance imaging study. Heart. 2009;95:1937–43.
20. DOH. Department of Health Reference Costs 2013–14. Department of Health Publications 2014:1–125 (Website: Febuary 2014, Accessed: June 2015).
21. Mather AN, Fairbairn TA, Artis NJ, Greenwood JP, Plein S. Timing of Cardiovascular MR Imaging after Acute Myocardial Infarction : Effect on Estimates of Infarct Characteristics and Prediction of Late Ventricular Remodeling. Radiology. 2011;261:116–26.

5

Local coronary wall eccentricity and endothelial function are closely related in patients with atherosclerotic coronary artery disease

Allison G. Hays[1*], Micaela Iantorno[1], Michael Schär[2], Monica Mukherjee[1], Matthias Stuber[2,3], Gary Gerstenblith[1] and Robert G. Weiss[1,2]

Abstract

Background: Coronary endothelial function (CEF) in patients with coronary artery disease (CAD) varies among coronary segments in a given patient. Because both coronary vessel wall eccentricity and coronary endothelial dysfunction are predictors of adverse outcomes, we hypothesized that local coronary endothelial dysfunction is associated with local coronary artery eccentricity.

Methods: We used 3 T coronary CMR to measure CEF as changes in coronary cross-sectional area (CSA) and coronary blood flow (CBF) during isometric handgrip exercise (IHE), a known endothelial-dependent stressor, in 29 patients with known CAD and 16 healthy subjects. Black-blood MRI quantified mean coronary wall thickness (CWT) and coronary eccentricity index (EI) and CEF was determined in the same segments.

Results: IHE-induced changes in CSA and CBF in healthy subjects (10.6 ± 6.6% and 38.3 ± 29%, respectively) were greater than in CAD patients 1.3 ± 7.7% and 6.5 ± 19.6%, respectively, $p < 0.001$ vs. healthy for both measures), as expected. Mean CWT and EI in healthy subjects (1.1 ± 0.3 mm 1.9 ± 0.5, respectively) were less than those in CAD patients (1.6 ± 0.4 mm, $p < 0.0001$; and 2.6 ± 0.6, $p = 0.006$ vs. healthy). In CAD patients, we observed a significant inverse relationship between stress-induced %CSA change and both EI ($r = -0.60$, $p = 0.0002$), and CWT ($r = -0.54$, $p = 0.001$). Coronary EI was independently and significantly related to %CSA change with IHE even after controlling for mean CWT (adjusted $r = -0.69$, $p = 0.0001$). For every unit increase in EI, coronary CSA during IHE is expected to change by -6.7 ± 9.4% (95% confidence interval: -10.3 to -3.0, $p = 0.001$).

Conclusion: There is a significant inverse and independent relationship between coronary endothelial macrovascular function and the degree of local coronary wall eccentricity in CAD patients. Thus anatomic and physiologic indicators of high-risk coronary vascular pathology are closely related. The noninvasive identification of coronary eccentricity and its relationship with underlying coronary endothelial function, a marker of vascular health, may be useful in identifying high-risk patients and culprit lesions.

Keywords: Coronary artery disease, Endothelium, Magnetic resonance imaging

* Correspondence: ahays2@jhmi.edu
[1]Department of Medicine, Division of Cardiology, Johns Hopkins University,
600 N Wolfe St., Baltimore, MD 21287, USA
Full list of author information is available at the end of the article

Background

Endothelial-dependent coronary artery vasoreactivity is an important indicator of vascular function and a predictor of future cardiovascular events [1–3]. Endothelial dysfunction in the coronary arteries is believed to play a critical role in the development and progression of local coronary atherosclerosis. Coronary endothelial function (CEF) is heterogeneous and varies among coronary segments in a given patient with coronary artery disease (CAD) for reasons that are incompletely understood [2, 4]. Likewise, coronary atherosclerosis is also a spatially-heterogeneous process with the extent and characteristics of atheroma varying extensively within a given CAD patient. Plaque eccentricity is common and is significantly related to features of lesion vulnerability and an increased risk of adverse clinical sequelae [5–7]. However, the assessment of both coronary functional and anatomic indices of disease traditionally required invasive techniques and therefore their relationship has not been well characterized in healthy and low-risk or stable populations [1, 8].

Both anatomic and functional changes of the coronaries can now be measured non-invasively using cardiovascular magnetic resonance imaging (CMR). Early anatomic changes associated with the development of atherosclerosis include outward arterial remodeling with preservation of the luminal size [9]. Because coronary vessel wall thickening precedes luminal narrowing, the degree of CAD may be underestimated with conventional imaging of the coronary lumen using x-ray angiography, CT or CMR [10]. However, early indices of coronary vessel wall remodeling including increased coronary wall thickness can be identified and reproducibly quantified using black blood CMR techniques [11–14], thereby enabling non-invasive detection and characterization of arterial remodeling and subclinical coronary atherosclerosis.

Likewise, coronary endothelial function (CEF), which is impaired early in the atherosclerotic process and is a predictor of subsequent cardiovascular events [2, 3, 15], can also be measured using non-invasive CMR methods. Recent studies demonstrate that CMR measures of CEF performed during isometric handgrip exercise (IHE) quantify nitric-oxide mediated coronary endothelial vasoreactivity [16] with excellent short- and longer-term reproducibility [17, 18].

Although invasive studies indicate that plaque composition may play an important role in atherosclerotic disease and coronary endothelial dysfunction [19], the underlying anatomic features of the coronary vessel wall (increased thickness and eccentricity) and their relationship to an early initiator of atherosclerotic disease, endothelial dysfunction, are not well characterized. Defining the presence of both in the same arterial segment, therefore, may enhance the non-invasive identification of those segments which are most vulnerable to the development and progression of disease. Moreover, because both plaque eccentricity and coronary endothelial dysfunction are associated with adverse outcomes [2, 3, 20], we used noninvasive CMR techniques to test the hypothesis that local coronary endothelial dysfunction is associated with local plaque eccentricity in patients with known CAD and in healthy age-matched subjects.

Methods

Participants

All participants provided written informed consent to a protocol approved by the Johns Hopkins School of Medicine Institutional Review Board. Subjects were outpatients at Johns Hopkins with no contraindications to CMR. Healthy subjects had no history of CAD or traditional CAD risk factors and, those over age 50 years had a <10 Agatston coronary artery calcium score on computed tomography (CT)[21] . CAD subjects were individuals without unstable coronary syndrome for at least 6 months, who were asymptomatic (no anginal symptoms) at the time of the study, and with a prior clinically indicated coronary x-ray angiography or coronary CTA (computed tomography angiography) documenting >30% luminal stenosis in at least one vessel. The data reported in this study are not a subset of prior published reports. Participants underwent CMR between February 2013 and March 2016.

Study protocol

CMR was performed on a commercial human 3 T CMR scanner (Achieva, Philips Healthcare, Best, NL) in the morning after an overnight fast. For endothelial function imaging, alternating anatomical and velocity-encoded images were collected at baseline and during approximately 5 min of continuous isometric handgrip exercise (IHE) as previously described [17, 22, 23]. Cross-sectional anatomical [24] and flow velocity encoded spiral CMR [25] were obtained using single breath-hold cine sequences [22, 26] with reproducibility of the techniques previously published [17, 18]. CMR parameters were: the temporal/spatial resolution for the anatomic images was: 15 ms/0.89×0.89×8.0 mm^3 and 34 ms/0.8×0.8×8 mm^3 for the flow velocity images (velocity encoding = 35 cm per second). Approximately 15–24 cardiac phases were acquired for the coronary flow scan, depending on heart rate. Radiofrequency excitation angle = 20°, 17 spiral interleaves were acquired, and all scans were prospectively triggered. The imaging plane for both endothelial function and wall thickness measurements was localized in a proximal or mid coronary segment that was straight, without branches and no more than mild luminal stenosis (≤30% luminal stenosis) over a distance of approximately 2 cm (based on prior coronary x-ray angiography or coronary CTA that was clinically indicated, and confirmed by visual assessment of 3D coronary MRA used to plan the 2D slices). In several cases, more than one 2D imaging plane was prescribed per subject. Black blood coronary vessel wall imaging was performed at rest using dual-inversion spiral imaging with a heart rate-dependent inversion time [27]. CMR parameters were: echo time = 0.84 ms, spectrally selective fat suppression, breath-hold duration approximately 15 to 24 s, acquisition window 21 ms, spatial resolution (acquired/reconstructed) = $0.6 \times 0.6 \times 8.00$ mm^3/$0.49 \times 0.49 \times 8.00$ mm^3 and a radiofrequency excitation angle = 45°. Linear volume shimming, localized to the intersection of the imaging slice and the heart, was performed to minimize off-resonance effects on spiral imaging; the readout durations of spiral interleaves were 13, 30, and 22 ms for anatomic, flow, and black blood sequences respectively. The total duration of the CMR exam was approximately 40–45 min. Heart rate and blood pressure were measured throughout the study using ECG and a noninvasive, CMR-compatible blood pressure monitor (Invivo, Orlando, FL). The rate pressure product (RPP) was calculated as systolic blood pressure x heart rate.

Image analysis

Images were analyzed for cross-sectional area (CSA) using a semi-automated software tool as previously reported [16, 22]. Semi-automated measurements of black-blood coronary cross sectional images were made (Soap Bubble version 4.5) to determine minimum, mean, and maximum coronary wall thicknesses (CWT) and eccentricity index (EI) (=the ratio of maximum to minimum CWT, Fig. 1) [28, 29]. For coronary flow velocity (CFV) and coronary blood flow (CBF) measurements, images were analyzed using semi-automated commercial software [22, 30].

Additional analyses were performed in all subjects to determine whether the combined effect of abnormal EI and abnormal CWT was associated with significantly greater impairment in CEF than was either variable alone. Coronary segments with both abnormal EI (defined as EI >1 SD above the mean EI of the healthy subjects) *and* abnormal mean CWT (defined as CWT >1 SD above the healthy mean CWT) had CEF quantified and compared with subjects with either abnormal EI alone, those with abnormal CWT alone, and those with neither abnormal CWR nor abnormal EI.

Statistical analysis

Data are expressed as mean values ± one standard deviation. The data were tested for normality using the Shapiro-Wilk test. Parametric (Student's t-test) and nonparametric testing (Wilcoxon signed rank test for paired data and Wilcoxon rank sum test for non-paired data) were used as appropriate. Linear regression analysis was performed to assess the relationship between continuous variables of coronary vasoreactivity and the anatomic atherosclerosis indices of coronary wall measurements. Multiple linear regression was employed to ascertain the relationship between EI and CEF after controlling for CWT (STATA version 13). Statistical significance was defined as a two-tailed p-value <0.05.

Results

All participants completed the study without complication. A total of 31 arterial segments in 29 CAD patients and 19 segments in 16 healthy subjects were analyzed. Baseline characteristics of the study population are presented in Table 1.

Hemodynamic effect of isometric handgrip stress

Isometric handgrip exercise (IHE) induced significant hemodynamic changes in both healthy subjects and patients. We observed a 30.1 ± 17.6% increase in the rate pressure product (RPP) with IHE stress in the healthy subjects and a 32.8 ± 17.2% increase in the CAD patients ($p < 0.0001$ stress vs. baseline, both groups). The absolute RPP during stress and the percent increase in RPP from

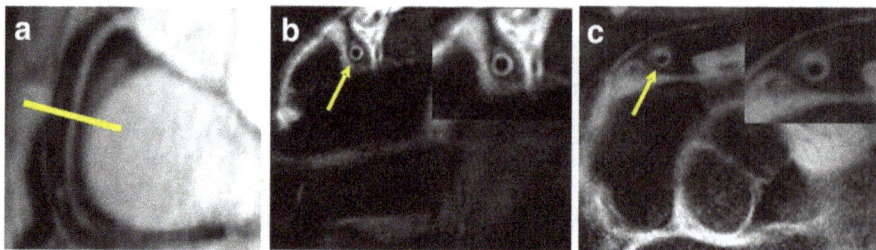

Fig. 1 CMR example of coronary black blood vessel wall imaging. Cross-sectional images in a young, healthy volunteer and in a patient with mild CAD. **a** A scout scan obtained along the right coronary artery (RCA) in a healthy subject is shown together with the location for cross-sectional imaging (*yellow line*). *Yellow arrows* denote RCA cross section. **b** The normal volunteer has an eccentricity index (maximum wall thickness/minimum wall thickness) of 1.3. **c** The CAD patient has an eccentricity index of 3.3, indicating eccentric arterial remodeling

Table 1 Characteristics of the subjects

	Healthy subjects (N = 16)	CAD patients (N = 29)	p-value
Age – years			
Mean ± SD	57 ± 21.2	58 ± 14.8	0.86
Range	25–80	37–83	
Male –no. (%)	8 (50)	21 (67)	0.37
Left Ventricular Ejection Fraction – %	N/A	59 ± 5.2	
Coronary artery imaged: Total segments	19	31	
RCA alone –no. (%)	11 (69)	20 (69)	NS
LAD alone–no. (%)	3 (19)	7 (24)	NS
Both RCA and LAD –no. (%)	2 (12)	2 (7)	NS
History of prior angioplasty	N/A	9 (31)	
History of CABG	N/A	1 (3)	
Significant multivessel CAD (>50% luminal stenosis in major epicardial coronary artery)	N/A	7 (24)	
Body Mass Index (Mean ± SD) (BMI, kg/m^2)	26.0 ± 5.2	27.1 ± 5.9	0.49
CAD risk factors[a] Mean ± SD	0	1.3 ± 0.8	<0.001
ACE-inhibitor use –no. (%)	0	12 (39)	<0.001
Beta-blocker use –no. (%)	0	15 (48)	<0.001
Statin use –no. (%)	0	20 (69)	<0.001

Abbreviations: *N/A* not applicable, *SD* standard deviation, *CAD* coronary artery disease, *RCA* right coronary artery, *LAD* left anterior descending artery, *ACE* angiotensin converting enzyme inhibitor, *NS* non-significant
[a]CAD risk factors excluding age and gender

baseline did not differ between the healthy subjects and CAD patients ($p = 0.48$, $p = 0.6$ respectively).

Coronary vasoreactivity

Baseline coronary cross-sectional area (CSA) was similar in healthy subjects and in patients with CAD (13.2 ± 4.5 mm^2 vs. 13.7 ± 5.8 mm^2, healthy vs CAD, $p = 0.8$). Coronary arteries dilated significantly more with IHE stress in the healthy subjects than those of CAD patients in that the percent change in stress-induced CSA was significantly higher in healthy age matched subjects (10.6 ± 6.6%) than in those with CAD (1.3 ± 7.7%, $p < 0.0001$, Fig. 2), consistent with prior reports [17, 22].

Coronary flow velocity and blood-flow measures

Peak diastolic CFV at baseline was similar in healthy subjects and patients with CAD (12.8 ± 3.8 cm/s vs. 14.0 ± 6.0 cm/s, healthy vs CAD, $p = 0.40$). The relative exercise-induced change in CFV was also greater in healthy subjects (+25.0 ± 24.7%) than in CAD patients (5.1 ± 17.9%, $p = 0.001$, Fig. 2). Likewise, baseline CBF was similar in healthy and CAD subjects (50.4 ± 19.2 ml/min vs 57.5 ± 31.7 ml/min, $p = 0.39$) but the CBF change with IHE stress was also significantly greater in the healthy group (+38.3 ± 29%) than in the

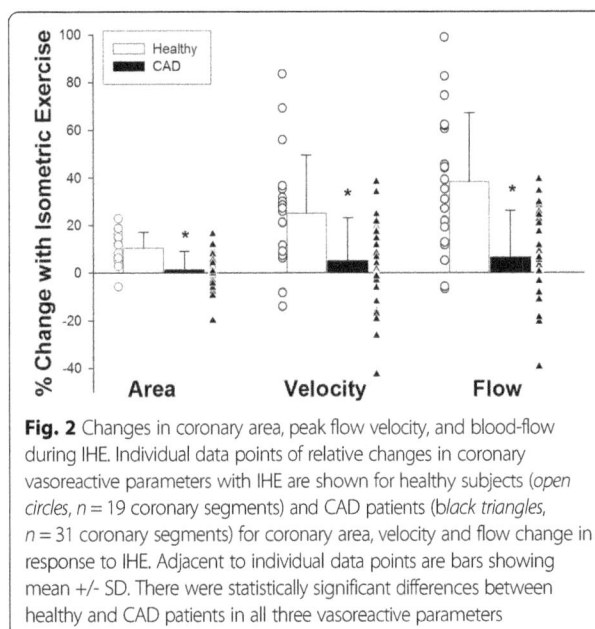

Fig. 2 Changes in coronary area, peak flow velocity, and blood-flow during IHE. Individual data points of relative changes in coronary vasoreactive parameters with IHE are shown for healthy subjects (*open circles*, n = 19 coronary segments) and CAD patients (*black triangles*, n = 31 coronary segments) for coronary area, velocity and flow change in response to IHE. Adjacent to individual data points are bars showing mean +/- SD. There were statistically significant differences between healthy and CAD patients in all three vasoreactive parameters

CAD group (+6.5 ± 19.6%, $p = 0.0001$). Figure 2 illustrates relative changes (%) in coronary area, velocity and flow with IHE in both groups.

Coronary wall measurements

Mean and maximum coronary wall thicknesses were 1.1 ± 0.3 mm and 1.9 ± 0.5 mm, respectively in the healthy subjects, and mean EI was 1.8 ± 0.5 in this group. Both mean and maximum CWT were higher in CAD patients (1.6 ± 0.4 mm and 2.6 ± 0.6 mm respectively $p < 0.0001$ healthy vs. CAD for both measures). Similarly, mean EI was significantly higher in the CAD group (2.3 ± 0.6, $p = 0.006$ vs. healthy group, Fig. 3) compared to the healthy group.

Relationship between coronary artery remodeling and endothelial-dependent coronary vasoreactivity

In healthy subjects, there was no significant relationship between measures of coronary wall remodeling (mean CWT or EI) and measures of CEF (Table 2). However, in CAD patients we observed a significant inverse relationship between mean CWT and %CSA change with stress (r = -0.54, $p = 0.001$, Fig. 5). Importantly, there was a significant inverse relationship between EI and %CSA change with IHE (r = -0.60, $p = 0.0002$, Fig. 5) in CAD patients. There was no significant relationship between CFV and either remodeling parameter (mean CWT and EI). Although we observed an inverse relationship between %CBF change and CWT in CAD patients, this was of borderline significance (r = -0.34, $p = 0.05$). There was no significant relationship between %CBF and EI (r = -0.27, $p = 0.13$, Fig. 5). Because mean CWT and EI were each inversely related to %CSA change with IHE (Fig. 5), we employed regression analysis to control for mean CWT and found that a significant relationship persisted between EI and %CSA change (adjusted r = -0.69, $p = 0.0001$), indicating that EI is independently associated with depressed (or impaired) CEF. For every unit increase in EI, coronary CSA with IHE is expected to decrease by -6.7 ± 1.7% (95% confidence interval: -10.3 to -3.0, $p = 0.001$). Using regression analysis, there was no significant relationship between the two coronary wall indices (mean CWT and EI, R = 0.27, $p = 0.13$, Fig. 3c). Furthermore, no significant interaction was detected between the variables CWT and EI (p value for interaction = 0.81).

To determine whether the combined effect of abnormal EI (defined as EI > 2.2 which is >1 SD above the healthy mean EI) and abnormal CWT (defined as CWT > 1.37 mm which is >1 SD above the healthy mean CWT) was associated with significantly greater impairment in CEF than either variable alone, we observed that coronary segments with both abnormal EI *and* abnormal mean CWT ($n = 10$ segments) had

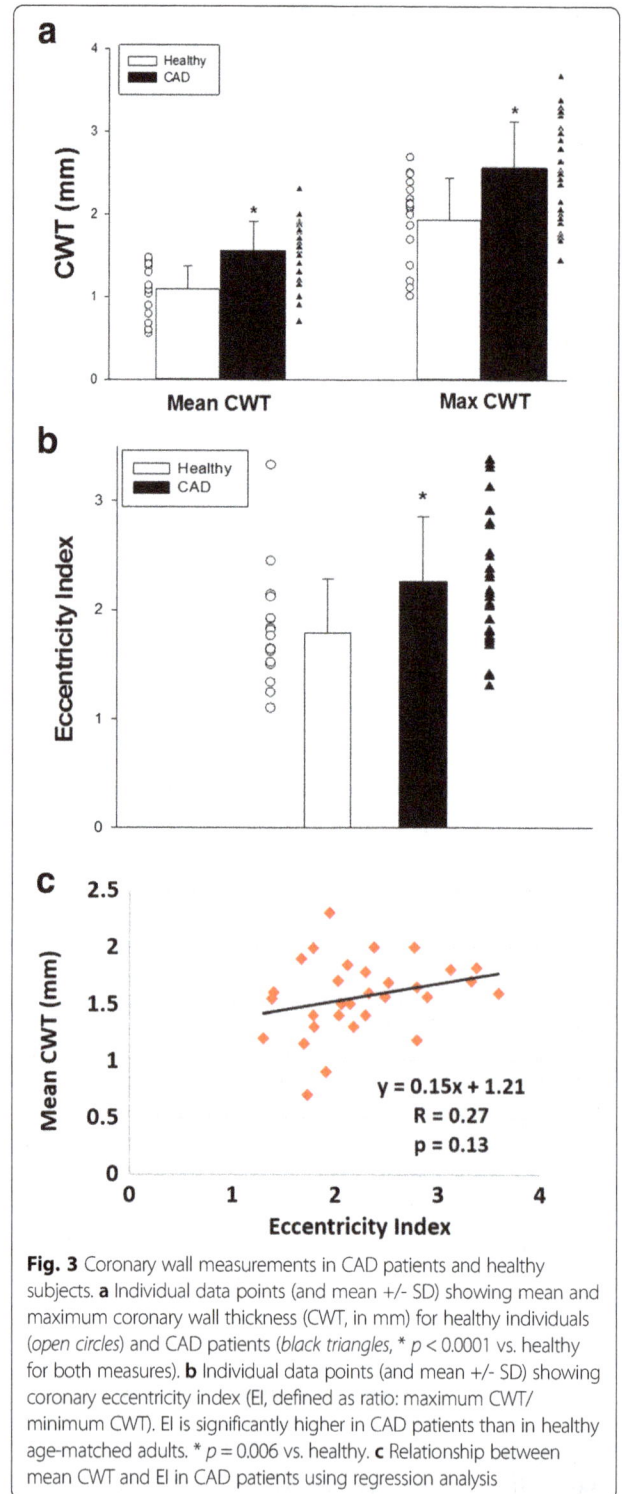

Fig. 3 Coronary wall measurements in CAD patients and healthy subjects. **a** Individual data points (and mean +/- SD) showing mean and maximum coronary wall thickness (CWT, in mm) for healthy individuals (*open circles*) and CAD patients (*black triangles*, * $p < 0.0001$ vs. healthy for both measures). **b** Individual data points (and mean +/- SD) showing coronary eccentricity index (EI, defined as ratio: maximum CWT/ minimum CWT). EI is significantly higher in CAD patients than in healthy age-matched adults. * $p = 0.006$ vs. healthy. **c** Relationship between mean CWT and EI in CAD patients using regression analysis

significantly reduced CEF (measured by %CSA change during IHE) as compared with subjects with abnormal EI alone ($n = 13$), those with abnormal CWT alone ($n = 12$), or neither ($n = 15$, for total of 50 segments in 29 CAD patient and 16 healthy subjects, Fig. 4).

Table 2 Relationship between coronary anatomic and functional measures

% Coronary Vasoreactive Change with IHE vs. Coronary Wall Measure:	% area change	% velocity change	% flow change
Healthy: Mean Coronary Wall Thickness	R = -0.17	R = 0.02	R = -0.02
	P = 0.46	P = 0.93	P = 0.92
Healthy: Eccentricity Index	R = 0.18	R = 0.08	R = 0.14
	P = 0.46	P = 0.74	P = 0.56
CAD: Mean Coronary Wall Thickness	R = -0.54	R = -0.11	R = -0.34
	P = 0.001	P = 0.51	P = 0.05
CAD: Eccentricity Index	R = -0.60	R = -0.06	R = -0.27
	P = 0.0002	P = 0.75	P = 0.13

Relationship between MRI measures of coronary remodeling (Coronary eccentricity index and mean coronary wall thickness) vs. coronary endothelial functional measures (% area change, % coronary peak velocity change and % coronary blood flow change with IHE) in healthy subjects and in patients with coronary artery disease using regression analysis
Italized items indicate statistically significant relationships

Discussion

The current study demonstrates the novel finding that an eccentric pattern of coronary wall remodeling is significantly and independently associated with abnormal local CEF in patients with mild CAD, and therefore that anatomic and physiologic early indicators of coronary vascular pathology are closely related. More specifically, coronary endothelial-dependent vasoreactivity was quantified with CMR-IHE testing and demonstrated a strong

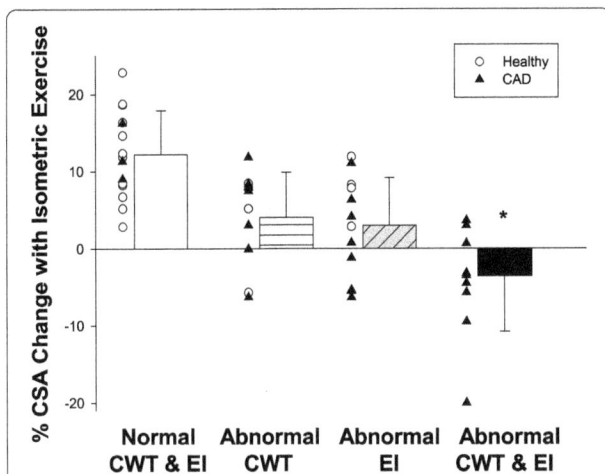

Fig. 4 Coronary area change with isometric handgrip stress in four groups. Individual data bars (mean +/- SD) are shown for the following groups: 1) Normal coronary wall thickness (CWT) and eccentricity index (EI) defined as values within one standard deviation of that of healthy subjects' values (*white bar*). 2) Coronary segments with abnormal CWT defined as CWT ≥1 standard deviation from the mean CWT of the healthy group (*white bar, horizontal lines*) 3) Segments with abnormal eccentricity index (EI, defined as EI ≥ 1 SD above the mean of the healthy group (*gray bar, diagonal lines*) and 4) Segments with *both* abnormal EI and abnormal CWT (*black bar*), illustrating that coronary endothelial function is more impaired in subjects with both abnormal CWT and abnormal EI than in those with either finding alone. Individual data points in *open circles* signify healthy subjects and those in *black triangles* signify CAD patients. * p < 0.05 (vs. Abnormal CWT group) and p < 0.05 (vs. Abnormal EI group)

inverse relationship between coronary macrovascular endothelial function, as measured by IHE-induced %CSA change, and the degree of local coronary wall eccentricity in patients with mild CAD. There was no relationship between the two indices in healthy control subjects. We previously reported that coronary endothelial function is closely related to the degree of coronary luminal stenosis and local coronary wall thickening [17, 22]. Although increased mean CWT and EI tend to occur in CAD patients and with aging, the two variables were not significantly related to one another in this population in the mild, non-stenotic vessels studied (Fig. 3). This novel noninvasive CMR approach combines functional (CEF) and anatomical imaging of the coronaries that were previously shown to be reproducible in the short and longer term [13, 14, 17, 18, 22], and may provide important insights in the pathophysiology of early atherosclerotic coronary disease.

The values for coronary wall thickening and coronary endothelial function reported here are similar to those previously reported using CMR [11, 31] and invasive techniques [2, 32, 33], although with different endothelial-dependent stressors. The values for CEF are similar to those obtained in our prior CMR studies, demonstrating a coronary vasodilatory response to IHE in the healthy subjects, and no vasodilatory response or a vasoconstrictor response in many CAD patients [16, 17, 22]. We previously showed that the administration of nitroglycerin, an endothelial independent stressor, caused normal vasodilatation in coronary segments with mild to severe CAD that exhibited abnormal responses to IHE. The finding that nitroglycerin dilated the same coronary artery segments in CAD patients that constricted by IHE demonstrated that endothelial-independent mechanisms were intact and, by inference, that the mechanism responsible for the impaired IHE-related coronary response in CAD is abnormal endothelial function rather than a mechanical disturbance such as may occur with heavy coronary calcification or increased vascular stiffness [17]. Although it is possible that severely calcified vessels may have mechanical properties that could limit dilatation, in the current paper we did not study patients with severe CAD and only studied segments with no more than mild CAD. Further, these findings confirm prior observations that mean coronary wall thickness is significantly higher in CAD patients than in healthy subjects which, in the presence of preserved luminal area, is indicative of positive arterial remodeling [9, 11]. We extend measures of wall eccentricity from other vascular beds [34, 35] to the coronary arteries and show that eccentricity of the coronary arteries of CAD patients with no significant luminal stenosis is greater than that of healthy age-matched individuals.

Although our study demonstrated a relationship between coronary macrovascular changes in CSA and coronary wall eccentricity index in CAD patients (Fig. 5a), there was no significant relationship between IHE-induced coronary velocity or flow change and EI in either the CAD or the healthy group (Fig. 5c,d). These findings suggest that *local* increased eccentricity is more closely related to measures of *local* coronary endothelial function (e.g. epicardial area change in a given coronary segment) rather than to more global endothelial function measures (velocity and flow) that also reflect changes in downstream microvascular vasoreactivity, distant from the eccentricity.

We previously reported that abnormal coronary endothelial function varied among arteries in a given CAD

patient and was related to the presence and degree of coronary wall thickening [22]. The observations here confirm that finding in different patients (Fig. 5) but also extend it, demonstrating that not only the degree but also the type of coronary wall remodeling (eccentric vs. concentric) is associated with impaired local coronary endothelial function in early coronary disease. Advances in CMR hardware (i.e. multitransmit radiofrequency) and software allow improved visualization of the coronary vessel wall, permitting a more detailed analysis of wall remodeling than was previously possible. The type of coronary wall remodeling (concentric vs. eccentric) may play an important role in local plaque progression or acute coronary syndrome [36]. Prior studies report that acute coronary syndromes tend to occur in vessels with angiographically mild disease [6]. One recent study determined that the presence in the coronary vessel wall of thin cap fibroatheromas (detected on intravascular ultrasound (IVUS)) and plaque burden are associated with an increased risk of acute coronary syndrome in the same vessel [37]. Non-invasive studies of coronary plaque composition may also play an important role in risk prediction [38, 39]. Therefore, based on these and other studies, the type and degree of coronary vessel remodeling and plaque composition [19] are important local factors that may potentially lead to unstable coronary syndromes.

Endothelial dysfunction is both a cause and a consequence of atherosclerosis, and thus, in terms of the

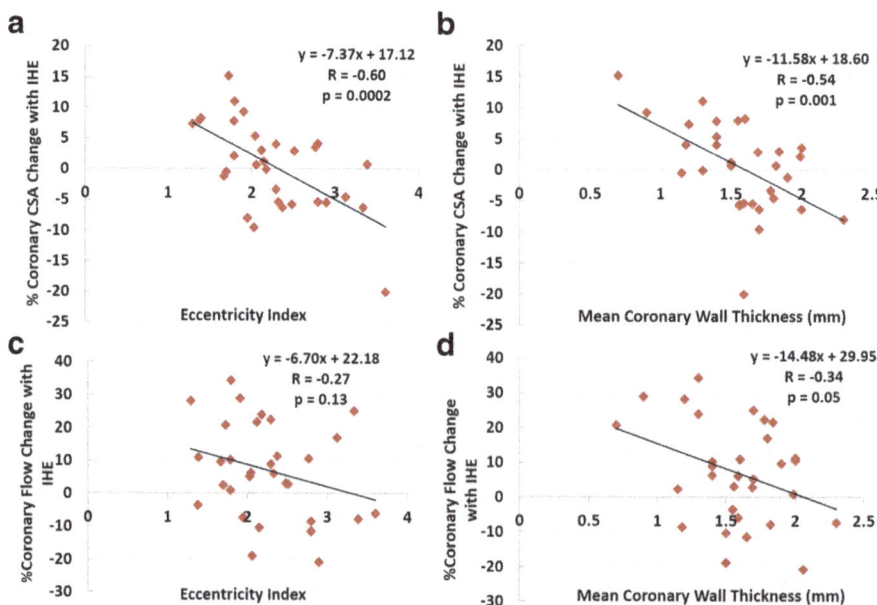

Fig. 5 CMR measures of coronary remodeling indices vs. measures of coronary endothelial function in CAD patients ($N = 31$ arterial segments in 29 subjects). **a** Coronary eccentricity index versus % coronary cross sectional area (CSA) change with isometric handgrip exercise (IHE). **b** Mean coronary wall thickness (CWT) versus %CSA change with IHE. **c** Coronary eccentricity index versus % coronary flow change with IHE. **d** Mean coronary wall thickness (CWT) versus % coronary flow change with IHE

correlation between local abnormal CEF and eccentricity observed here, it is difficult to determine whether depressed CEF contributes to coronary wall thickening/eccentricity, vice versa or both. It is clear that local factors contribute to the focal development of atherosclerosis and that local differences in three-dimensional coronary blood flow affect endothelial shear stress which, in turn, both modulates endothelial cell function and biochemistry [40] and drives plaque formation [41]. Eccentric lesions are associated with inflammation and are prone to rupture, which results in clinical events [35]. Others have suggested that changes in eccentricity over time may also be a strong predictor of future plaque rupture [40] and this noninvasive CMR approach is well suited to serial studies over time as well.

Recently, coronary endothelial function, eccentricity, wall shear stress, and plaque burden were measured invasively in patients with chest pain referred for angiography [42]. Wall shear stress was directly related to macrovascular CEF and inversely related to EI. Segments with the most plaque burden and lowest wall shear stress manifested impaired CEF and greater plaque eccentricity [42]. Unfortunately in that IVUS study the authors did not report whether there was a relationship between eccentricity and depressed CEF, as studied here for the first time. Taken together, the prior invasive studies and the current noninvasive report demonstrate that abnormal CEF varies regionally throughout the coronary vasculature and is related locally to plaque characteristics (amount, composition, and eccentricity/geometry) that were previously associated with adverse outcomes. Because acute vascular events tend to occur in areas of eccentric atherosclerosis [20, 35], the identification of areas of wall eccentricity and the correlation with underlying coronary endothelial function may be critically important in identifying potential high risk culprit lesions.

One limitation to the current study is that CMR imaging of the coronaries cannot distinguish separate layers of the vessel wall or measure coronary plaque components due to limits of spatial resolution. Although IVUS and optical coherence tomography are more sensitive at detecting and characterizing early vessel wall disease than CMR, they are invasive. Although multi-detector computed tomography (MDCT) has been used to assess coronary remodeling and plaque [43], the exposure to ionizing radiation and contrast media limit its application in low risk populations and in repeated studies. In addition, MDCT cannot directly measure coronary velocity or flow for the complete assessment of CEF. Although we primarily focused on proximal and mid coronary segments to evaluate stress-induced area changes, the ability to also measure coronary velocity and flow permits a more global assessment of downstream endothelial function that complements the measures of local epicardial vasoreactivity. Now that the relationship between local CEF and eccentricity has been identified, future work is needed to expand these noninvasive measures to longer coronary artery segments and the circumflex artery distribution as well as long-term studies to relate these measures to subsequent outcomes in large populations. The current coronary scan coverage is limited and this merits further improvement. Nevertheless, these coronary CMR CEF methods enable reproducible, noninvasive measures of coronary vasoreactivity that are NO-dependent [16] and that have been reported in a wide range of healthy subjects and patients with coronary artery disease.

Conclusions

In summary, the present findings demonstrate that the degree of coronary wall eccentricity is inversely related to local macrovascular CEF in patients with mild CAD. Moreover, the relationship between coronary eccentricity and local CEF is independent of coronary wall thickness. These findings indicate that an eccentric pattern of coronary wall remodeling is associated with abnormal local CEF, and therefore that anatomic and physiologic early indicators of coronary vascular pathology are closely related in early atherosclerotic disease. This novel imaging approach may offer important insights into the pathobiology of atherosclerosis, the local progression of CAD, and the identification of high-risk patients and possibly high-risk coronary lesions.

Abbreviations
ACE: Angiotensin converting enzyme; BMI: Body mass index; CABG: Coronary artery bypass graft; CAD: Coronary artery disease; CBF: Coronary blood flow; CEF: Coronary endothelial function; CFV: Coronary flow velocity; CSA: Coronary cross sectional area; CTA: Computed tomography angiography; CWT: Coronary wall thickness; EI: Eccentricity index; IHE: Isometric handgrip exercise; IVUS: Intravascular ultrasound; LAD: Left anterior descending; MDCT: Multi-detector computed tomography; NO: Nitric oxide; RCA: Right coronary artery; RPP: Rate-pressure product

Funding
This work was supported by the National Institutes of Health (HL120905, HL125059, HL61912), the American Heart Association (11SDG5200004), the Swiss National Science Foundation Grant 320030-143923, the Johns Hopkins PJ Schafer Award, and the Clarence Doodeman Endowment of Johns Hopkins.

Authors' contributions
Conceived and designed the experiments: RGW, AGH, GG, M Stuber, M Schär. Software development: M Schär, M Stuber. Performed the experiments: AGH, MI, M Schär, SS, RGW. Analyzed the data: AGH, MI, M Schär, MM. Contributed reagents/materials/analysis tools: M Schär, M Stuber. Wrote/edited the paper: AGH, RGW, M Stuber, M Schär, GG, MI, MM. All authors read and approved the final manuscript.

Competing interests
The authors declare that they have no competing interests.

Consent for publication

Not applicable.

Author details

[1]Department of Medicine, Division of Cardiology, Johns Hopkins University, 600 N Wolfe St., Baltimore, MD 21287, USA. [2]Department of Radiology, Division of Magnetic Resonance Research, Johns Hopkins University, 600 N. Wolfe St., Baltimore, MD 21287, USA. [3]Department of Radiology, Centre Hospitalier Universitaire Vaudois, Center for Biomedical Imaging (CIBM), University of Lausanne, Lausanne, Switzerland.

References

1. Deanfield JE, Halcox JP, Rabelink TJ. Endothelial function and dysfunction: testing and clinical relevance. Circulation. 2007;115:1285–95.
2. Schachinger V, Britten MB, Zeiher AM. Prognostic impact of coronary vasodilator dysfunction on adverse long-term outcome of coronary heart disease. Circulation. 2000;101:1899–906.
3. Suwaidi JA, Hamasaki S, Higano ST, Nishimura RA, Holmes Jr DR, Lerman A. Long-term follow-up of patients with mild coronary artery disease and endothelial dysfunction. Circulation. 2000;101:948–54.
4. Manginas A, Voudris V, Pavlides G, Karatasakis G, Athanassopoulos G, Cokkinos DV. Effect of plaque burden on coronary vasoreactivity in early atherosclerosis. Am J Cardiol. 1998;81:401–6.
5. Yamagishi M, Terashima M, Awano K, Kijima M, Nakatani S, Daikoku S, Ito K, Yasumura Y, Miyatake K. Morphology of vulnerable coronary plaque: insights from follow-up of patients examined by intravascular ultrasound before an acute coronary syndrome. J Am Coll Cardiol. 2000;35:106–11.
6. Fuster V. 50th anniversary historical article. Acute coronary syndromes: the degree and morphology of coronary stenoses. J Am Coll Cardiol. 1999;34:1854–6.
7. Virmani R, Burke AP, Farb A, Kolodgie FD. Pathology of the vulnerable plaque. J Am Coll Cardiol. 2006;47:C13–8.
8. Ganz P, Vita JA. Testing endothelial vasomotor function: nitric oxide, a multipotent molecule. Circulation. 2003;108:2049–53.
9. Glagov S, Weisenberg E, Zarins CK, Stankunavicius R, Kolettis GJ. Compensatory enlargement of human atherosclerotic coronary arteries. N Engl J Med. 1987;316:1371–5.
10. Hodgson JM, Reddy KG, Suneja R, Nair RN, Lesnefsky EJ, Sheehan HM. Intracoronary ultrasound imaging: correlation of plaque morphology with angiography, clinical syndrome and procedural results in patients undergoing coronary angioplasty. J Am Coll Cardiol. 1993;21:35–44.
11. Fayad ZA, Fuster V, Fallon JT, Jayasundera T, Worthley SG, Helft G, Aguinaldo JG, Badimon JJ, Sharma SK. Noninvasive in vivo human coronary artery lumen and wall imaging using black-blood magnetic resonance imaging. Circulation. 2000;102:506–10.
12. Kim WY, Stuber M, Bornert P, Kissinger KV, Manning WJ, Botnar RM. Three-dimensional black-blood cardiac magnetic resonance coronary vessel wall imaging detects positive arterial remodeling in patients with nonsignificant coronary artery disease. Circulation. 2002;106:296–9.
13. Desai MY, Lai S, Barmet C, Weiss RG, Stuber M. Reproducibility of 3D free-breathing magnetic resonance coronary vessel wall imaging. Eur Heart J. 2005;26:2320–4.
14. Hazirolan T, Gupta SN, Mohamed MA, Bluemke DA. Reproducibility of black-blood coronary vessel wall MR imaging. J Cardiovasc Magn Reson. 2005;7:409–13.
15. Nitenberg A, Chemla D, Antony I. Epicardial coronary artery constriction to cold pressor test is predictive of cardiovascular events in hypertensive patients with angiographically normal coronary arteries and without other major coronary risk factor. Atherosclerosis. 2004;173:115–23.
16. Hays AG, Iantorno M, Soleimanifard S, Steinberg A, Schar M, Gerstenblith G, Stuber M, Weiss RG. Coronary vasomotor responses to isometric handgrip exercise are primarily mediated by nitric oxide: a noninvasive MRI test of coronary endothelial function. Am J Physiol Heart Circ Physiol. 2015;308:H1343–50.
17. Hays AG, Hirsch GA, Kelle S, Gerstenblith G, Weiss RG, Stuber M. Noninvasive visualization of coronary artery endothelial function in healthy subjects and in patients with coronary artery disease. J Am Coll Cardiol. 2010;56:1657–65.
18. Hays AG, Stuber M, Hirsch GA, Yu J, Schar M, Weiss RG, Gerstenblith G, Kelle S. Non-invasive detection of coronary endothelial response to sequential handgrip exercise in coronary artery disease patients and healthy adults. PLoS ONE. 2013;8:e58047.
19. Choi BJ, Prasad A, Gulati R, Best PJ, Lennon RJ, Barsness GW, Lerman LO, Lerman A. Coronary endothelial dysfunction in patients with early coronary artery disease is associated with the increase in intravascular lipid core plaque. Eur Heart J. 2013;34:2047–54.
20. Higuma T, Soeda T, Abe N, Yamada M, Yokoyama H, Shibutani S, Vergallo R, Minami Y, Ong DS, Lee H, et al. A Combined Optical Coherence Tomography and Intravascular Ultrasound Study on Plaque Rupture, Plaque Erosion, and Calcified Nodule in Patients With ST-Segment Elevation Myocardial Infarction: Incidence, Morphologic Characteristics, and Outcomes After Percutaneous Coronary Intervention. JACC Cardiovasc Interv. 2015;8:1166–76.
21. Agatston AS, Janowitz WR, Hildner FJ, Zusmer NR, Viamonte Jr M, Detrano R. Quantification of coronary artery calcium using ultrafast computed tomography. J Am Coll Cardiol. 1990;15:827–32.
22. Hays AG, Kelle S, Hirsch GA, Soleimanifard S, Yu J, Agarwal HK, Gerstenblith G, Schar M, Stuber M, Weiss RG. Regional coronary endothelial function is closely related to local early coronary atherosclerosis in patients with mild coronary artery disease: pilot study. Circ Cardiovasc Imaging. 2012;5:341–8.
23. Weiss RG, Bottomley PA, Hardy CJ, Gerstenblith G. Regional myocardial metabolism of high-energy phosphates during isometric exercise in patients with coronary artery disease. N Engl J Med. 1990;323:1593–600.
24. Meyer CH, Hu BS, Nishimura DG, Macovski A. Fast spiral coronary artery imaging. Magn Reson Med. 1992;28:202–13.
25. Keegan J, Gatehouse PD, Yang GZ, Firmin DN. Spiral phase velocity mapping of left and right coronary artery blood flow: correction for through-plane motion using selective fat-only excitation. J Magn Reson Imaging. 2004;20:953–60.
26. Terashima M, Meyer CH, Keeffe BG, Putz EJ, de la Pena-Almaguer E, Yang PC, Hu BS, Nishimura DG, McConnell MV. Noninvasive assessment of coronary vasodilation using magnetic resonance angiography. J Am Coll Cardiol. 2005;45:104–10.
27. Fleckenstein JL, Archer BT, Barker BA, Vaughan JT, Parkey RW, Peshock RM. Fast short-tau inversion-recovery MR imaging. Radiology. 1991;179:499–504.
28. Mintz GS, Popma JJ, Pichard AD, Kent KM, Satler LF, Chuang YC, DeFalco RA, Leon MB. Limitations of angiography in the assessment of plaque distribution in coronary artery disease: a systematic study of target lesion eccentricity in 1446 lesions. Circulation. 1996;93:924–31.
29. Miao C, Chen S, Macedo R, Lai S, Liu K, Li D, Wasserman BA, Vogel-Claussen J, Lima JA, Bluemke DA. Positive remodeling of the coronary arteries detected by magnetic resonance imaging in an asymptomatic population: MESA (Multi-Ethnic Study of Atherosclerosis). J Am Coll Cardiol. 2009;53:1708–15.
30. Doucette JW, Corl PD, Payne HM, Flynn AE, Goto M, Nassi M, Segal J. Validation of a Doppler guide wire for intravascular measurement of coronary artery flow velocity. Circulation. 1992;85:1899–911.
31. Botnar RM, Stuber M, Kissinger KV, Kim WY, Spuentrup E, Manning WJ. Noninvasive coronary vessel wall and plaque imaging with magnetic resonance imaging. Circulation. 2000;102:2582–7.
32. von Birgelen C, Klinkhart W, Mintz GS, Papatheodorou A, Herrmann J, Baumgart D, Haude M, Wieneke H, Ge J, Erbel R. Plaque distribution and vascular remodeling of ruptured and nonruptured coronary plaques in the same vessel: an intravascular ultrasound study in vivo. J Am Coll Cardiol. 2001;37:1864–70.
33. Ludmer PL, Selwyn AP, Shook TL, Wayne RR, Mudge GH, Alexander RW, Ganz P. Paradoxical vasoconstriction induced by acetylcholine in atherosclerotic coronary arteries. N Engl J Med. 1986;315:1046–51.
34. Li F, McDermott MM, Li D, Carroll TJ, Hippe DS, Kramer CM, Fan Z, Zhao X, Hatsukami TS, Chu B, et al. The association of lesion eccentricity with plaque morphology and components in the superficial femoral artery: a high-spatial-resolution, multi-contrast weighted CMR study. J Cardiovasc Magn Reson. 2010;12:37.
35. Ohara T, Toyoda K, Otsubo R, Nagatsuka K, Kubota Y, Yasaka M, Naritomi H, Minematsu K. Eccentric stenosis of the carotid artery associated with ipsilateral cerebrovascular events. AJNR Am J Neuroradiol. 2008;29:1200–3.
36. Puri R, Nicholls SJ, Brennan DM, Andrews J, Liew GY, Carbone A, Copus B, Nelson AJ, Kapadia SR, Tuzcu EM, et al. Coronary atheroma composition and its association with segmental endothelial dysfunction in non-ST segment elevation myocardial infarction: novel insights with radiofrequency (iMAP)

intravascular ultrasonography. Int J Cardiovasc Imaging. 2015;31:247–57.

37. Stone GW, Maehara A, Lansky AJ, de Bruyne B, Cristea E, Mintz GS, Mehran R, McPherson J, Farhat N, Marso SP, et al. A prospective natural-history study of coronary atherosclerosis. N Engl J Med. 2011;364:226–35.

38. Ito H, Motoyama S, Sarai M, Kawai H, Harigaya H, Kan S, Kato S, Anno H, Takahashi H, Naruse H, et al. Characteristics of plaque progression detected by serial coronary computed tomography angiography. Heart Vessels. 2014;29:743–9.

39. Kaul S, Narula J. In search of the vulnerable plaque: is there any light at the end of the catheter? J Am Coll Cardiol. 2014;64:2519–24.

40. Papafaklis MI, Takahashi S, Antoniadis AP, Coskun AU, Tsuda M, Mizuno S, Andreou I, Nakamura S, Makita Y, Hirohata A, et al. Effect of the local hemodynamic environment on the de novo development and progression of eccentric coronary atherosclerosis in humans: insights from PREDICTION. Atherosclerosis. 2015;240:205–11.

41. Wentzel JJ, Chatzizisis YS, Gijsen FJ, Giannoglou GD, Feldman CL, Stone PH. Endothelial shear stress in the evolution of coronary atherosclerotic plaque and vascular remodelling: current understanding and remaining questions. Cardiovasc Res. 2012;96:234–43.

42. Puri R, Leong DP, Nicholls SJ, Liew GY, Nelson AJ, Carbone A, Copus B, Wong DT, Beltrame JF, Worthley SG, Worthley MI. Coronary artery wall shear stress is associated with endothelial dysfunction and expansive arterial remodelling in patients with coronary artery disease. EuroIntervention. 2015; 10:1440–8.

43. Achenbach S, Ropers D, Hoffmann U, MacNeill B, Baum U, Pohle K, Brady TJ, Pomerantsev E, Ludwig J, Flachskampf FA, et al. Assessment of coronary remodeling in stenotic and nonstenotic coronary atherosclerotic lesions by multidetector spiral computed tomography. J Am Coll Cardiol. 2004;43:842–7.

6

Nonenhanced MR angiography of the pulmonary arteries using single-shot radial quiescent-interval slice-selective (QISS)

Robert R. Edelman[1,2*], Robert I. Silvers[1,3], Kiran H. Thakrar[1,3], Mark D. Metzl[1,3], Jose Nazari[1,3], Shivraman Giri[4] and Ioannis Koktzoglou[1,3]

Abstract

Background: For evaluation of the pulmonary arteries in patients suspected of pulmonary embolism, CT angiography (CTA) is the first-line imaging test with contrast-enhanced MR angiography (CEMRA) a potential alternative. Disadvantages of CTA include exposure to ionizing radiation and an iodinated contrast agent, while CEMRA is sensitive to respiratory motion and requires a gadolinium-based contrast agent. The primary goal of our technical feasibility study was to evaluate pulmonary arterial conspicuity using breath-hold and free-breathing implementations of a recently-developed nonenhanced approach, single-shot radial quiescent-interval slice-selective (QISS) MRA.

Methods: Breath-hold and free-breathing, navigator-gated versions of radial QISS MRA were evaluated at 1.5 Tesla in three healthy subjects and 11 patients without pulmonary embolism or arterial occlusion by CTA. Images were scored by three readers for conspicuity of the pulmonary arteries through the level of the segmental branches. In addition, one patient with pulmonary embolism was imaged.

Results: Scan time for a 54-slice acquisition spanning the pulmonary arteries was less than 2 minutes for breath-hold QISS, and less than 3.4 min using free-breathing QISS. Pulmonary artery branches through the segmental level were conspicuous with either approach. Free-breathing scans showed only mild blurring compared with breath-hold scans. For both readers, less than 1% of pulmonary arterial segments were rated as "not seen" for breath-hold and navigator-gated QISS, respectively. In subjects with atrial fibrillation, single-shot radial QISS consistently depicted the pulmonary artery branches, whereas navigator-gated 3D balanced steady-state free precession showed motion artifacts. In one patient with pulmonary embolism, radial QISS demonstrated central pulmonary emboli comparably to CEMRA and CTA. The thrombi were highly conspicuous on radial QISS images, but appeared subtle and were not prospectively identified on scout images acquired using a single-shot bSSFP acquisition.

Conclusions: In this technical feasibility study, both breath-hold and free-breathing single-shot radial QISS MRA enabled rapid, consistent demonstration of the pulmonary arteries through the level of the segmental branches, with only minimal artifacts from respiratory motion and cardiac arrhythmias. Based on these promising initial results, further evaluation in patients with suspected pulmonary embolism appears warranted.

Keywords: Radial, Quiescent-interval slice-selective, Breath-holding, Navigator-gated, Cardiac

* Correspondence: Redelman999@gmail.com
[1]Department of Radiology, NorthShore University HealthSystem, 2650 Ridge Avenue, Evanston, IL 60201, USA
[2]Feinberg School of Medicine, Northwestern University, Chicago, USA
Full list of author information is available at the end of the article

Background

Patients presenting with suspected pulmonary embolism (PE) are routinely evaluated by computed tomography angiography (CTA) [1]. The risk of having a pulmonary embolism doubles for each 10 years after age 60 [https://www.nhlbi.nih.gov/health/health-topics/topics/pe/atrisk]. Given the nearly 40% prevalence of chronic kidney disease among patients over the age of 60 years [2] and the potentially nephrotoxic effects of iodinated contrast agents, there is a substantial need for a safer imaging option in this patient group. First-pass contrast-enhanced MR angiography (CEMRA) of the pulmonary arteries is a promising alternative to CTA that avoids exposure to iodinated contrast agents and ionizing radiation [3]. However, potential challenges include the requirement for breath-holding, which may be problematic for dyspneic patients, and incomplete pulmonary artery opacification due to mistiming of the data acquisition with respect to the gadolinium bolus. Moreover, gadolinium-based contrast agents are absolutely contraindicated in pregnant patients and relatively contraindicated in those with severe renal impairment [4]. For patients with contraindications to CTA or CEMRA, a nonenhanced MRA (NEMRA) alternative would be useful.

Recently, a radial quiescent-interval slice-selective (QISS) technique was described for breath-hold imaging of the coronary arteries [5]. Radial k-space trajectories provide several advantages over Cartesian trajectories including reduced motion sensitivity, more flexible control over temporal and spatial resolution, and higher undersampling factors [6, 7]. For coronary artery QISS, two or more shots are typically required to achieve sufficiently high temporal resolution, on the order of 150 msec or less, to minimize blurring from coronary motion. Such high temporal resolution is not needed for imaging of the pulmonary arteries, which allows the use of a more efficient single-shot radial QISS acquisition. Not only does the use of a single-shot acquisition at least double the number of slices that can be acquired in each breath-hold, it avoids artifacts from shot-to-shot signal variations caused by respiratory motion or cardiac arrhythmias. Given its high imaging efficiency and resistance to motion artifacts, single-shot radial QISS could have potential utility as a nonenhanced option for evaluating patients with suspected pulmonary embolism. As an initial step, we performed a technical feasibility study to evaluate pulmonary arterial conspicuity using breath-hold and free-breathing implementations of single-shot radial QISS.

Methods

This investigational review board (IRB)-approved study was conducted on a 1.5 Tesla scanner (MAGNETOM Avanto, Siemens Healthcare, Erlangen, Germany). Two groups of subjects were studied: (1) 3 healthy subjects; and (2) 11 patients (10 male, age range 50–73 years) who were scheduled for pulmonary vein isolation due to recurrent or persistent atrial fibrillation and had recently undergone CTA for anatomical evaluation of the pulmonary veins and heart. This patient cohort additionally provided the opportunity to evaluate the robustness of the radial QISS technique with respect to cardiac arrhythmias, since six patients were in atrial fibrillation at the time of the MR exam. Retrospective approval from the IRB was obtained for one additional patient: a 68-year-old male with shortness of breath and suspected peri-valvular leak following mitral valve repair, who underwent cardiac MR which revealed clinically unsuspected central pulmonary emboli. This patient subsequently underwent a chest CTA that confirmed the MR findings.

Imaging parameters for radial QISS were developed empirically from prior studies in volunteers and patients. Typical QISS imaging parameters included: electrocardiographic gating (ECG), one slice acquired per RR interval, radial balanced steady-state free precession (bSSFP) readout with 98 views, flip angle for the bSSFP RF excitation = 120 degrees, chemical shift-selective fat suppression, in-plane inversion using a frequency offset corrected inversion (FOCI) RF pulse with thickness = 4.5 mm, TI ~ 600 msec, in-plane resolution ~1.6-mm (or 0.8-mm after interpolation), field of view ~260-mm, slice thickness ~ 3.1-mm with 30% slice overlap, number of slices ~54, equidistant azimuthal view angle increment, readout bandwidth = 1359 Hz/pixel, bSSFP repetition time (TR) ~ 2.9 msec. Breath-hold scans were acquired over 3 breath-holds (~18 slices per breath-hold) with 10 to12 seconds between breath-holds. Free-breathing radial QISS used navigator gating with a 3-mm acceptance window and both leading and trailing cross-pair navigators. In total, all 14 subjects were imaged with breath-hold QISS, while only 13 of these subjects were imaged with navigator-gated QISS. Scans were acquired in tilted coronal and axial planes.

Navigator-gated, T2-prepared fat-saturated 3D bSSFP scans were obtained using a Cartesian k-space trajectory, bSSFP RF excitation flip angle = 90 degrees, ~72 3-mm thick slices (1.5-mm after interpolation), in-plane resolution ~1–2-mm (before interpolation), 25 segments, readout bandwidth = 1313 Hz/pixel, bSSFP TR ~ 3.1 msec. Due to time constraints, navigator-gated 3D scans were only obtained in eight subjects (1 volunteer, 7 patients).

First-pass CEMRA used a breath-hold fluoro-triggered technique with scan time = 17 s, flip angle = 23 degrees, TR = 2.7 msec, TE = 1.0 msec, spatial resolution = 2-mm × 1.1-mm × 1.0-mm, ipat acceleration factor = 4, 6/8 partial Fourier in slice and phase directions. CTA was done using a standard high-pitch retrospective-ECG gated spiral protocol on a dual-source scanner (Siemens

MAGNETOM Flash, Erlangen, Germany) with 0.6-mm slice thickness.

Image Analysis: Radial QISS source images and thin multi-planar reconstructions from the three healthy volunteers and 11 patients were evaluated by three radiologists, each with more than 5 years' experience in the interpretation of pulmonary CTA and body MRA. The pulmonary arterial tree was divided into 25 segments per Jackson and Huber [8], and vessel conspicuity was rated as: 1 = vessel seen, sharp margins, negligible artifacts; 2 = vessel seen, mildly blurred margins, mild artifacts; 3 = vessel seen, markedly blurred margins, moderate artifacts; 4 = vessel not seen, severe artifacts. To determine which pulmonary artery segments were evaluable for the image analysis, CEMRA was the reference in healthy volunteers and CTA the reference in patients. Subsegmental arterial branches, as well as segments not evaluable by CEMRA (in volunteers) or CTA (in patients) were excluded from the analysis.

Statistical Analysis: Differences in image quality ratings between the three nonenhanced protocols were assessed using Friedman tests. Gwet's AC1 was used to assess inter-reader agreement for vessels proximal to the segmental arteries, and for the segmental branches. Bonferroni-corrected P values <0.05 were considered statistically significant. Analyses were performed in R software (version 3.3.2, R Foundation for Statistical Computing, Vienna, Austria).

Results

Typical breath-hold times were ~15–20 s for an 18-slice radial QISS scan, depending on the heart rate. A 54-slice, three breath-hold acquisition spanning the pulmonary arteries was completed in less than 2 min in all subjects. Scan times for a 54-slice navigator-gated QISS scan ranged from 2.0 to 3.4 min. Pulmonary artery branches were conspicuous using either breath-hold or navigator-gated radial QISS, with only mild if any

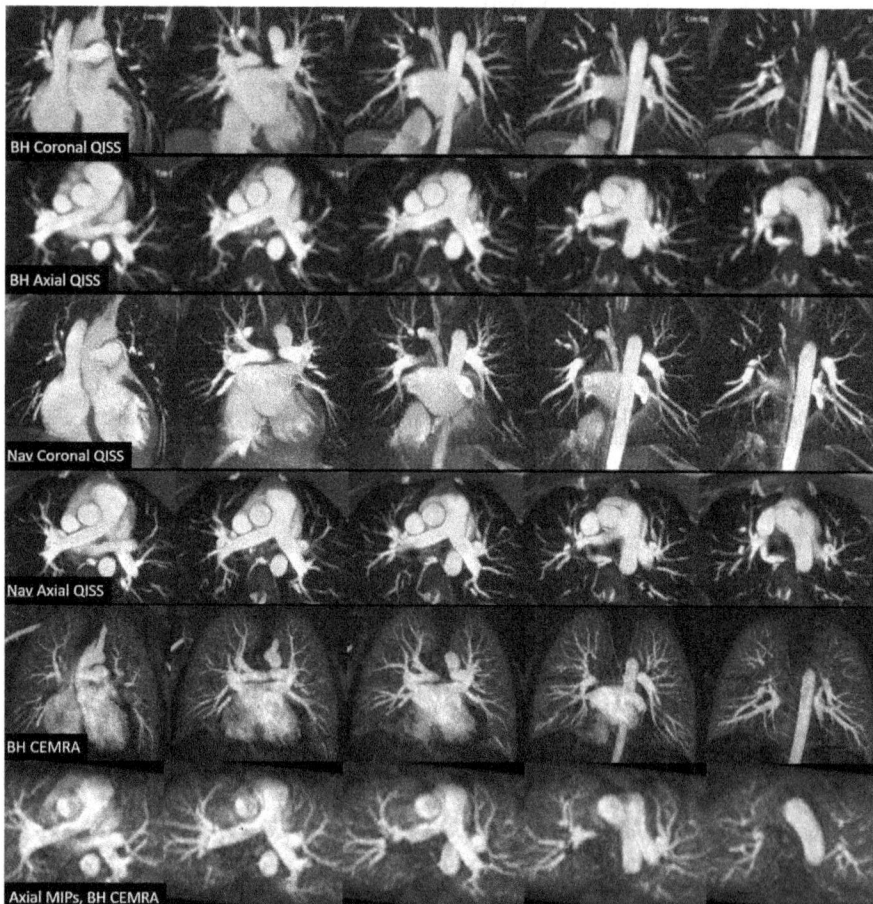

Fig. 1 Comparison of 12-mm thick maximum intensity projections from coronal and axial breath-hold single-shot radial QISS, coronal and axial navigator-gated single-shot radial QISS, and breath-hold coronal CEMRA in a healthy subject. For radial QISS, the maximum intensity projections were reconstructed in the same orientation as the scan. For CEMRA, coronal and axial maximum intensity projections were reconstructed from a coronal scan. Both breath-hold and free-breathing QISS provided comparable depiction of pulmonary arterial anatomy to CEMRA

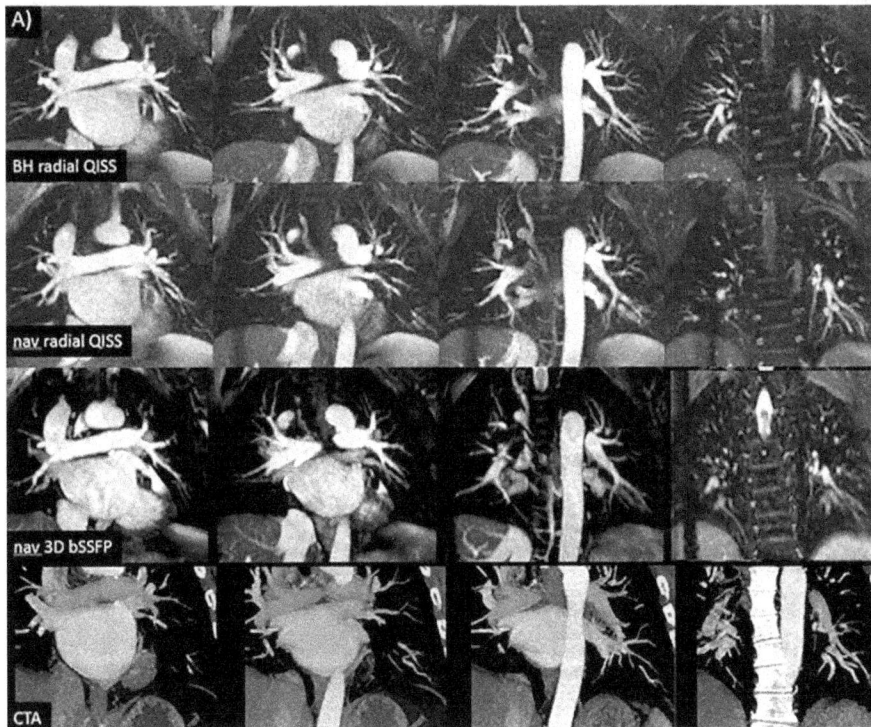

Fig. 2 50-year-old male scheduled for pulmonary vein isolation, who was in sinus rhythm at the time of the CMR exam. **a** 12-mm thick maximum intensity projection images from coronal breath-hold radial QISS, navigator-gated radial QISS, navigator-gated 3D bSSFP, and CTA. Image quality is excellent with all MRA pulse sequences. Scan time was 3.4 min for navigator-gated QISS versus 10.3 min for navigator-gatd 3D bSSFP

blurring apparent on the free-breathing images (Figs. 1 and 2). Compared with navigator-gated 3D, vessels generally appeared sharper with navigator-gated radial QISS and there was less signal from pericardial fluid (Fig. 3). In patients with an irregular cardiac rhythm due to atrial fibrillation, the pulmonary artery branches were conspicuous on radial QISS images, but were degraded with navigator-gated 3D (Fig. 4).

Contrast-enhanced MRA in the volunteers and CTA in the patients demonstrated patency of all scored pulmonary arterial segments, with no evidence of pulmonary embolism or pulmonary artery occlusion down to the segmental level. The mean conspicuity of evaluable pulmonary arterial segments was rated in the acceptable range (1 to 3) by all three readers for both breath-hold and navigator-gated single-shot radial QISS (Table 1). Across the three readers, only 0.57% (2/350) and 0.62% (2/325) of pulmonary arterial segments were rated as "not seen" for breath-hold and navigator-gated QISS, respectively. By comparison, 31.0% (62/200) pulmonary arterial segments were rated as "not seen" during navigator-gated, T2-prepared fat-saturated 3D bSSFP. Friedman testing revealed significant differences in image quality scores between the three nonenhanced protocols ($P < 0.05$). Mean image quality scores for breath-hold QISS, navigator-gated QISS and T2-

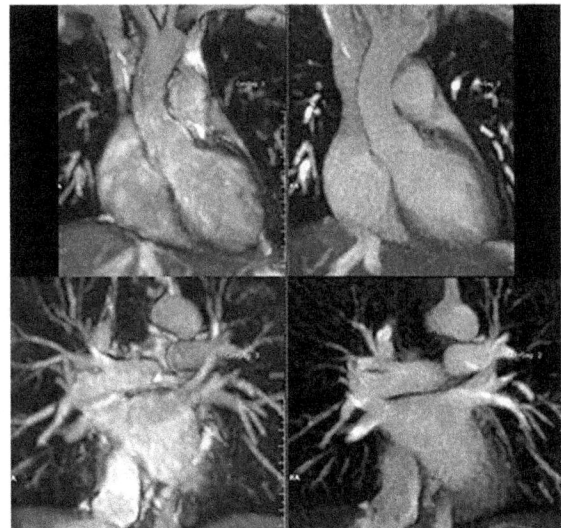

Fig. 3 Comparison of 12-mm thick maximum intensity projections from navigator-gated 3D bSSFP (left) and navigator-gated single-shot radial QISS (right) in a healthy subject. Scans were acquired with identical spatial resolution, navigator positioning, and navigator acceptance window. Compared with 3D bSSFP, single-shot radial QISS shows better suppression of signal from pericardial fluid and less sensitivity to flow and respiratory motion artifacts, resulting in more uniform vessel signal and improved vessel sharpness

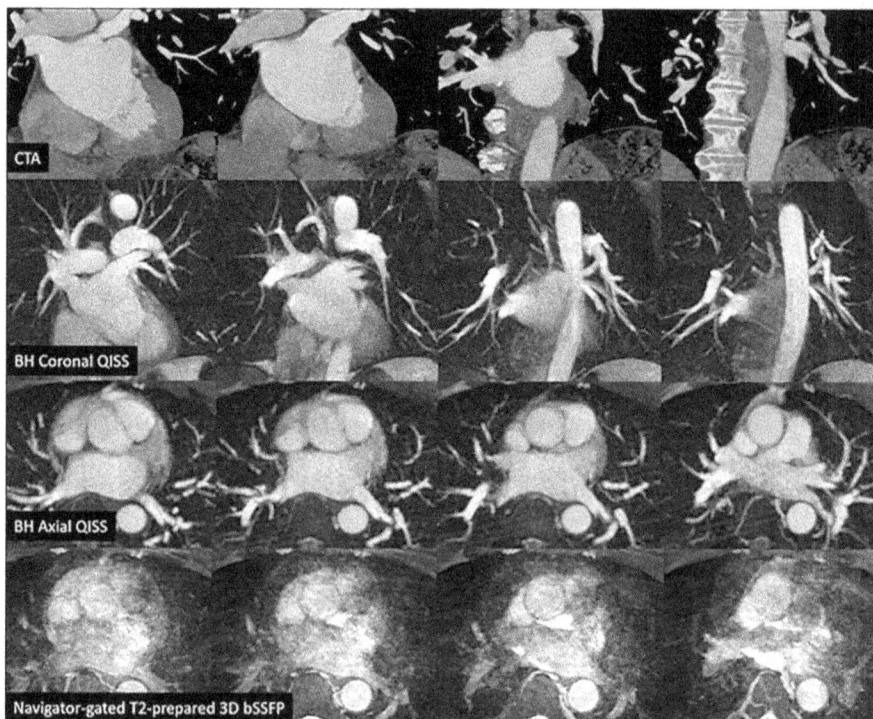

Fig. 4 64-year-old male with poorly controlled atrial fibrillation and a rapid, variable RR interval (~480 ms) who underwent CTA and MRA prior to pulmonary vein isolation. All images are 12-mm thick maximum intensity projections. Single-shot radial QISS (*middle rows*) provided excellent depiction of the pulmonary arteries and veins in coronal and axial orientations despite the uncontrolled arrhythmia, whereas the navigator-gated 3D bSSFP images (*bottom row*) show severe artifacts

prepared fat-saturated 3D bSSFP were 2.1, 2.3 and 2.7 respectively ($P < 0.001$ across nonenhanced protocols), and 2.0 for CEMRA. In general, breath-hold QISS provided better image quality than CEMRA for the pulmonary arteries through the level of the lobar branches, while the converse was true for the segmental branches. However, the number of subjects with CEMRA was too small for statistically meaningful comparison.

For the pulmonary arteries through the level of the lobar branches, inter-reader agreement was substantial for breath-hold QISS (AC1 = 0.62, $P < 0.001$), moderate for navigator-gated QISS (AC1 = 0.47, $P < 0.001$) and T2-prepared fat-saturated 3D bSSFP (AC1 = 0.45, $P < 0.001$), and poor for CEMRA (AC1 = 0.15, $P < 0.01$). For segmental branches, inter-reader agreement was fair for breath-hold QISS (AC1 = 0.24, $P < 0.001$), navigator-gated QISS (AC1 = 0.37, $P < 0.001$), T2-prepared fat-saturated 3D bSSFP (AC1 = 0.22, $P < 0.001$), and CEMRA (AC1 = 0.25, $P < 0.001$).

In one patient with clinically unsuspected pulmonary embolism, radial QISS demonstrated the central pulmonary thrombi comparably to CEMRA and CTA (Fig. 5). The thrombi were highly conspicuous on radial QISS images, but appeared subtle and were not prospectively identified on scout images acquired using an ECG-gated single-shot bSSFP acquisition.

Discussion

Nonenhanced MRA provides a risk-free imaging alternative to CTA and CEMRA. For instance, navigator-gated 3D bSSFP is a well-described free-breathing technique that has been used to image the coronary arteries, pulmonary arteries and other great vessels in the chest [9–12]. However, no NEMRA technique has yet provided the combination of image quality, spatial resolution, scan speed, and resistance to artifacts from cardiac and respiratory motion needed to reliably evaluate the pulmonary arteries. To date, NEMRA has shown only modest sensitivity and specificity in clinical trials for pulmonary embolism [13, 14].

In this prospective technical feasibility study, breath-hold single-shot radial QISS MRA demonstrated pulmonary arterial anatomy from the main pulmonary artery through the level of the segmental branches in less than 2 min. Navigator-gated acquisitions were only slightly slower with scan times of 3.4 min or less, despite the use of both leading and trailing navigators to minimize blurring from respiration. Navigator-gated QISS tended to show slight blurring compared with breath-hold scans, but all pulmonary artery segments were adequately visualized.

In one patient, single-shot QISS clearly demonstrated multiple pulmonary emboli, whereas single-shot bSSFP

Table 1 Image quality ratings

Segment	Nonenhanced QISS BH	Nonenhanced QISS Nav	Nonenhanced 3D Nav bSSFP	Friedman *P*-value	CEMRA
Main Pulmonary Artery	1.0	1.1	1.6	NS	1.4
Right Pulmonary Artery	1.1	1.2	1.6	NS	1.4
Left Pulmonary Artery	1.1	1.2	1.6	NS	1.4
Right Upper Lobar Artery	1.3	1.6	2.0	NS	1.6
Right Lower Lobar Artery	1.3	1.5	2.0	NS	1.7
Left Upper Lobar Artery	1.7	1.7	2.3	NS	1.4
Left Lower Lobar Artery	1.3	1.7	2.0	NS	1.4
RUL-Apical	2.5	2.7	3.0	<0.01	1.9
RUL-Anterior	2.6	2.7	3.0	NS	2.1
RUL-Posterior	2.5	2.7	3.0	<0.01	2.1
RML-Lateral	2.6	2.7	3.1	<0.01	2.1
RML-Medial	2.6	2.7	3.0	<0.01	2.1
RLL-Superior	2.6	2.7	3.0	<0.01	2.1
RLL-Medial Basal	2.5	2.7	3.0	<0.05	2.1
RLL-Anterior Basal	2.5	2.7	3.0	<0.01	2.1
RLL-Lateral Basal	2.6	2.7	3.1	<0.05	2.1
RLL-Posterior Basal	2.4	2.7	3.1	<0.01	2.1
LUL-Apicoposterior	2.4	2.7	3.0	<0.05	2.1
LUL-Anterior	2.4	2.7	3.0	<0.05	2.2
LUL-Superior Lingular	2.5	2.7	3.0	<0.01	2.4
LUL-Inferior Lingular	2.5	2.7	3.0	<0.05	2.4
LLL-Superior	2.5	2.7	3.0	<0.01	2.4
LLL-Anteromedial Basal	2.5	2.7	3.0	<0.01	2.4
LLL-Lateral Basal	2.4	2.6	3.1	<0.01	2.2
LLL-Posterior Basal	2.2	2.4	3.1	<0.001	2.2
All Segments	2.1	2.3	2.7	<0.001	2.0

Values are means across the three readers. *BH* breath-hold, *Nav* navigator-gated, *bSSFP* balanced steady-state free precession, *RUL* right upper lobe, *RML* right middle lobe, *RLL* right lower lobe, *LUL* left upper lobe, *LLL* left lower lobe, *NS* not significant

showed poor conspicuity of the emboli. This case highlights that QISS, unlike bSSFP, is a highly flow-dependent imaging technique. A potential concern with QISS is saturation of in-plane flow, which is a common source of artifacts with conventional 2D time-of-flight MRA. However, we did not observe a significant degree of in-plane saturation in the pulmonary arteries through the segmental level. To maximize flow contrast, the QISS technique applies an in-plane inversion pulse prior to a quiescent interval of a few hundred milliseconds, which is then followed by a single-shot bSSFP readout. QISS differs from 2D time-of-flight MRA in that rapid systolic flow during the quiescent interval will tend to wash out saturated spins, even when the slice and vessel orientations are substantially aligned.

Cardiac arrhythmias are common in older patients due to hypertension and other co-morbidities [15]. We found that single-shot radial QISS, in contrast to navigator-gated 3D bSSFP, is resistant to motion artifacts

from atrial fibrillation. The sub-second (~284 msec) readout duration for each single-shot radial QISS image effectively freezes cardiac motion and thereby avoids image artifacts. On the other hand, a navigator-gated 3D bSSFP acquisition accumulates data over dozens of cardiac cycles, so that beat-to-beat variations in cardiac dimensions and tissue signal cause image artifacts.

Compared with CEMRA, radial QISS eliminates the possibility of artifacts from imaging too early or late during the contrast infusion. The ability to repeat the scan and tailor scan planes and spatial resolution as needed, along with the capability for free-breathing acquisitions, represent other potential advantages over CEMRA, where flexibility is limited by the need to acquire all data during the first pass of contrast agent.

Further improvements in radial QISS image quality should be readily obtainable. For instance, given that these images are sparse and undersampled, iterative reconstruction techniques such as non-Cartesian SENSE

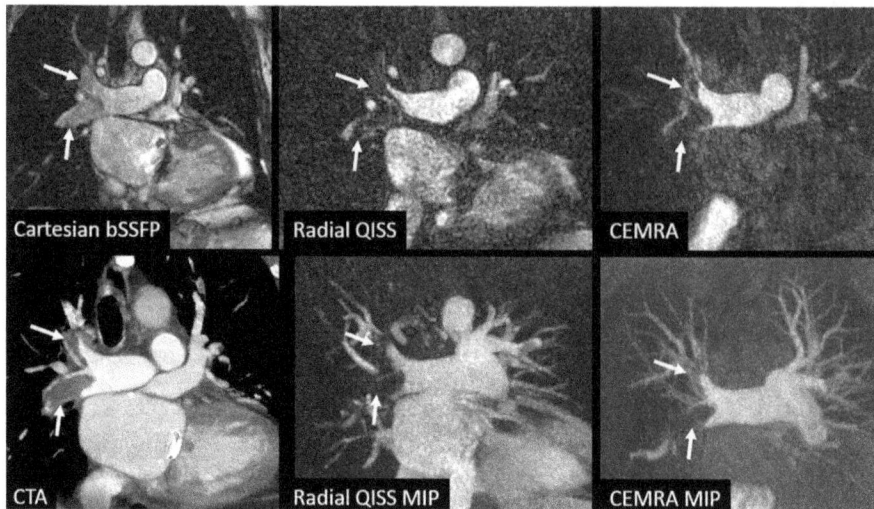

Fig. 5 68-year-old male with shortness of breath and suspected peri-valvular leak following mitral valve repair, who underwent CMR which revealed clinically unsuspected central pulmonary emboli. *Top row*: source images from scout scan acquired using ECG-gated single-shot Cartesian bSSFP (*left*), single-shot radial QISS (*middle*), and CEMRA (*right*), *Bottom row*: multi-planar reconstruction from CTA performed immediately following the MR exam (*left*), 64-mm maximum intensity projection from radial QISS (*middle*), 64-mm maximum intensity projection from CEMRA (*right*). The pulmonary emboli are well shown by radial QISS and CEMRA. Note that the thrombi are much more conspicuous with radial QISS than with bSSFP

or compressed sensing can be used to improve image quality [16, 17]. Simultaneous multi-slice imaging techniques can further shorten scan time, although to date most efforts have been directed to Cartesian rather than radial imaging [18].

There are several limitations to our study design. While radial QISS consistently demonstrated the pulmonary arteries down to the segmental level, imaging of smaller subsegmental branches could prove challenging due to the impact of off-resonance effects within the lung parenchyma relating to the use of a bSSFP readout. As more powerful gradient systems become available, it should be possible to shorten the bSSFP TR, thereby reducing off-resonance artifacts and improving the conspicuity of distal pulmonary arterial branches. The quality of the B0 shim is more critical with QISS, which uses a bSSFP readout, than with CEMRA, which uses a short-TE 3D spoiled gradient-echo readout. Only a small number of subjects were evaluated, and only one had significant pulmonary arterial pathology. While pulmonary emboli were anecdotally demonstrated using QISS in one patient, no assumptions can be made about the diagnostic accuracy of the technique.

Conclusions

In summary, this technical feasibility study has demonstrated that both breath-hold and free-breathing radial QISS can rapidly and consistently depict normal pulmonary arterial anatomy down to the segmental level with an exam time on the order of a few minutes. The technique unambiguously detected central pulmonary emboli in one patient, with much improved contrast compared with standard bSSFP. Further study will be required to determine the accuracy and utility of the radial QISS technique in patients suspected of pulmonary embolism.

Abbreviations
bSSFP: Balanced steady-state free precession; CE: Contrast enhanced; CTA: Computed tomography angiography; ECG: Electrocardiogram; MRA: Magnetic resonance angiography; PE: Pulmonary embolism; QISS: Quiescent-interval slice-selective

Acknowledgements
We would like to thank Dr. Wei Li for assisting with data collection and analysis.

Funding
Research support, NIH grants R01 HL130093 and R21 HL126015. Research support, Siemens Healthcare. Research support, Department of Radiology, NorthShore University HealthSystem.

Authors' contributions
RE participated in all aspects of the study and is the guarantor of study integrity. RS assisted with image analysis and manuscript review. KT assisted with image analysis and manuscript review. MM assisted with patient recruitment and manuscript review. JN assisted with patient recruitment and manuscript review. SG assisted with pulse sequence implementation and manuscript review. IK assisted with pulse sequence implementation, statistical analysis and manuscript review. All authors read and approved the manuscript.

Authors' information
None.

Competing interests
RE: Research support and invention licensing agreement, Siemens Healthcare.
SG: Employee, Siemens Healthcare.
There were no non-financial conflicts of interest for any of the authors.

Consent for publication

Consent for publication of their individual details and accompanying images in this manuscript was prospectively provided in 13 subjects, the need for consent was retrospectively waived by the IRB in one patient. No protected health information for any subject is given in this manuscript.

Author details

[1]Department of Radiology, NorthShore University HealthSystem, 2650 Ridge Avenue, Evanston, IL 60201, USA. [2]Feinberg School of Medicine, Northwestern University, Chicago, USA. [3]The University of Chicago Pritzker School of Medicine, Chicago, USA. [4]Siemens Medical Solutions USA, Inc., Chicago, USA.

References

1. Lapner ST, Kearon C. Diagnosis and management of pulmonary embolism. BMJ. 2013 Feb 20;346:f757. doi:10.1136/bmj.f757.
2. Coresh J, Astor BC, Greene T, Eknoyan G, Levey AS. Prevalence of chronic kidney disease and decreased kidney function in the adult US population. Third National Health and nutrition examination survey. Am J Kidney Dis. 2003;41:1–12.
3. Nagle SK, Schiebler ML, Repplinger MD, François CJ, Vigen KK, Yarlagadda R, et al. Contrast enhanced pulmonary magnetic resonance angiography for pulmonary embolism: building a successful program. Eur J Radiol. 2016; 85(3):553–63. doi:10.1016/j.ejrad.2015.12.018. Epub 2015 Dec 29
4. Semelka RC, Ramalho M, AlObaidy M, Ramalho J. Gadolinium in humans: a family of disorders. AJR Am J Roentgenol. 2016;207(2):229–33. doi:10.2214/AJR.15.15842. Epub 2016 May 25
5. Edelman RR, Giri S, Pursnani A, Botelho MPF, Li W, Koktzoglou I. Breath-hold imaging of the coronary arteries using quiescent-interval slice-selective (QISS) magnetic resonance angiography: pilot study at 1.5 Tesla and 3 Tesla. J Cardiovasc Magn Reson. 2015;17:101. PMID 26597281
6. Glover GH, Pauly JM. Projection reconstruction techniques for reduction of motion effects in MRI. Magn Reson Med. 1992;28:275–89.
7. Edelman RR, Botelho M, Pursnani A, Giri S, Koktzoglou I. Improved dark blood imaging of the heart using radial balanced steady-state free precession. J Cardiovasc Magn Reson. 2016 Oct 19;18(1):69.
8. Jackson CL, Huber JF. Correlated applied anatomy of the bronchial tree and lungs with a system of nomenclature. Dis Chest. 1943;9:319–26.
9. François CJ, Tuite D, Deshpande V, Jerecic R, Weale P, Carr JC. Pulmonary vein imaging with unenhanced three-dimensional balanced steady-state free precession MR angiography: initial clinical evaluation. Radiology. 2009; 250(3):932–9. doi:10.1148/radiol.2502072137. Epub 2009 Jan 22
10. Hui BK, Noga ML, Gan KD, Wilman AH. Navigator-gated three-dimensional MR angiography of the pulmonary arteries using steady-state free precession. J Magn Reson Imaging. 2005 Jun;21(6):831–5.
11. Gebker R, Gomaa O, Schnackenburg B, Rebakowski J, Fleck E, Nagel E. Comparison of different MRI techniques for the assessment of thoracic aortic pathology: 3D contrast enhanced MR angiography, turbo spin echo and balanced steady state free precession. Int J Cardiovasc Imaging. 2007 Dec;23(6):747–56.
12. Tomasian A, Lohan DG, Laub G, Singhal A, Finn JP, Krishnam MS. Noncontrast 3D steady state free precession magnetic resonance angiography of the thoracic central veins using nonselective radiofrequency excitation over a large field of view. Investig Radiol. 2008;43:306–13. PubMed: 18424951
13. Kluge A, Mueller C, Strunk J, Lange U, Bachmann G. Experience in 207 combined MRI examinations for acute pulmonary embolism and deep vein thrombosis. AJR Am J Roentgenol. 2006 Jun;186(6):1686–96.
14. Kalb B, Sharma P, Tigges S, et al. MR imaging of pulmonary embolism: diagnostic accuracy of contrast-enhanced 3D MR pulmonary angiography, contrast-enhanced low-flip angle 3D GRE, and nonenhanced free-induction FISP sequences. Radiology. 2012 Apr;263(1):271–8. doi:10.1148/radiol.12110224.
15. Chow GV, Marine JE, Fleg JL. Epidemiology of arrhythmias and conduction disorders in older adults. Clin Geriatr Med. 2012 Nov;28(4):539–53.
16. Wright KL, Hamilton JI, Griswold MA, Gulani V, Seiberlich N. Non-Cartesian parallel imaging reconstruction. J Magn Reson Imaging. 2014;40(5):1022–40. doi:10.1002/jmri.24521. Epub 2014 Jan 10
17. Akçakaya M, Hu P, Chuang ML, et al. Accelerated noncontrast-enhanced pulmonary vein MRA with distributed compressed sensing. J Magn Reson Imaging. 2011 May;33(5):1248–55. doi:10.1002/jmri.22559.
18. Barth M, Breuer F, Koopmans PJ, Norris DG, Poser BA. Simultaneous multislice (SMS) imaging techniques. Magn Reson Med. 2016;75(1):63–81. doi:10.1002/mrm.25897. Epub 2015 Aug 26

7

Diagnostic performance of image navigated coronary CMR angiography in patients with coronary artery disease

Markus Henningsson[1*], Joy Shome[1], Konstantinos Bratis[1], Miguel Silva Vieira[1], Eike Nagel[1,2,3] and Rene M. Botnar[1,4]

Abstract

Background: The use of coronary MR angiography (CMRA) in patients with coronary artery disease (CAD) remains limited due to the long scan times, unpredictable and often non-diagnostic image quality secondary to respiratory motion artifacts. The purpose of this study was to evaluate CMRA with image-based respiratory navigation (iNAV CMRA) and compare it to gold standard invasive x-ray coronary angiography in patients with CAD.

Methods: Consecutive patients referred for CMR assessment were included to undergo iNAV CMRA on a 1.5 T scanner. Coronary vessel sharpness and a visual score were assigned to the coronary arteries. A diagnostic reading was performed on the iNAV CMRA data, where a lumen narrowing >50% was considered diseased. This was compared to invasive x-ray findings.

Results: Image-navigated CMRA was performed in 31 patients (77% male, 56 ± 14 years). The iNAV CMRA scan time was 7 min:21 s ± 0 min:28 s. Out of a possible 279 coronary segments, 26 segments were excluded from analysis due to stents or diameter less than 1.5 mm, resulting in a total of 253 coronary segments. Diagnostic image quality was obtained for 98% of proximal coronary segments, 94% of middle segments, and 91% of distal coronary segments. The sensitivity and specificity was 86% and 83% per patient, 80% and 92% per vessel and 73% and 95% per segment.

Conclusion: In this study, iNAV CMRA offered a very good diagnostic performance when compared against invasive x-ray angiography. Due to the short and predictable scan time it can add clinical value as a part of a comprehensive CAD assessment protocol.

Keywords: Coronary MR angiography, Image navigators, Respiratory motion correction, Coronary artery disease

Background

Whole-heart coronary magnetic resonance angiography (CMRA) allows for non-invasive and ionizing radiation free detection of lumen narrowing coronary artery disease (CAD) [1]. Nevertheless, CMRA in patients with CAD remains limited due to the long scan times as well as unpredictable and often non-diagnostic CMRA image quality. The most common image degradation in CMRA is caused by image blurring and ghosting from respiratory motion [2]. This is due to the necessity of acquiring high-resolution whole-heart CMRA during free-breathing.

* Correspondence: markus.henningsson@kcl.ac.uk
Dr. Debiao Li served as the Guest Editor for this manuscript.
[1]Division of Biomedical Engineering and Imaging Sciences, King's College London, London, UK
Full list of author information is available at the end of the article

Conventional motion compensation for CMRA involves interleaving a one-dimensional diaphragmatic 'navigator' acquisition to track the lung-liver interface in foot-head direction. This allows prospective correction (typically assuming a fixed linear relationship between motion of the diaphragm and that of the heart) and gating, which narrows down the range of acceptable motion to end-expiration at the expense of prolonging scan time [3].

In the last decade, a number of navigator techniques have been described which allow direct measurement and correction of respiratory induced motion of the heart. These include self-navigation, which extract the motion information from the CMRA data itself [4, 5], and image-based navigation where real-time images are used to estimate bulk respiratory motion of the heart

[6–9]. In addition to directly tracking respiratory motion of the heart, self-navigation simplifies CMRA ease-of-use compared to other navigator approaches, as no dedicated navigator scan planning is necessary. Self-navigation and image-based navigation can be combined with affine [10, 11] and non-linear [12, 13] correction which aims to correct for all respiratory motion, leading to CMRA data across the whole respiratory cycle and shorter scan time compared to a gated scan. However, these advanced correction strategies require computationally expensive offline post-processing.

More recently, respiratory motion compensation using image-based navigation (iNAV) has been proposed for CMRA, and allows for accurate, direct tracking of the respiratory motion of the heart and can be implemented with inline correction [14]. In conjunction with efficient respiratory gating such as constant respiratory efficiency using single end-expiratory threshold (CRUISE), CMRA can be acquired with high image quality, with inline processing and in a clinically acceptable scan time [15].

The purpose of this study was to evaluate iNAV-CRUISE motion compensation for CMRA and compare it to gold standard invasive x-ray coronary angiography in patients with CAD.

Methods

Patient selection

Between February 2014 and October 2014, based on the availability of the research team, consecutive patients referred for CMR were considered for inclusion in this prospective study. The study was approved by the institutional ethics committee and all participants provided written informed consent. Patients were excluded from the study if they had pace makers, defibrillators or other general contraindications to CMR such as claustrophobia.

CMR protocol

All experiments were performed on a 1.5 T clinical CMR scanner (Achieva, Philips Healthcare, Best, The Netherlands) using a 32-channel cardiac coil. The patients underwent a protocol consisting of multi-slice cine stack, first-pass perfusion, multi-slice late gadolinium enhancement stack and iNAV CMRA. For the late gadolinium enhancement, contrast medium was used (Gadobutrol, Gadovist®, Bayer AG, Leverkusen, Germany, dose: 0.2 mmol/kg). The CMRA scan was performed after contrast administration using bolus injection for the first-pass perfusion and before the late gadolinium enhancement scans. No specific patient preparation was performed, such as administration of β-blockers or nitroglycerine, for the CMRA scan.

Image navigated CMRA

Image navigator correction and gating was implemented for CMRA respiratory motion compensation. The iNAV was acquired using 10 startup echoes of the balanced steady state free precesion (bSSFP) sequence, as previously described [16]. A region-of-interest encompassing the whole heart was tracked in foot-head (FH) and left-right (LR) direction, and selected using the local shim geometry. The iNAV reference was defined as the first acquired navigator to which all subsequent iNAVs were registered using normalised cross-correlation. The 2D translational correction was applied to the CMRA k-space raw data by modulating its phase. Respiratory gating was implemented using CRUISE. In brief, this approach acquires twice as much data as needed to fill CMRA k-space (resulting in exactly 50% gating efficiency) and only the half acquired at the most end-expiratory was used to reconstruct the gated image [15]. Both iNAV correction and gating was performed in real-time on the scanner, and no post-processing was required.

The CMRA protocol consisted of a bSSFP sequence with the following imaging parameters: FOV = 330 × 330 × 110 mm^3, Δx = 1.3 × 1.3 × 1.3 mm^3, repetition time/echo time = 3.9/1.95 ms, flip angle = 70°, coronal orientation, and parallel imaging acceleration factor = 2.5 (in-plane phase encoding direction). Electrocardiogram triggering was used to minimize cardiac motion, with subject-specific trigger delays and acquisition windows. To improve CMRA contrast, T2 prep (echo time = 35 ms) and fat suppression pre-pulses were used. The nominal scan time, including respiratory gating with 50% efficiency, was 7 min and 16 s, assuming a heart rate of 60 beats per minute and an acquisition window of 120 ms.

Image analysis

All CMRA images were reformatted using dedicated software to visualize the right coronary artery (RCA), left main and left anterior descending coronary artery (LAD), and left circumflex coronary artery (LCX). To objectively and subjectively assess CMRA image quality, vessel sharpness measurements and visual score were performed on all datasets. Vessel sharpness was calculated on the first 4 cm of all coronary arteries, as a percentage where 0% equals no edge and 100% a step edge, using dedicated software [17]. For the patient data, vessel sharpness was assessed by an expert (Reviewer 1, with 8 years of experience in CMRA). Vessel sharpness was repeated on 10 random datasets 3 months later to assess intra-observer variability, compounding the vessel sharpness of the RCA, LAD and LCX. A second expert (Reviewer 2, with 4 years of experience in CMRA) performed vessel sharpness measurements on 10 random patient datasets to evaluate inter-observer variability, again, compounding sharpness values from the three coronary arteries.

A visual score was used, based on a previous CMRA patient study [1], to qualitatively assess coronary artery image quality based on the following scale: 0 – coronary artery not visible, 1 – visible but with marked blurring, 2 – visible with moderate blurring, 3 – visible with mild blurring, and 4 – visible with sharp edges. Visual score of 2 or higher was considered diagnostic quality. A segmental analysis was performed using a 9 coronary segment model, previously used in CMRA studies [18]. With this model the following segments were analysed: the left main (LM) artery, proximal, mid and distal segments of the LAD, proximal and mid segments of the LCX, and proximal mid and distal segments of the RCA. Coronary segments were excluded from analysis if they had previous stents or if the diameter was less than 1.5 mm. The visual scoring was performed independently by two experts, blinded to the patient's information.

To assess diagnostic performance significant coronary stenosis was visually defined as luminal narrowing of more than 50% in each of the 9 segments using an intention-to-treat approach. The findings from the diagnostic reading of the coronary segments were compared to gold standard coronary x-ray angiographies, which were performed within 6 months of the CMRA scan. The diagnostic reading was performed by two expert readers, blinded to the x-ray angiography results. Disagreements between the readers were settled with a consensus reading. The likelihood of stenosis was graded according to the following scale: 1 – absent, 2 – probably absent, 3 – possibly present, 4 – probably present and 5 – definitely present [19].

Statistical analysis

All statistical analyses were performed using MATLAB (The Mathworks Inc., Natick, MA USA) statistics toolbox. For the continuous variables vessel sharpness and scan time, a two-tailed t-test was performed to evaluate statistical significance. Continuous variables are presented as mean ± standard deviation. For the categorical variable (visual score) a Wilcoxon signed rank test was performed to evaluate statistical significance. Categorical variables are presented as median, 75th percentile, 25th percentile. A P value smaller than 0.05 was considered statistically significant. To evaluate intra-and inter-observer variability intra-class correlation coefficient was calculated for the different measurements. Additionally, the mean difference and standard deviation for the intra and inter-observer measurements were calculated. Inter-observer agreement of the visual scores was performed using Cohen's kappa coefficient where a coefficient less than 0.4 was considered poor, between 0.4 and 0.75 good, and higher than 0.75 excellent agreement.

The visual scores for coronary segments were divided into proximal (proximal RCA, LM, proximal LAD, and proximal LCX), middle (middle RCA, LAD and LCX) and distal (distal RCA and LAD) segments to evaluate image quality between segments. This analysis included a Kruskal-Wallis one-way analysis of variance to determine any difference between the three groups, using a $P < 0.05$ to signify statistical difference. If a statistically significant difference was found, post hoc multiple Mann Whitney U tests were performed with a $P < 0.017$ considered statistically significant. The smaller significance threshold is due to the Bonferroni correction for multiple comparisons (0.05/3 = 0.017).

To assess whether patient variables such as age, heart rate, and body mass index (BMI) were correlated with vessel sharpness, bivariate analysis was performed. A linear regression model was calculated and Pearson's correlation coefficient calculated to investigate if these variables could predict coronary vessel sharpness. The coronary vessel sharpness score was averaged across the RCA, LAD and LCX for each patient to obtain a single vessel sharpness score.

Results

In total, 31 patients were recruited for the study and their characteristics are summarized in Table 1. Of the 31 CMRA datasets, coronary stents precluded analysis in 8 coronary arteries. In total, out of a possible 279 coronary segments, 26 segments (8 proximal, 9 middle and 9 distal segments) were excluded from analysis due to stents or diameter less than 1.5 mm, resulting in a total of 253 coronary segments. The effective duration for the 31 patient scans was 7:21 ± 0:28 (min:sec). The CMRA acquisition was performed in systole in 19% of 6 patients (6 of 31) (heart rate = 78 ± 12 beats/min; acquisition window = 85 ± 22 ms; imaging time = 8:30 ± 0:33 min:sec) and diastole in 81% of patients (25 of 31) (heart rate = 63 ± 15 beats/min; acquisition window = 118 ± 38 ms;

Table 1 Patient characteristics

Total no of patients	31
Age (y)	56.4 ± 14.7
Men	24 (77.4%)
Heart rate (bpm)	66.4 ± 10.9
BMI (kg/m^2)	27.3 ± 4.0
Hypertension	17 (55.8%)
Hyperlipidaemia	13 (41.9%)
Smoker	10 (32.2%)

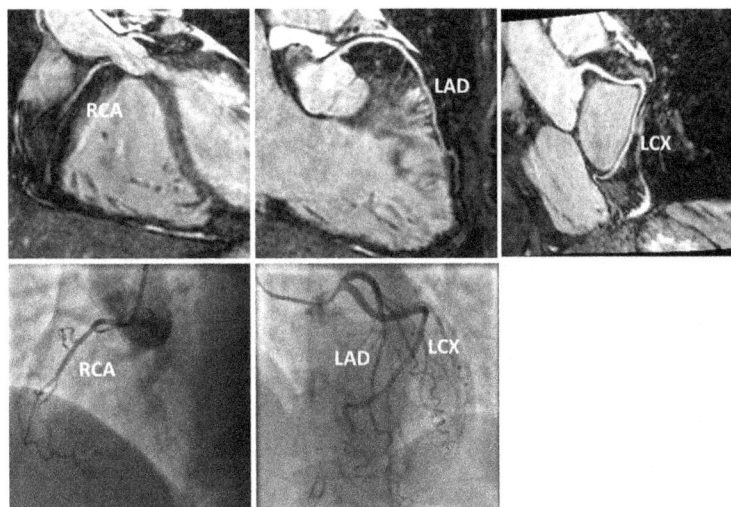

Fig. 1 Reformatted CMRA datasets (top row) from a patient without coronary artery disease but non dominant right coronary artery (RCA). Coronary x-ray angiography in the same patient (bottom row). LAD = left anterior descending artery; LCX = left circumflex artery

imaging time = 7:13 ± 0:18 min:sec). An example CMRA dataset from a patient without CAD but non dominant RCA which precluded analysis of mid and distal segments of the RCA is shown in Fig. 1.

CMRA image quality

The distribution of the visual scores of the 253 coronary segments, divided into proximal, middle and distal segments is shown in Fig. 2. The Kruskal-Wallis test, comparing distributions of visual scores for proximal, middle and distal segments, revealed a statistically significant

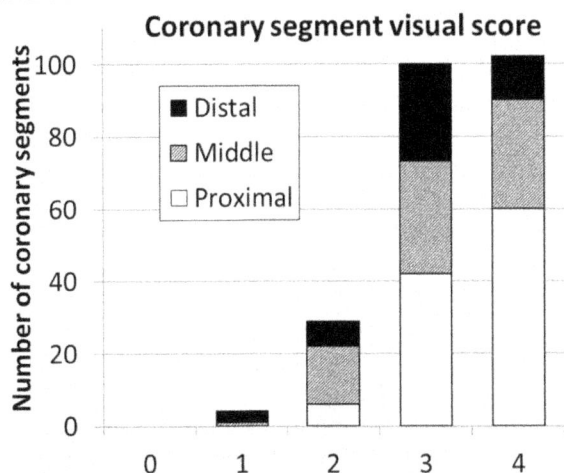

Fig. 2 Distribution of visual scores of coronary segments, partitioned into proximal, middle and distal segments. A score of 0 is considered a non-visible coronary segment and 5 a visible segment with sharp edges. Visual scores of 2 or higher are considered to be of diagnostic image quality

difference ($P < 0.01$). Post-hoc Mann Whitney U test showed a statistically significant difference between visual scores for proximal and mid segments (proximal: 4,4,3 vs mid: 3,4,3, $P < 0.01$) and proximal and distal segments (proximal: 4,4,3 vs distal: 3,3,3 $P < 0.001$). Diagnostic image quality, defined as having a visual score of 2 or more, was obtained in 98% of all proximal coronary segments (113/115), 94% of middle segments (79/84), and 91% of distal coronary segments (49/54). In two patients, with significant arrhythmia, non-diagnostic image quality was found in 9 coronary segments, which corresponded to 75% of the total number of non-diagnostic segments. There was a good agreement between observers for the visual scoring, with a kappa coefficient of 0.71.

Vessel sharpness for the RCA was 53.9% ± 9.5%, LAD 56.2% ± 7.2% and LCX 51.9% ± 6.9%. Both intra- and inter-observer variability showed good agreement. The intra-observer mean difference was found to be −0.05% with a 95% confidence interval of 1.8% to −1.9%. The inter-observer mean difference was 0.23% and 95% confidence interval of 3.2% to −2.8%. The correlation analysis between patient characteristics and coronary vessel sharpness is shown in Fig. 3. None of the variables including age, BMI or heart rate predicted coronary sharpness on the multiple regression analysis ($R^2 = 0.10$, p = N.S.).

Diagnostic performance

Seven patients (24%) were found to have significant CAD based on coronary x-ray angiography. This included 8 diseased proximal segments, four diseased middle segments and three diseased distal segments. The

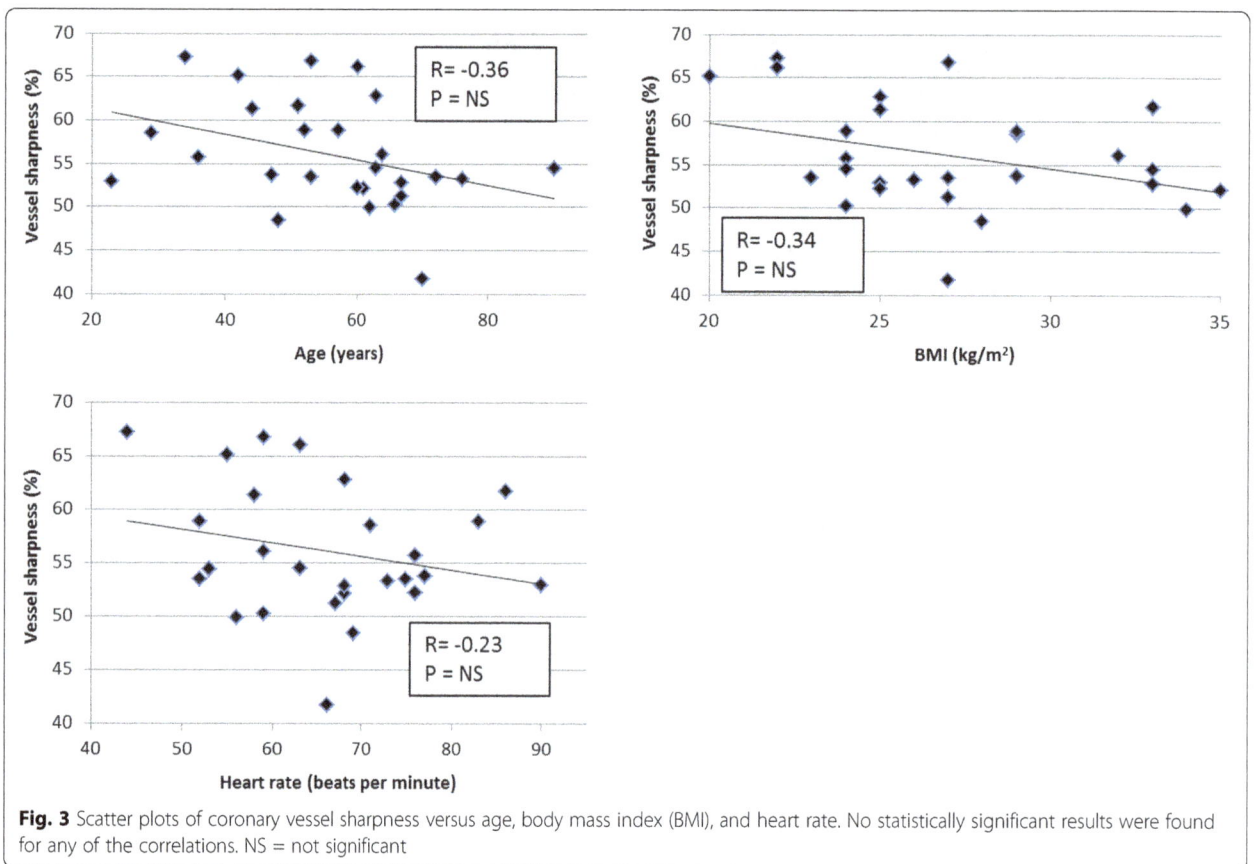

Fig. 3 Scatter plots of coronary vessel sharpness versus age, body mass index (BMI), and heart rate. No statistically significant results were found for any of the correlations. NS = not significant

receiver-operator characteristics curves for the CMRA per patient, vessel and segment are shown in Fig. 4. The per-patient, vessel and segment area under the curve was 0.91% (95% CI: 79% to 100%), 93% (95% CI: 81% to 100%) and 92% (95% CI: 84% to 99%), respectively. CMRA was able to detect significant CAD in 6 out of 7 patients (86%), 8 out of 10 vessels (80%), and 11 out of 15 segments (73%). The sensitivity, specificity, positive predictive value and negative predictive value for the-per patient, vessel and segmental analysis are summarized in Table 2. Example images from three patients with coronary artery disease, where the diagnosis was identified from the CMRA and confirmed in the coronary X-ray angiography, are shown in Fig. 5.

Discussion

In this work, we have evaluated a new approach for respiratory motion compensated CMRA using image navigator motion correction and gating. Compared to conventional CMRA motion compensation using a diaphragmatic navigator, the proposed approach reduces operator dependence as no dedicated respiratory navigator scan planning is required. The inline motion compensation allowed CMRA reconstruction at the scanner console and visualization of coronary arteries to aid

diagnosis without interrupting the clinical workflow. A high percentage (241 of 253; 95%) of coronary artery segments was of diagnostic image quality, suggesting the proposed iNAV CMRA approach is a robust and reliable tool with additive clinical value.

In recent years, there have been a few studies in patients with CAD using CMRA with conventional respiratory motion compensation. In a multi-center trial Kato et al. [19] reported a per-patient sensitivity and specificity of 88% and 72%, respectively, using 1.5 T scanners with Cartesian bSSFP acquisition and a spatial resolution similar to iNAV CMRA. Yang et al. [20] obtained a sensitivity of 94% and specificity of 82% using a 3 T scanner and slow-infusion contrast enhanced gradient echo acquisition. While the diagnostic performance in these studies was comparable to iNAV CMRA, the scan time was approximately 2 min longer, with a large distribution of values reflecting the unpredictability of scan times using the conventional navigator approach. Furthermore, the reported failure rate in these studies was 8–10%, while the completion rate of iNAV CMRA was 100%.

A further two studies have reported on the use of advanced respiratory motion compensation strategies in patients with CAD. Piccini et al. used a radial k-space

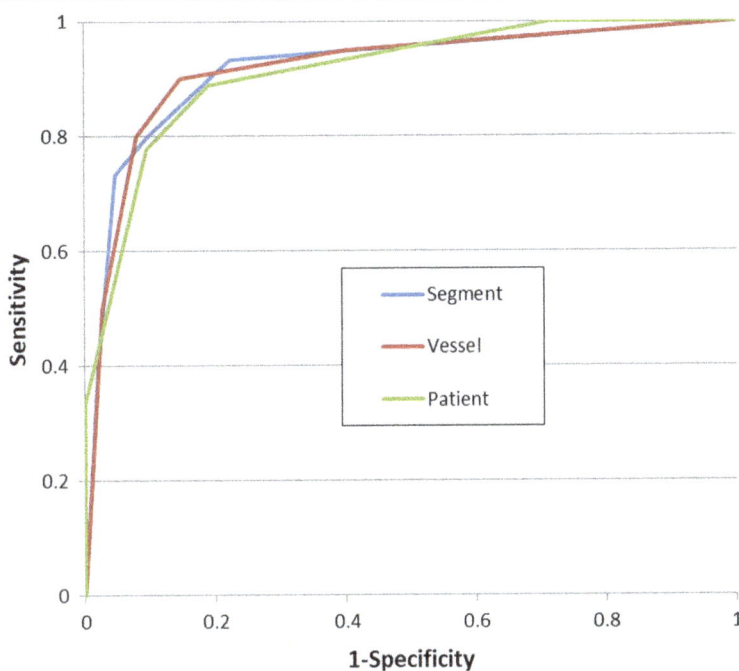

Fig. 4 A receiver operator characteristic curves of iNAV CMRA for detecting significant coronary artery stenosis

trajectory with translational correction and 100% gating efficiency, and obtained a per-patient sensitivity and specificity of 71% and 62%, respectively [21]. Differences in navigator acquisition approach may explain the differences in diagnostic performance compared to iNAV CMRA, where Piccini et al. used a one-dimensional projection navigator to detect motion, which may include static tissue leading to motion under-estimation. In comparison, the spatially resolved iNAV avoids this problem, allowing for accurate motion estimation even with only a few phase encoding steps [16]. Furthermore, a constant 50% gating efficiency was implemented for iNAV CMRA. This effectively discards the most motion corrupted data which may have been corrupted by large translations and n'on-rigid motion. Despite the scan time penalty introduced by the respiratory gating, the mean scan time using iNAV (7:21 min:sec) was shorter compared to Piccini et al. (7:50 min:sec) This is likely

due to the use of parallel imaging with a factor of 2.5, as well as the lower spatial resolution. Similar to Piccini et al., He et al. [18] used a radial trajectory with 100% respiratory gating efficiency but more advanced 3D affine motion correction and reported a per-patient sensitivity and specificity was 96% and 69%, respectively. Apart from the technical differences in strategies for respiratory motion correction, a higher field strength (3 T) and higher spatial resolution (1 mm isotropic), He et al. used a stricter exclusion criteria which encompassed patients with arrhythmia. However, this criterion was not applied in the current study and affected the diagnostic performance as a majority of non-diagnostic segments were found in two patients with significant arrhythmia, which led to false positive diagnosis, lower specificity and PPV. Compared to the technique developed by He et al. iNAV CMRA does not require offline, retrospective postprocessing. To account for non-rigid motion without the use of respiratory gating could involve implementing image registration and correction with more degrees of freedom, such as affine or non-linear motion models. However, this is technically challenging to perform in real-time due to the increased computational complexity. Furthermore, the spatial resolution of the navigator also has to be sufficiently high to capture this motion, whereas the proposed iNAV has limited resolution in LR direction and is a projection of the heart in anterior-posterior direction. Recently, techniques have been proposed to enable motion estimation from high resolution

Table 2 Diagnostic performance. Data are % (raw data) [95% confidence interval]. PPV = positive predictive value; NPV = negative predictive values

	Patient	Vessel	Segment
Sensitivity	86 (6/7) [42–99]	80 (8/10) [44–97]	73 (11/15) [45–92]
Specificity	83 (21/24) [62–95]	92 (68/72) [83–97]	95 (227/238) [92–98]
PPV	60 (6/10) [37–79]	57 (8/14) [34–75]	50 (11/22) [34–66]
NPV	95 (20/21) [76–99]	97 (68/70) [91 99]	98 (227/231) [96–99]

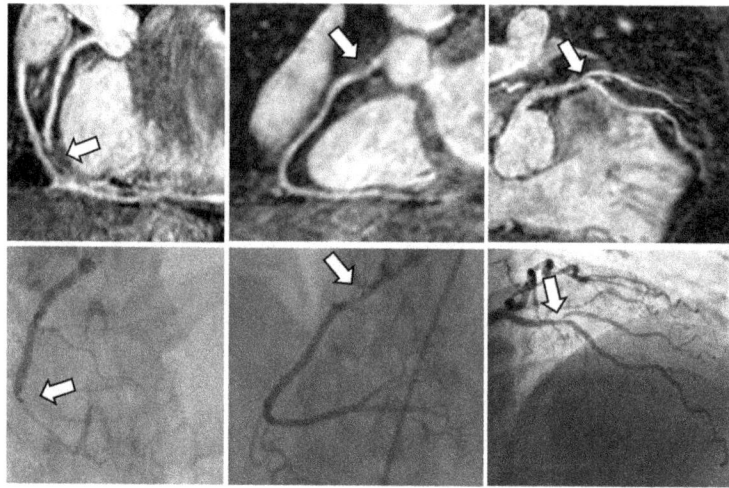

Fig. 5 Images from three patients with coronary artery disease, diagnosed using coronary magnetic resonance angiography (top row) and confirmed with coronary x-ray angiography (bottom row)

navigators, by combining data from multiple cardiac cycles but the same respiratory state [18, 22–24]. A drawback of attempting to estimate and correct motion with more degrees of freedom is the inclusion of additional noise associated with these measurements. Robust registration algorithms are required to minimize this source of noise. The use of global motion models to correct for all respiratory motion also risk introducing motion artifacts arising from tissue within the FOV which has different respiratory motion characteristics than the heart.

A robust CMRA sequence with short and predictable scan time would allow integrating CMRA into routine CMR scanning. CMRA has been used as part of a standard protocol in scientific studies [25] but not implemented in clinical scanning due to unpredictable scan time and image quality. Integrating CMRA would have a number of advantages in comparison to invasive angiography or coronary CT angiography, as it is non-invasive, not limited by the presence of coronary calcifications, does not use ionizing radiation and uses well tolerated and not nephrotoxic contrast agents. Additionally, the visualization of coronary morphology using CMRA can be integrated into a comprehensive evaluation of patients with angina symptoms, which also integrates optimal assessment of cardiac function, myocardial perfusion and viability and tissue characterization [26], therefore extending the diagnostic spectrum to include other causes of angina-like symptomatology [27]. Since the presence of stents systematically leads to metal artifacts and prohibiting the assessment of the coronary lumen these patients may be less well suited. The high negative predictive value of CMRA (similar to CTA studies) may increase the utilization of CMR as a first line tool in patients with low to intermediate pretest likelihood for significant coronary artery disease. Due to the excellent performance of CMR perfusion imaging in diagnosing significant ischemia [25] as well as guide patient management [28] CMR would offer a complete package in a wide range of patients.

This study has a number of limitations. It contains relatively few patients with low prevalence of CAD (24%) and thus resulted in a wide 95% confidence interval. From a technical perspective the technique is currently incompatible with the conventional arrhythmia rejection algorithm which renders it unsuitable for patients with frequent arrhythmias.

Conclusions

In this work we have demonstrated that iNAV is a robust approach for mitigating motion artefacts for CMRA in patients with suspected CAD. Due to the short and predictable scan time it can add clinical value as a part of a comprehensive CAD assessment protocol.

Abbreviations
2D: Two-dimensional; 3D: Three-dimensional; bSSFP: Balanced steady-state free precession; CAD: Coronary artery disease; CI: Confidence interval; CMRA: Coronary magnetic resonance angiography; CRUISE: Constant respiratory efficiency using single end-expiratory threshold; FOV: Field-of-view; iNAV: With image-based navigation; LAD: Left anterior descending coronary artery; LCX: Left circumflex coronary artery; LM: Left main coronary artery; RCA: Right coronary artery

Acknowledgements
On this occasion there is no one we wish to acknowledge.

Funding
This work was supported by the Department of Health through the National Institute for Health Research (NIHR) comprehensive Biomedical Research Centre award to Guy's & St Thomas' NHS Foundation Trust in partnership with King's College London and King's College Hospital NHS Foundation Trust. The Division of Imaging Sciences receives also support as the Centre of Excellence in Medical Engineering (funded by the Welcome Trust and EPSRC; grant number WT 088641/Z/09/Z) as well as the BHF Centre of Excellence (British Heart Foundation award RE/08/03).

Authors' contribution
MH conceived of the study, developed the sequence, acquired data, performed processing and analysis and drafted the manuscript. RMB, EN and KB contributed to study design and data collection. JS and MSV performed data processing and analysis. All authors participated in revising the manuscript, read and approved the final manuscript.

Consent for publication
Written informed consent was obtained from patients for publication of their individual details and accompanying images in this manuscript. The consent form is held in the patients' clinical notes and is available for review by the Editor-in-Chief.

Competing interests
The authors declare that they have no competing interests.

Author details
[1]Division of Biomedical Engineering and Imaging Sciences, King's College London, London, UK. [2]Institute for Experimental and Translational Cardiovascular Imaging, Goethe University, Frankfurt/Main, Germany. [3]DZHK (German Centre for Cardiovascular Research, Standort RheinMain), Berlin, Germany. [4]Escuela de Ingeniería, Pontificia Universidad Católica de Chile, Santiago, Chile.

References
1. Kim WY, et al. Coronary magnetic resonance angiography for the detection of coronary stenoses. N Engl J Med. 2001;345:1863–9.
2. Henningsson M, Botnar RM. Advanced respiratory motion compensation for coronary MR angiography. Sensors (Basel). 2013;13:6882–99.
3. Oshinski JN, Hofland L, Mukundan S Jr, Dixon WT, Parks WJ, Pettigrew RI. Two-dimensional coronary MR angiography without breath holding. Radiology. 1996;201:737–43.
4. Stehning C, Bornert P, Nehrke K, Eggers H, Stuber M. Free-breathing whole-heart coronary MRA with 3D radial SSFP and self-navigated image reconstruction. Magn Reson Med. 2005;54:476–80.
5. Piccini D, Littmann A, Nielles-Vallespin S, Zenge MO. Respiratory self-navigation for whole-heart bright-blood coronary MRI: methods for robust isolation and automatic segmentation of the blood pool. Magn Reson Med. 2012;68:571–9.
6. Henningsson M, Smink J, Razavi R, Botnar RM. Prospective respiratory motion correction for coronary MR angiography using a 2D image navigator. Magn Reson Med. 2013;69:486–94.
7. Wu HH, Gurney PT, Hu BS, Nishimura DG, McConnell MV. Free-breathing multiphase whole-heart coronary MR angiography using image-based navigators and three-dimensional cones imaging. Magn Reson Med. 2013;69:1083–93.
8. Scott AD, Keegan J, Firmin DN. Beat-to-beat respiratory motion correction with near 100% efficiency: a quantitative assessment using high-resolution coronary artery imaging. Magn Reson Imaging. 2011;29:568–78.
9. Moghari MH, Roujol S, Henningsson M, Kissinger KV, Annese D, Nezafat R, Manning WJ, Geva T, Powell AJ. Three-dimensional heart locator for whole-heart coronary magnetic resonance angiography. Magn Reson Med. 2014;71:2118–26.
10. Pang J, Bhat H, Sharif B, Fan Z, Thomson LE, LaBounty T, Friedman JD, Min J, Berman DS, Li D. Whole-heart coronary MRA with 100% respiratory gating efficiency: self-navigated three-dimensional retrospective image-based motion correction (TRIM). Magn Reson Med. 2014;71:67–74.
11. Aitken AP, Henningsson M, Botnar RM, Schaeffter T, Prieto C. 100% efficient three-dimensional coronary MR angiography with two-dimensional beat-to-beat translational and bin-to-bin affine motion correction. Magn Reson Med. 2015;74:756–64.
12. Schmidt JF, Buehrer M, Boesiger P, Kozerke S. Nonrigid retrospective respiratory motion correction in whole-heart coronary MRA. Magn Reson Med. 2011 Dec;66(6):1541–9.
13. Cruz G, Atkinson D, Henningsson M, Botnar RM, Prieto C. Highly efficient nonrigid motion-corrected 3D whole-heart coronary vessel wall imaging. Magn Reson Med. 2017;77:1894–908.
14. Henningsson M, Hussain T, Vieira MS, Greil GF, Smink J, Ensbergen GV, Beck G, Botnar RM. Whole-heart coronary MR angiography using image-based navigation for the detection of coronary anomalies in adult patients with congenital heart disease. J Magn Reson Imaging. 2016;43:947–55.
15. Henningsson M, Smink J, van Ensbergen G. Botnar R. Magn Reson Med: Coronary MR angiography using image-based respiratory motion compensation with inline correction and fixed gating efficiency; 2017.
16. Henningsson M, Koken P, Stehning C, Razavi R, Prieto C, Botnar RM. Whole-heart coronary MR angiography with 2D self-navigated image reconstruction. Magn Reson Med. 2012;67:437–45.
17. Etienne A, Botnar RM, Van Muiswinkel AM, Boesiger P, Manning WJ, Stuber M. "soap-bubble" visualization and quantitative analysis of 3D coronary magnetic resonance angiograms. Magn Reson Med. 2002;48:658–66.
18. He Y, Pang J, Dai Q, Fan Z, An J, Li D. Diagnostic performance of self-navigated whole-heart contrast-enhanced coronary 3-T MR angiography. Radiology. 2016 Nov;281(2):401–8.
19. Kato S, Kitagawa K, Ishida N, Ishida M, Nagata M, Ichikawa Y, Katahira K, Matsumoto Y, Seo K, Ochiai R, Kobayashi Y, Sakuma H. Assessment of coronary artery disease using magnetic resonance coronary angiography: a national multicenter trial. J Am Coll Cardiol. 2010;56(12):983–91.
20. Yang Q, Li K, Liu X, Bi X, Liu Z, An J, Zhang A, Jerecic R, Li D. Contrast-enhanced whole-heart coronary magnetic resonance angiography at 3.0-T: a comparative study with X-ray angiography in a single center. J Am Coll Cardiol. 2009;54(1):69–76.
21. Piccini D, et al. Respiratory self-navigated postcontrast whole-heart coronary MR angiography: initial experience in patients. Radiology. 2014;270(2):378–86.
22. Schmidt JF, Buehrer M, Boesiger P, Kozerke S. Nonrigid retrospective respiratory motion correction in whole-heart coronary MRA. Magn Reson Med. 2011;66:1541–9.
23. Henningsson M, Prieto C, Chiribiri A, Vaillant G, Razavi R, Botnar RM. Whole-heart coronary MRA with 3D affine motion correction using 3D image-based navigation. Magn Reson Med. 2014;71:173–81.
24. Aitken AP, Henningsson M, Botnar RM, Schaeffter T, Prieto C. 100% efficient three-dimensional coronary MR angiography with two-dimensional beat-to-beat translational and bin-to-bin affine motion correction. Magn Reson Med. 2015;74(3):756–64.
25. Greenwood JP, Motwani M, Maredia N, Brown JM, Everett CC, Nixon J, Bijsterveld P, Dickinson CJ, Ball SG, Plein S. Comparison of cardiovascular magnetic resonance and single-photon emission computed tomography in women with suspected coronary artery disease from the Clinical Evaluation of Magnetic Resonance Imaging in Coronary Heart Disease (CE-MARC) Trial. Circulation. 2014;129:1129–38.
26. Plein S, Ridgway JP, Jones TR, Bloomer TN, Sivananthan MU. Coronary artery disease: assessment with a comprehensive MR imaging protocol–initial results. Radiology. 2002;225:300–7.
27. Dastidar AG, Rodrigues JC, Ahmed N, Baritussio A, Bucciarelli-Ducci C. The role of cardiac MRI in patients with troponin-positive chest pain and unobstructed coronary arteries. Curr Cardiovasc Imaging Rep. 2015;8:28.
28. Hussain ST, Paul M, Plein S, McCann GP, Shah AM, Marber MS, Chiribiri A, Morton G, Redwood S, MacCarthy P, Schuster A, Ishida M, Westwood MA, Perera D, Nagel E. Design and rationale of the MR-INFORM study: stress perfusion cardiovascular magnetic resonance imaging to guide the management of patients with stable coronary artery disease. J Cardiovasc Magn Reson. 2012;14:65.

8

Representation of cardiovascular magnetic resonance in the AHA/ACC guidelines

Florian von Knobelsdorff-Brenkenhoff[1,2,3*], Guenter Pilz[1] and Jeanette Schulz-Menger[2,3]

Abstract

Background: Whereas evidence supporting the diagnostic value of cardiovascular magnetic resonance (CMR) has increased, there exists significant worldwide variability in the clinical utilization of CMR. A recent study demonstrated that CMR is represented in the majority of European Society for Cardiology (ESC) guidelines, with a large number of specific recommendations in particular regarding coronary artery disease. To further investigate the gap between the evidence and clinical use of CMR, this study analyzed the role of CMR in the guidelines of the American College of Cardiology (ACC) and American Heart Association (AHA).

Methods: Twenty-four AHA/ACC original guidelines, updates and new editions, published between 2006 and 2017, were screened for the terms "magnetic", "MRI", "CMR", "MR" and "imaging". Non-cardiovascular MR examinations were excluded. All CMR-related paragraphs and specific recommendations for CMR including the level of evidence (A, B, C) and the class of recommendation (I, IIa, IIb, III) were extracted.

Results: Twelve of the 24 guidelines (50.0%) contain specific recommendations regarding CMR. Four guidelines (16.7%) mention CMR in the text only, and 8 (33.3%) do not mention CMR. The 12 guidelines with recommendations for CMR contain in total 65 specific recommendations (31 class-I, 23 class-IIa, 6 class-IIb, 5 class-III). Most recommendations have evidence level C (44/65; 67.7%), followed by level B (21/65; 32.3%). There are no level A recommendations. 22/65 recommendations refer to vascular imaging, 17 to congenital heart disease, 8 to cardiomyopathies, 8 to myocardial stress testing, 5 to left and right ventricular function, 3 to viability, and 2 to valvular heart disease.

Conclusions: CMR is represented in two thirds of the AHA/ACC guidelines, which contain a number of specific recommendations for the use of CMR. In a simplified comparison with the ESC guidelines, CMR is less represented in the AHA/ACC guidelines in particular in the field of coronary artery disease.

Keywords: Cardiac magnetic resonance, Guideline, Cardiology, Reimbursement

Background

The body of evidence supporting the beneficial utilization of cardiovascular magnetic resonance (CMR) has grown significantly over the last decade [1, 2]. A recent analysis exhibited that CMR is already incorporated into 88% of the guidelines published by the European Society of Cardiology, in many as specific recommendations, and in most at least by mention in the text passages [3]. Hence, CMR commonly plays a role in evidence based diagnostic and therapeutic pathways, and can even be considered mandatory in a number of clinical scenarios. However, in the experience of the authors, the integration of CMR into clinical medicine appears to still be limited relative to the growing evidence supporting its benefits. This discrepancy may be attributed to a number of factors, such as limited access to scanners equipped for CMR, lack of people with the necessary skills to run and interpret a CMR study, relatively high costs, competing diagnostic modalities, and inadequate reimbursement. The guidelines published by the American Heart Association (AHA) and the American College of Cardiology (ACC) are often used as the basis

* Correspondence: florian.vonknobelsdorff@khagatharied.de
[1]Department of Cardiology, Clinic Agatharied, Ludwig-Maximilians-University Munich, Norbert-Kerkel-Platz, 83734 Hausham, Germany
[2]Charité – Universitätsmedizin Berlin, corporate member of Freie Universität Berlin, Humboldt-Universität zu Berlin, and Berlin Institute of Health, DZHK (German Centre for Cardiovascular Research), partner site Berlin, Berlin, Germany
Full list of author information is available at the end of the article

for clinical decision making and therefore can have a high impact on utilization of technology such as CMR. This analysis systematically summarizes the representation of CMR in the AHA/ACC guidelines to stimulate the discussion about future needs for training, distribution of equipment, and reimbursement of CMR worldwide.

Methods

All AHA/ACC guidelines published between 2006 and June 2017 and listed on the AHA and ACC websites were collected (Table 1). If more than one guideline for the same topic was published during this period, the most recent was included in the analysis. If a guideline was updated, both the full guideline and the update were analyzed in combination. The documents were screened for the terms "magnetic", "MRI", "CMR", "MR" and "imaging". MRI in the context of non-cardiovascular examinations, such as brain MRI, was not included. The main conclusions were extracted, and if available, the class of recommendation and the level of evidence were given. The class of recommendation (i.e., the strength of the recommendation) encompasses the anticipated magnitude and certainty of benefit in proportion to risk (Table 2). The level of evidence rates evidence on the basis of the type, quality, quantity, and consistency of data from clinical trials and other reports (Table 3) [4]. Whereas recent guidelines separate levels B and C into sublevels, earlier guidelines did not. In this analysis, the level as provided in each guideline is given. The number in parenthesis behind the citation provides the page number of the full text guideline. If a recommendation refers to "imaging" in general, it was registered only if the context included CMR. This analysis was performed twice for every guideline to assure that no relevant information was missed. The absolute number of recommendations was then summarized. The guidelines are listed in chronologic order beginning with the most recent. Only USA-guidelines published by the AHA and ACC were included; AHA/ACC position statements, and guidelines published by other organizations, were not included to guarantee consistency.

Results

In total 24 AHA/ACC guidelines were analyzed. For five guidelines, more recent updates were included in a combined analysis with the full guidelines (heart failure update 2017 and 2016 [5, 6], valve disease update 2017 [7], stable ischemic heart disease update 2014 [8], device-based therapy of cardiac rhythm abnormalities update 2012 [9]). There is one update from 2015 incorporating the previous STEMI and PCI guidelines [10–12]. In this case, all three documents were analyzed together, and the guidelines were counted as two separate cases. Two updates on secondary prevention were published during the inclusion

period (2011 and 2006 [13, 14]), but no explicit original guideline. Both updates were analyzed and counted as one guideline. The "Guidelines on perioperative cardiovascular evaluation and care for non-cardiac surgery" were published twice (2014 and 2007 [15, 16]), but only the more recent version entered the quantitative analysis.

Of the 24 analyzed AHA/ACC guidelines, 12 (50.0%) contain specific recommendations regarding the use of CMR (Table 1). Four guidelines (16.7%) principally mention scenarios in which CMR may be used, but without giving specific recommendations. Eight guidelines (33.3%) do not mention CMR at all. (Fig. 1).

The 12 guidelines with recommendations regarding the use of CMR contain in total 65 specific recommendations. These are 31 class-I recommendations, 23 class-IIa recommendations, 6 class-IIb recommendations and 5 class-III recommendations (Fig. 1). The 5 class-III recommendations stem from the guidelines concerning lower peripheral artery disease ($n = 1$) [4], stable ischemic heart disease ($n = 3$) [8, 17], and risk assessment in asymptomatic adults ($n = 1$) [18].

Most of the CMR recommendations have evidence level C (44/65; 67.7%), followed by level B (21/65; 32.3%). No CMR recommendations have evidence level A.

The four guidelines that contained the most recommendations for CMR, were the guidelines on adults with congenital heart disease ($n = 17$) [19], extracranial carotid and vertebral artery disease ($n = 9$) [20], thoracic aortic disease ($n = 8$) [21], and stable ischemic heart disease ($n = 8$) [8, 17].

Twenty-two of the 65 recommendations refer to vascular imaging, 17 recommendations refer to congenital heart disease, 8 to myocardial stress testing, 8 to cardiomyopathies, 5 to LV and RV function assessment, 3 to viability and 2 to valvular heart disease (Fig. 1).

Table 4 lists the 65 recommendations categorized by clinical scenario and diagnosis (following the style of the ESC guideline summary [3]).

- 2017 ACC/AHA/HFSA Focused Update of the 2013 ACCF/AHA Guideline for the Management of Heart Failure [5]
- 2016 ACC/AHA/HFSA Focused Update on New Pharmacological Therapy for Heart Failure: An Update of the 2013 ACCF/AHA Guideline for the Management of Heart Failure [6]
- 2013 ACCF/AHA Guideline for the Management of Heart Failure - A Report of the American College of Cardiology Foundation/American Heart Association Task Force on Practice Guidelines [22]

The most recent full AHA/ACC guideline regarding heart failure was published in 2013 and updated in 2016 and 2017. In the 2013 full version, under the topic

Table 1 List of AHA/ACC guidelines used for the analysis. +++ = guideline contains specific recommendations regarding the use of CMR; ++ = guideline mentions scenarios in which CMR may be used, but without giving any specific recommendation; + = guideline does not mention CMR at all

Nr.	Title	Year	Role of CMR	I	IIa	IIb	III
1	• ACC/AHA/HFSA Focused Update of the 2013 ACCF/AHA Guideline for the Management of Heart Failure [5] • ACC/AHA/HFSA Focused Update on New Pharmacological Therapy for Heart Failure: An Update of the 2013 ACCF/AHA Guideline for the Management of Heart Failure [6] • ACCF/AHA Guideline for the Management of Heart Failure [22]	2017 2016 2013	+++	0	2	2	0
2	• AHA/ACC Focused Update of the 2014 AHA/ACC Guideline for the Management of Patients With Valvular Heart Disease [7] • AHA/ACC Guideline for the Management of Patients With Valvular Heart Disease [23]	2017 2014	+++	5	0	1	0
3	• ACC/AHA/HRS Guideline for Evaluation and Management of Patients With Syncope [24]	2017	+++	0	1	1	0
4	• AHA/ACC Guideline on the Management of Patients With Lower Extremity Peripheral Artery Disease [4]	2016	+++	1	0	0	1
5	• ACC/AHA/HRS Guideline for the Management of Adult Patients With Supraventricular Tachycardia [25]	2015	+				
6	• ACC/AHA/SCAI Focused Update on Primary Percutaneous Coronary Intervention for Patients With ST-Elevation Myocardial Infarction: An Update of the 2011 ACCF/AHA/SCAI Guideline for Percutaneous Coronary Intervention and the 2013 ACCF/AHA Guideline for the Management of ST-Elevation Myocardial Infarction [10] • ACCF/AHA Guideline for the Management of ST-Elevation Myocardial Infarction [11]	2015 2013	+				
7	• ACCF/AHA/SCAI Guideline for Percutaneous Coronary Intervention [12]	2011	++				
8	• ACC/AHA Guideline on Perioperative Cardiovascular Evaluation and Management of Patients Undergoing Noncardiac Surgery [15] • ACC/AHA Guidelines on Perioperative Cardiovascular Evaluation and Care for Noncardiac Surgery [16]	2014 2007	++				
9	• ACC/AHA/AATS/PCNA/SCAI/STS Focused Update of the Guideline for the Diagnosis and Management of Patients With Stable Ischemic Heart Disease [8] • ACCF/AHA/ACP/AATS/PCNA/SCAI/STS Guideline for the Diagnosis and Management of Patients With Stable Ischemic Heart Disease [17]	2014 2012	+++	1	4	0	3
10	• AHA/ACC Guideline for the Management of Patients With Non–ST-Elevation Acute Coronary Syndromes [26]	2014	+++	1	0	0	0
11	• AHA/ACC/HRS Guideline for the Management of Patients With Atrial Fibrillation [27]	2014	++				
12	• AHA/ACC/TOS Guideline for the Management of Overweight and Obesity in Adults [28]	2013	+				
13	• AHA/ACC Guideline on Lifestyle Management to Reduce Cardiovascular Risk [29]	2013	+				
14	• ACC/AHA Guideline on the Treatment of Blood Cholesterol to Reduce Atherosclerotic Cardiovascular Risk in Adults [30]	2013	+				
15	• ACC/AHA Guideline on the Assessment of Cardiovascular Risk [31]	2013	+				
16	• ACCF/AHA/HRS Focused Update Incorporated Into the ACCF/AHA/HRS 2008 Guidelines for Device-Based Therapy of Cardiac Rhythm Abnormalities [9] • ACC/AHA/HRS Guidelines for Device-Based Therapy of Cardiac Rhythm Abnormalities [32]	2012 2008	++				
17	• ACCF/AHA Guideline for the Diagnosis and Treatment of Hypertrophic Cardiomyopathy [33]	2011	+++	2	1	3	0
18	• ACCF/AHA Guideline for Coronary Artery Bypass Graft Surgery [34]	2011	+				
19	• AHA/ACCF Secondary Prevention and Risk Reduction Therapy for Patients With Coronary and Other Atherosclerotic Vascular Disease: 2011 Update [13] • AHA/ACC Guidelines for Secondary Prevention for Patients With Coronary and Other Atherosclerotic Vascular Disease: 2006 Update [14]	2011 2006	+				
20	• ASA/ACCF/AHA/AANN/AANS/ACR/ASNR/CNS/ SAIP/SCAI/SIR/SNIS/SVM/SVS Guideline on the Management of Patients With Extracranial Carotid and Vertebral Artery [20]	2011	+++	4	4	1	0
21	• ACCF/AHA/AATS/ACR/ASA/SCA/SCAI/SIR/STS/SVM Guidelines for the Diagnosis and Management of Patients With Thoracic Aortic Disease [21]	2010	+++	3	5	0	0
22	• ACCF/AHA Guideline for Assessment of Cardiovascular Risk in Asymptomatic Adults [18]	2010	+++	0	0	0	1
23	• ACC/AHA Guidelines for the Management of Adults With Congenital Heart Disease [19]	2008	+++	14	2	1	0
24	• ACC/AHA/ESC Guidelines for Management of Patients With Ventricular Arrhythmias and the Prevention of Sudden Cardiac Death [35]	2006	+++	0	1	0	0

"Initial and serial evaluation of the heart failure patient", specific recommendations for the use of CMR are defined, in particular regarding assessment of LV function, perfusion and viability (Table 5). CMR is additionally mentioned as an alternative to echocardiography, as CMR "assesses LV volume and EF measurements at least

Table 2 Class (Strength) of Recommendation [4]

Class of recommendation	Definition	Suggested phrases for writing recommendations

Class I (strong)	Benefit >> > Risk	• is recommended
		• is indicated / useful / effective / beneficial
		• should be performed / administered / other
		• Comparative-Effectiveness phrases:
		  – Treatment / strategy A is recommended / indicated in preference to treatment B
		  – Treatment A should be chosen over treatment B

Class IIa (Moderate)	Benefit > > Risk	• Is reasonable
		• Can be useful / effective / beneficial
		• Comparative-Effectiveness phrases
		  – Treatment / strategy A is probably recommended / indicated in preference to treatment B
		  – It is reasonable to choose treatment A over treatment B

Class IIb (Weak)	Benefit ≥ Risk	• May / might be reasonable • May / might be considered • Usefulness / effectiveness is unknown / unclear / uncertain or not well established
Class III: No benefit (Moderate)	Benefit = Risk	• Is not recommended • Is not indicated / useful / effective / beneficial • Should not be performed / administered / other
Class III: Harm (Strong)	Risk > Benefit	• Potentially harmful • Causes harm • Associated with excess morbidity / mortality • Should not be performed / administered / other

as accurately as echocardiography" (page 19). Furthermore, its potential to provide "additional information about myocardial perfusion, viability, and fibrosis can help identify heart failure etiology and assess prognosis" (page 19) is highlighted. Finally, the use of CMR in known or suspected congenital heart diseases is indicated as "CMR provides high anatomical resolution of all aspects of the heart and surrounding structure" (page 19). Under the heading "Cardiac structural abnormalities and other causes of heart failure", CMR is recommended in subjects with known or suspected cardiac sarcoidosis, as CMR "can identify cardiac involvement with patchy areas of myocardial inflammation and fibrosis" (page 14).

- 2017 AHA/ACC Focused Update of the 2014 AHA/ACC Guideline for the Management of Patients With Valvular Heart Disease [7]
- 2014 AHA/ACC Guideline for the Management of Patients With Valvular Heart Disease [23]

In patients with suspected valvular heart disease, echocardiography is the cornerstone of the diagnostic algorithm. The guideline adds that generally "Other ancillary testing such as transesophageal echocardiography (TEE), computed tomography (CT) or cardiac magnetic resonance (CMR) imaging, stress testing, and diagnostic hemodynamic cardiac catheterization may

Table 3 Level of Evidence [4]

Level	Definition
Level A	• High quality evidence from more than 1 randomized controlled trial • Meta-analyses of high-quality randomized controlled trials • One or more randomized controlled trial corroborated by high-quality registry studies
Level B-R (randomized)	• Moderate-quality evidence from 1 or more randomized controlled trial • Meta-analyses of moderate-quality randomized controlled trials
Level B-NR (nonrandomized)	• Moderate-quality evidence from 1 or more well-designed well-executed nonrandomized studies, observational studies, or registry studies • Meta-analyses of such studies
Level C-LD (limited data)	• Randomized or nonrandomized observational or registry studies with limitations of design or execution • Meta-analyses of such studies • Physiological or mechanistic studies in human subjects
Level C-EO (expert opinion)	• Consensus of expert opinion based on clinical experience

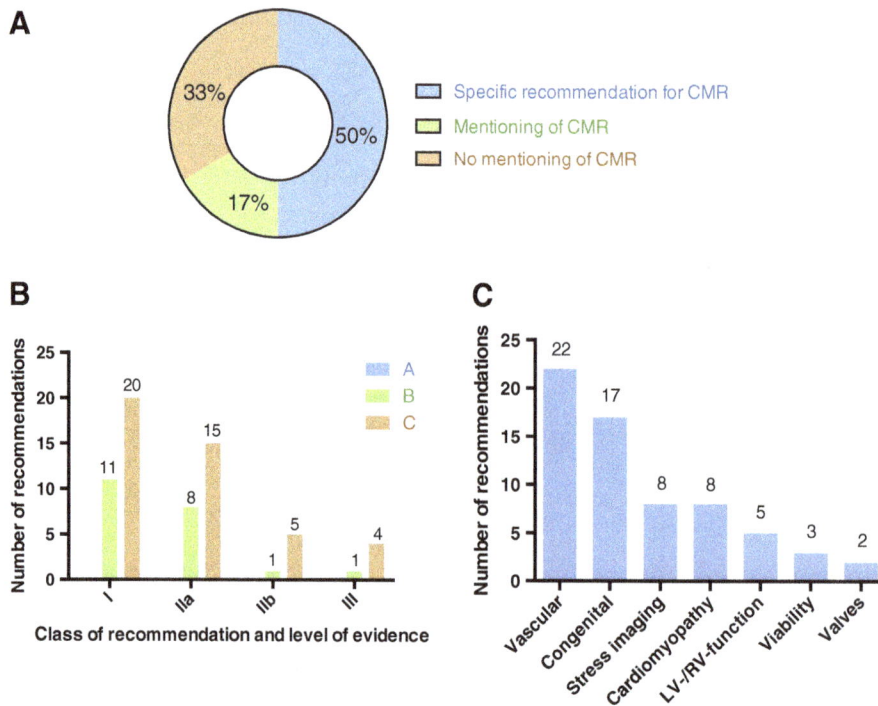

Fig. 1 Panel **a** Categorization of the 24 analyzed AHA/ACC guidelines regarding the role of CMR. Panel **b** Distribution of the 65 specific recommendations for CMR in the 24 AHA/ACC guidelines regarding "class of recommendations" and "level of evidence". Panel **c** Categorization of the 65 specific recommendations in the 24 AHA/ACC guidelines regarding the diagnostic target

be required to determine the optimal treatment for a patient with valvular heart disease" (page 7).

Specifically, in *aortic stenosis*, "CMR imaging shows promise for evaluation of severity of aortic stenosis, but is not widely available" (page 17). In *aortic regurgitation*, "CMR imaging provides accurate measures of regurgitant volume and regurgitant fraction... as well as assessment of aortic morphology, LV volume, and LV systolic function. In addition to its value in patients with suboptimal echocardiographic data, CMR is useful for evaluating patients in whom there is discordance between clinical assessment and severity of aortic regurgitation by echocardiography. CMR measurement of regurgitant severity is less variable than echocardiographic measurement" (page 29). This approach is expressed as a Class I, Level B-recommendation (Table 6). In subjects with aortic regurgitation and chronic aortic disease, "CMR imaging is useful ..., but is rarely used in unstable patients with suspected dissection" (page 27). For the subset of patients with bicuspid aortic valve disease, the guideline defines several specific recommendations about the use of CMR to assess the thoracic aorta (Table 6). In this context, the guideline states that "Magnetic resonance angiography or chest CT angiography provide accurate diameter measurements when aligned perpendicular to the long axis of the aorta. Advantages of magnetic resonance angiography and CT angiography

compared with TTE include higher spatial (but lower temporal) resolution and the ability to display a 3D reconstruction of the entire length of the aorta"(page 33). Furthermore, the guideline emphasizes that "Magnetic resonance angiography imaging is preferred over CT angiography imaging, when possible, because of the absence of ionizing radiation exposure in patients who likely will have multiple imaging studies over their lifetime" (page 33).

In *mitral regurgitation (MR)*, "in cases where TTE image quality is poor, CMR may be of value in MR evaluation. CMR produces highly accurate data on LV volumes, RV volumes, and LVEF, and an estimation of MR severity, but outcome data using CMR volumes is pending. CMR is less helpful in establishing mitral pathoanatomy" (pages 43–44; Table 6). Furthermore, "Three-dimensional echocardiography, strain imaging, or CMR may add more accurate assessment of the LV response in the future" (page 43).

In *tricuspid regurgitation*, "Both CMR and real-time 3D echocardiography may provide more accurate assessment of right ventricular volumes and systolic function, as well as annular dimension and the degree of leaflet tethering. CMR may be the ideal modality in young asymptomatic patients with severe tricuspid regurgitation to assess initial and serial measurements of right ventricular size and systolic function" (Table 6).

Table 4 Summary of clinical scenarios / diagnosis groups, where the AHA/ACC guidelines make recommendations regarding CMR

	Class	Level	Guideline
Suspected / stable coronary artery disease			
Noninvasive imaging to detect myocardial ischemia and viability is reasonable in heart failure and coronary artery disease	IIa	C	Heart failure [5, 6, 22]
Noninvasive imaging (stress nuclear/positron emission tomography, CMR, or stress echocardiography), cardiac CT angiography, or cardiac catheterization, including coronary arteriography, is useful to establish etiology of chronic secondary MR (stages B to D) and/or to assess myocardial viability, which in turn may influence management of functional MR.	I	C	Valve disease [7, 23]
Pharmacological stress with CMR can be useful for patients with an intermediate to high pretest probability of obstructive ischemic heart disease, who have an uninterpretable ECG and at least moderate physical functioning or no disabling comorbidity.	IIa	B	Stable CAD [8]
Pharmacological stress CMR is reasonable for patients with an intermediate to high pretest probability of ischemic heart disease, who are incapable of at least moderate physical functioning or have disabling comorbidity.	IIa	B	Stable CAD [8]
Echocardiography, radionuclide imaging, CMR, and cardiac CT are not recommended for routine assessment of LV function in patients with a normal ECG, no history of myocardial infarction, no symptoms or signs suggestive of heart failure, and no complex ventricular arrhythmias.	III	C	Stable CAD [8]
Routine reassessment (<1 year) of LV function with technologies such as echocardiography, radionuclide imaging, CMR, or cardiac CT is not recommended in patients with no change in clinical status and for whom no change in therapy is contemplated.	III	C	Stable CAD [8]
CMR with pharmacological stress is reasonable for risk assessment in patients with stable ischemic heart disease who are able to exercise to an adequate workload but have an uninterpretable ECG.	IIa	B	Stable CAD [8]
Pharmacological stress imaging (nuclear MPI, echocardiography, or CMR) or CCTA is not recommended for risk assessment in patients with stable ischemic heart disease who are able to exercise to an adequate workload and have an interpretable ECG.	III	C	Stable CAD [8]
Pharmacological stress CMR is reasonable for risk assessment in patients with stable ischemic heart disease who are unable to exercise to an adequate workload regardless of interpretability of ECG.	IIa	B	Stable CAD [8]
Acute coronary syndrome			
Imaging with ventriculography, echocardiography, or magnetic resonance imaging should be performed to confirm or exclude the diagnosis of stress (Takotsubo) cardiomyopathy.	I	B	NSTEMI [26]
Before coronary revascularization			
Viability assessment is reasonable before revascularization in heart failure patients with coronary artery disease	IIa	B	Heart failure [5, 6, 22]
Either exercise or pharmacological stress with imaging (nuclear MPI, echocardiography, or CMR) is recommended for risk assessment in patients with stable ischemic heart disease, who are being considered for revascularization of known coronary stenosis of unclear physiological significance.	I	B	Stable CAD [8]
Heart failure			
Radionuclide ventriculography or MRI can be useful to assess LVEF and volume	IIa	C	Heart failure [5, 6, 22]
MRI is reasonable when assessing myocardial infiltration or scar	IIa	B	Heart failure [5, 6, 22]
Ventricular arrhythmia			
MRI, cardiac computed tomography (CT), or radionuclide angiography can be useful in patients with ventricular arrhythmias when echocardiography does not provide accurate assessment of LV and RV function and/or evaluation of structural changes.	IIa	B	Ventricular arrhythmias [35]
Hypertrophic cardiomyopathy			
CMR imaging is indicated in patients with suspected HCM when echocardiography is inconclusive for diagnosis.	I	B	HCM [33]
CMR imaging is indicated in patients with known HCM when additional information that may have an impact on management or decision making regarding invasive management, such as magnitude and distribution of hypertrophy or anatomy of the mitral valve apparatus or papillary muscles, is not adequately defined with echocardiography.	I	B	HCM [33]
CMR imaging is reasonable in patients with HCM to define apical hypertrophy and/or aneurysm if echocardiography is inconclusive.	IIa	B	HCM [33]
In selected patients with known HCM, when SCD risk stratification is inconclusive after documentation of the conventional risk factors, CMR imaging with assessment of late gadolinium enhancement (LGE) may be considered in resolving clinical decision making.	IIb	C	HCM [33]

Table 4 Summary of clinical scenarios / diagnosis groups, where the AHA/ACC guidelines make recommendations regarding CMR *(Continued)*

The usefulness of the following potential SCD risk modifiers is unclear but might be considered in selected patients with HCM for whom risk remains borderline after documentation of conventional risk factors: CMR imaging with LGE.	IIb	C	HCM [33]

Athlete's heart

Extended monitoring (including MRI) can be beneficial for athletes with unexplained exertional syncope after an initial cardiovascular evaluation.	IIa	C-LD	Syncope [24]

Storage disease

CMR imaging may be considered in patients with LV hypertrophy and the suspicion of alternative diagnoses to HCM, including cardiac amyloidosis, Fabry disease, and genetic phenocopies such as LAMP2 cardiomyopathy.	IIb	C	HCM [33]

Vascular disease

Aortic magnetic resonance angiography or CT angiography is indicated in patients with a bicuspid aortic valve when morphology of the aortic sinuses, sinotubular junction, or ascending aorta cannot be assessed accurately or fully by echocardiography. (Level of Evidence: C)	I	C	Valve disease [7, 23]
Serial evaluation of the size and morphology of the aortic sinuses and ascending aorta by echocardiography, CMR, or CT angiography is recommended in patients with a bicuspid aortic valve and an aortic diameter greater than 4.0 cm, with the examination interval determined by the degree and rate of progression of aortic dilation and by family history. In patients with an aortic diameter greater than 4.5 cm, this evaluation should be performed annually.	I	C	Valve disease [7, 23]
Duplex ultrasound, computed tomography angiography (CTA), or magnetic resonance angiography (MRA) of the lower extremities is useful to diagnose anatomic location and severity of stenosis for patients with symptomatic peripheral artery disease in whom revascularization is considered	I	B-NR	Peripheral Artery Disease [4]
Invasive and noninvasive angiography (ie, CTA, MRA) should not be performed for the anatomic assessment of patients with asymptomatic peripheral artery disease.	III	B-R	Peripheral Artery Disease [4]
In patients with acute, focal ischemic neurological symptoms corresponding to the territory supplied by the left or right internal carotid artery, magnetic resonance angiography (MRA) or computed tomography angiography (CTA) is indicated to detect carotid stenosis when sonography either cannot be obtained or yields equivocal or otherwise nondiagnostic results.	I	C	Carotid and vertebral artery [20]
When an extracranial source of ischemia is not identified in patients with transient retinal or hemispheric neurological symptoms of suspected ischemic origin, CTA, MRA, or selective cerebral angiography can be useful to search for intracranial vascular disease.	IIa	C	Carotid and vertebral artery [20]
When the results of initial noninvasive imaging are inconclusive, additional examination by use of another imaging method is reasonable. In candidates for revascularization, MRA or CTA can be useful when results of carotid duplex ultrasonography are equivocal or indeterminate.	IIa	C	Carotid and vertebral artery [20]
When intervention for significant carotid stenosis detected by carotid duplex ultrasonography is planned, MRA, CTA, or catheter-based contrast angiography can be useful to evaluate the severity of stenosis and to identify intrathoracic or intracranial vascular lesions that are not adequately assessed by duplex ultrasonography.	IIa	C	Carotid and vertebral artery [20]
MRA without contrast is reasonable to assess the extent of disease in patients with symptomatic carotid atherosclerosis and renal insufficiency or extensive vascular calcification.	IIa	C	Carotid and vertebral artery [20]
When complete carotid arterial occlusion is suggested by duplex ultrasonography, MRA, or CTA in patients with retinal or hemispheric neurological symptoms of suspected ischemic origin, catheter-based contrast angiography may be considered to determine whether the arterial lumen is sufficiently patent to permit carotid revascularization.	IIb	C	Carotid and vertebral artery [20]
Noninvasive imaging by CTA or MRA for detection of vertebral artery disease should be part of the initial evaluation of patients with neurological symptoms referable to the posterior circulation and those with subclavian steal syndrome.	I	C	Carotid and vertebral artery [20]
In patients whose symptoms suggest posterior cerebral or cerebellar ischemia, MRA or CTA is recommended rather than ultrasound imaging for evaluation of the vertebral arteries.	I	C	Carotid and vertebral artery [20]
Contrast-enhanced CTA, MRA, and catheter-based contrast angiography are useful for diagnosis of cervical artery dissection.	I	C	Carotid and vertebral artery [20]
Urgent and definitive imaging of the aorta using transesophageal echocardiogram, computed tomographic imaging, or magnetic resonance imaging is recommended to identify or exclude thoracic aortic dissection in patients at high risk for the disease by initial screening.	I	B	Thoracic aorta [21]
The initial evaluation of Takayasu arteritis or giant cell arteritis should include thoracic aorta and branch vessel computed tomographic imaging or magnetic resonance imaging to inves- tigate the possibility of aneurysm or occlusive disease in these vessels.	I	C	Thoracic aorta [21]

Table 4 Summary of clinical scenarios / diagnosis groups, where the AHA/ACC guidelines make recommendations regarding CMR *(Continued)*

For patients with isolated aortic arch aneurysms less than 4.0 cm in diameter, it is reasonable to reimage using computed tomographic imaging or magnetic resonance imaging, at 12- month intervals, to detect enlargement of the aneurysm.	IIa	C	Thoracic aorta [21]
For patients with isolated aortic arch aneurysms 4.0 cm or greater in diameter, it is reasonable to reimage using computed tomographic imaging or magnetic resonance imaging, at 6-month intervals, to detect en largement of the aneurysm.	IIa	C	Thoracic aorta [21]
For imaging of pregnant women with aortic arch, descending, or abdominal aortic dilatation, magnetic resonance imaging (without gadolinium) is recommended over computed tomographic imaging to avoid exposing both the mother and fetus to ionizing radiation. Transesophageal echocardiogram is an option for imaging of the thoracic aorta.	I	C	Thoracic aorta [21]
Computed tomographic imaging or magnetic resonance imaging of the thoracic aorta is reasonable after a Type A or B aortic dissection or after prophylactic repair of the aortic root/ ascending aorta.	IIa	C	Thoracic aorta [21]
Computed tomographic imaging or magnetic resonance imaging of the aorta is reasonable at 1, 3, 6, and 12 months postdissection and, if stable, annually thereafter so that any threatening enlargement can be detected in a timely fashion.	IIa	C	Thoracic aorta [21]
If a thoracic aortic aneurysm is only moderate in size and remains relatively stable over time, magnetic resonance imaging instead of computed tomographic imaging is reasonable to minimize the patient's radiation exposure.	IIa	C	Thoracic aorta [21]
MRI for detection of vascular plaque is not recommended for cardiovascular risk assessment in asymptomatic adults.	III	C	Risk assessment [18]
Valvular heart disease			
CMR is indicated in patients with moderate or severe AR (stages B, C, and D) and suboptimal echocardiographic images for the assessment of LV systolic function, systolic and diastolic volumes, and measurement of AR severity.	I	B	Valve disease [7, 23]
CMR is indicated in patients with chronic primary MR to assess LV and RV volumes, function, or MR severity and when these issues are not satisfactorily addressed by TTE.	I	B	Valve disease [7, 23]
CMR or real-time 3D echocardiography may be considered for assessment of right ventricular systolic function and systolic and diastolic volumes in patients with severe tricuspid regurgitation (stages C and D) and suboptimal 2D echocardiograms.	IIb	C	Valve disease [7, 23]
Congenital heart disease			
Diagnostic and interventional procedures, including imaging (ie, echocardiography, MRI, or CT, advanced cardiac catheterization, and electrophysiology procedures for adults with complex and moderate CHD should be performed in a regional ACHD center with appropriate experience in CHD and in a laboratory with appropriate personnel and equipment. Personnel performing such procedures should work as part of a team with expertise in the surgical and transcatheter management of patients with CHD.	I	C	Congenital heart disease [19]
(In bicuspid aortic valve disease) MRI/CT can be beneficial to add important information about the anatomy of the thoracic aorta.	IIa	C	Congenital heart disease [19]
(In bicuspid aortic valve disease) MRI may be beneficial in quantifying aortic regurgitation when other data are ambiguous or borderline.	IIb	C	Congenital heart disease [19]
(In supravalvular aortic stenosis) TTE and/or TEE with Doppler and either MRI or CT should be performed to assess the anatomy of the LVOT, the ascending aorta, coronary artery anatomy and flow, and main and branch pulmonary artery anatomy and flow.	I	C	Congenital heart disease [19]
Every patient with coarctation (repaired or not) should have at least 1 cardiovascular MRI or CT scan for complete evaluation of the thoracic aorta and intracranial vessels.	I	B	Congenital heart disease [19]
Evaluation of the coarctation repair site by MRI/CT should be performed at intervals of 5 years or less, depending on the specific anatomic findings before and after repair.	I	C	Congenital heart disease [19]
Patients with suspected supravalvular, branch, or peripheral pulmonary stenosis should have baseline imaging with echocardiography-Doppler plus 1 of the following: MRI angiography, CT angiography, or contrast angiography.	I	C	Congenital heart disease [19]
(In congenital coronary anomalies of ectopic arterial origin) CT or MRA is useful as the initial screening method in centers with expertise in such imaging.	I	B	Congenital heart disease [19]
(In suspicion of a coronary arteriovenous fistula), if a continuous murmur is present, its origin should be defined either by echocardiography, MRI, CT angiography, or cardiac catheterization.	I	C	Congenital heart disease [19]
The evaluation of all ACHD patients with suspected pulmonary arterial hypertension should include noninvasive assessment of cardiovascular anatomy and potential shunting, as detailed below: Diagnostic cardiovascular imaging via TTE, TEE, MRI, or CT as appropriate.	I	C	Congenital heart disease [19]

Table 4 Summary of clinical scenarios / diagnosis groups, where the AHA/ACC guidelines make recommendations regarding CMR (Continued)

Patients with tetralogy of Fallot should have echocardiographic examinations and/or MRIs performed by staff with expertise in ACHD.	I	C	Congenital heart disease [19]
Additional imaging with TEE, CT, or MRI, as appropriate, should be performed in a regional ACHD center to evaluate the great arteries and veins, as well as ventricular function, in patients with prior atrial baffle repair of d-TGA.	I	B	Congenital heart disease [19]
Periodic MRI or CT can be considered appropriate to evaluate the anatomy and hemodynamics in more detail in patients with prior arterial switch operation.	IIa	C	Congenital heart disease [19]
(In congenitally corrected transposition of the great arteries), echocardiography-Doppler study and/or MRI should be performed yearly or at least every other year by staff trained in imaging complex CHD.	I	C	Congenital heart disease [19]
The following diagnostic evaluations are recommended for patients with congenitally corrected transposition of the great arteries: ECG, chest x-ray, echocardiography-Doppler study, MRI, exercise testing.	I	C	Congenital heart disease [19]
(In patients with prior repair of congenitally corrected transposition of the great arteries), echocardiography-Doppler study and/or MRI should be performed yearly or at least every other year by staff trained in imaging complex CHD.	I	C	Congenital heart disease [19]
All patients with prior Fontan type of repair should have periodic echocardiographic and/or magnetic resonance examinations performed by staff with expertise in ACHD.	I	C	Congenital heart disease [19]
Syncope			
Computed tomography (CT) or magnetic resonance imaging (MRI) may be useful in selected patients presenting with syncope of suspected cardiac etiology.	IIb	B-NR	Syncope [24]

Class = class of recommendation
Level = level of evidence
NSTEMI = non-ST-elevation myocardial infarction
CAD = coronary artery disease
HCM = hypertrophic cardiomyopathy

- 2017 ACC/AHA/HRS Guideline for the Evaluation and Management of Patients With Syncope [24]

"Imaging modalities, including CT and MRI, are usually reserved for selected patients presenting with syncope, especially when other noninvasive means are inadequate or inconclusive. These modalities offer superior spatial resolution in delineating cardiovascular anatomy (e.g., in patients with structural, infiltrative, or congenital heart disease. ... MRI is useful when there is a suspicion of ARVC or cardiac sarcoidosis" (page 25). In athletes, "imaging may include echocardiography or MRI as required" (page 64). The specific

recommendations for CMR in patients with syncope are shown in Table 7.

- 2016 AHA/ACC Guideline on the management of patients with lower extremity peripheral artery disease [4]

This guideline contains two recommendations for CMR under the heading "3.3. Imaging for anatomic assessment" (Table 8). Furthermore, Fig. 1 in the guideline ("Diagnostic testing for suspected peripheral artery disease") and figure 2 in the guideline ("Diagnostic testing for suspected critical limb ischemia") include CMR as part of the diagnostic algorithm.

For symptomatic patients with peripheral artery disease, in whom revascularization is considered, additional imaging with duplex ultrasonography, CTA, or MRA is useful to develop an individualized treatment plan. The guidelines state, "all 3 of these noninvasive imaging methods have good sensitivity and specificity as compared with invasive angiography" (page 24). CMR is characterized by superior spatial resolution compared to ultrasound. The guideline also discusses the issue that gadolinium contrast, used frequently in CMR angiography studies, can confer risk of nephrogenic systemic sclerosis in patients with advanced renal dysfunction. Generally, the choice of the examination should be determined in an individualized approach to the

Table 5 Recommendations for CMR in heart failure

Recommendations for non-invasive cardiac imaging in heart failure	Class[a]	Level[b]	Page
Radionuclide ventriculography or MRI can be useful to assess LVEF and volume	IIa	C	18
Noninvasive imaging to detect myocardial ischemia and viability is reasonable in heart failure and coronary artery disease	IIa	C	18
Viability assessment is reasonable before revascularization in heart failure patients with coronary artery disease	IIa	B	18
MRI is reasonable when assessing myocardial infiltration or scar	IIa	B	18

[a]Class of recommendation
[b]Level of evidence

Table 6 Recommendations for CMR in valvular heart disease

	Class[a]	Level[b]	Page
Aortic regurgitation			
CMR is indicated in patients with moderate or severe AR (stages B, C, and D) and suboptimal echocardiographic images for the assessment of LV systolic function, systolic and diastolic volumes, and measurement of AR severity.	I	B	29
Bicuspid aortic valve disease			
Aortic magnetic resonance angiography or CT angiography is indicated in patients with a bicuspid aortic valve when morphology of the aortic sinuses, sinotubular junction, or ascending aorta cannot be assessed accurately or fully by echocardiography.	I	C	32
Serial evaluation of the size and morphology of the aortic si- nuses and ascending aorta by echocardiography, CMR, or CT angiography is recommended in patients with a bicuspid aortic valve and an aortic diameter greater than 4.0 cm, with the examination interval determined by the degree and rate of progression of aortic dilation and by family history. In patients with an aortic diameter greater than 4.5 cm, this evaluation should be performed annually.	I	C	33
Mitral regurgitation			
CMR is indicated in patients with chronic primary MR to assess LV and RV volumes, function, or MR severity and when these issues are not satisfactorily addressed by TTE.	I	B	43
Noninvasive imaging (stress nuclear/positron emission tomog- raphy, CMR, or stress echocardiography), cardiac CT angiography, or cardiac catheterization, including coronary arteriography, is useful to establish etiology of chronic secondary MR (stages B to D) and/or to assess myocardial viability, which in turn may influence management of functional MR.	I	C	50
Tricuspid regurgitation			
CMR or real-time 3D echocardiography may be considered for assessment of right ventricular systolic function and systolic and diastolic volumes in patients with severe tricuspid regurgitation (stages C and D) and suboptimal 2D echocardiograms.	IIb	C	54

[a]Class of recommendation
[b]Level of evidence

anatomic assessment for each patient, including risk-benefit assessment of each study type (page 24).

Furthermore, the guideline emphasized that angiography, either noninvasive or invasive, should not be performed for the anatomic assessment of patients with peripheral artery disease without leg symptoms because delineation of anatomy will not change treatment for this population (page 25), expressed as a III-B recommendation.

- 2015 ACC/AHA/HRS Guideline for the management of adult patients with supraventricular tachycardia [25]

This guideline does not mention CMR.

- 2015 ACC/AHA/SCAI Focused Update on Primary Percutaneous Coronary Intervention for Patients With ST-Elevation Myocardial Infarction: An Up-date of the 2011 ACCF/AHA/SCAI Guideline for Percutaneous Coronary Intervention and the 2013 ACCF/AHA Guideline for the Management of ST-Elevation Myocardial Infarction [10]
- 2013 ACCF/AHA Guideline for the Management of ST-Elevation Myocardial Infarction [11]
- 2011 ACCF/AHA/SCAI Guideline for Percutaneous Coronary Intervention [12]

The 2015 update and the 2013 STEMI guideline do not mention CMR. In the 2011 percutaneous coronary intervention guideline, CMR is mentioned in the text as a diagnostic tool to detect periprocedural myocardial infarction (page 40).

- 2014 ACC/AHA Guideline on Perioperative Cardiovascular Evaluation and Management of Patients Undergoing Noncardiac Surgery [15]
- 2007 ACC/AHA Guidelines on Perioperative Cardiovascular Evaluation and Care for Noncardiac Surgery [16]

Table 7 Recommendations for cardiac imaging in syncope

Recommendations for cardiac imaging in syncope	Class[a]	Level[b]	Page
Computed tomography (CT) or magnetic resonance imaging (MRI) may be useful in selected patients presenting with syncope of suspected cardiac etiology.	IIb	B-NR	25
Extended monitoring (including MRI) can be beneficial for athletes with unexplained exertional syncope after an initial cardiovascular evaluation.	IIa	C-LD	64

[a]Class of recommendation
[b]Level of evidence

Table 8 Recommendations for CMR in peripheral artery disease

Recommendations for imaging for anatomic assessment	Class[a]	Level[b]	Page
Duplex ultrasound, computed tomography angiography (CTA), or magnetic resonance angiography (MRA) of the lower extremities is useful to diagnose anatomic location and severity of stenosis for patients with symptomatic peripheral artery disease in whom revascularization is considered	I	B-NR	24
Invasive and noninvasive angiography (ie, CTA, MRA) should not be performed for the anatomic assessment of patients with asymptomatic peripheral artery disease.	III	B-R	25

[a]Class of recommendation
[b]Level of evidence

In subjects undergoing non-cardiac surgery, the appropriate preoperative use of non-invasive stress testing is discussed. There are several specific recommendations in the guideline covering different clinical scenarios. The only recommended stress (exercise or pharmacology) tests with imaging are nuclear myocardial perfusion and dobutamine stress echocardiography (pages 18–20). Regarding CMR it is stated, "There are insufficient data to support the use of dobutamine stress magnetic resonance imaging in preoperative risk assessment" (page 20). Under the heading "future research directions", the document states, "Diagnostic cardiovascular testing continues to evolve, with newer imaging modalities being developed, such as ... cardiac magnetic resonance imaging. The value of these modalities in preoperative screening is uncertain and warrants further study" (page 35).

- 2014 ACC/AHA/AATS/PCNA/SCAI/STS Focused Update of the Guideline for the Diagnosis and Management of Patients With Stable Ischemic Heart Disease [8]
- 2012 ACCF/AHA/ACP/AATS/PCNA/SCAI/STS Guideline for the Diagnosis and Management of Patients With Stable Ischemic Heart Disease [17]

In the 2014 update, CMR is not mentioned. One of the central aspects of the 2012 full guideline is the appropriate use of noninvasive stress testing to assess coronary artery disease. Nuclear perfusion imaging and stress-echocardiography are generally regarded as first choices; however, CMR is included both in the text and in the diagnostic algorithms and in the specific recommendations, underlying its increasing importance.

The guideline is separated into several parts, with the first part focusing on the initial diagnosis of stable ischemic heart disease. Stress CMR is included both in figure 2

of the guideline (page 12) illustrating the diagnostic algorithm, and in table 11 of the guideline (page 23) that summarizes the recommendation level for all available diagnostic tests. Two specific recommendations for stress CMR are expressed (Table 9). A subchapter (page 25) summarizes the current evidence regarding the diagnostic accuracy of pharmacological stress CMR wall motion / perfusion imaging, and underlines the complementary information provided by late gadolinium enhancement scar imaging. In addition, under the subheading "cost effectiveness", data from the EuroCMR registry are mentioned, which provided evidence that "CMR can improve patient management" by reducing the number of indicated coronary angiographies (page 22). Finally, the idea of imaging the coronary anatomy by CMR angiography is discussed in a subchapter (page 26), pointing at the principal feasibility in studies, but also underlining its variable diagnostic accuracy and limited widespread use. On page 21, potential limitations of CMR (claustrophobia, implanted devices, nephrogenic systemic fibrosis) are mentioned.

A second part of the guideline deals with risk stratification in known coronary artery disease. The comprehensive information gained by CMR is pronounced: CMR "accurately measures LV performance and provides insight into myocardial and valvular structures. Use of delayed hyperenhancement techniques can identify otherwise undetected scarred as well as viable myocardium." (page 30). The use of CMR to risk stratify subjects with coronary artery disease is integrated both in figure 3 of the guideline (page 13) containing the corresponding diagnostic algorithm, in table 12 of the guideline (page 31) that summarizes the recommendation level for all diagnostic tests and in tables 20 and 21 of the guideline (page 77–78) that summarize the tests for follow-up. Several scenarios where CMR is or is not recommended are reflected in specific recommendations (Table 10). A subchapter summarizes the evidence for

Table 9 Recommendations for CMR for the diagnosis of stable coronary artery disease

Diagnosis stable coronary artery disease	Class[a]	Level[b]	Page
Pharmacological stress with CMR can be useful for patients with an intermediate to high pretest probability of obstructive ischemic heart disease, who have an uninterpretable ECG and at least moderate physical functioning or no disabling comorbidity.	IIa	B	22
Pharmacological stress CMR is reasonable for patients with an intermediate to high pretest probability of ischemic heart disease, who are incapable of at least moderate physical functioning or have disabling comorbidity.	IIa	B	24

[a]Class of recommendation
[b]Level of evidence

Table 10 Recommendations for CMR for risk stratification and follow-up in stable coronary artery disease

	Class[a]	Level[b]	Page
Resting imaging to assess cardiac structure and function			
Echocardiography, radionuclide imaging, CMR, and cardiac CT are not recommended for routine assessment of LV function in patients with a normal ECG, no history of myocardial infarction, no symptoms or signs suggestive of heart failure, and no complex ventricular arrhythmias.	III	C	29
Routine reassessment (<1 year) of LV function with technologies such as echocardiography, radionuclide imaging, CMR, or cardiac CT is not recommended in patients with no change in clinical status and for whom no change in therapy is contemplated.	III	C	31
Risk assessment in patients able to exercise			
CMR with pharmacological stress is reasonable for risk assessment in patients with stable ischemic heart disease who are able to exercise to an adequate workload but have an uninterpretable ECG.	IIa	B	30
Pharmacological stress imaging (nuclear MPI, echocardiography, or CMR) or CCTA is not recommended for risk assessment in patients with stable ischemic heart disease who are able to exercise to an adequate workload and have an interpretable ECG.	III	C	30
Risk assessment in patients unable to exercise			
Pharmacological stress CMR is reasonable for risk assessment in patients with stable ischemic heart disease who are unable to exercise to an adequate workload regardless of interpretability of ECG.	IIa	B	30
Risk assessment regardless of patients' ability to exercise			
Either exercise or pharmacological stress with imaging (nuclear MPI, echocardiography, or CMR) is recommended for risk assessment in patients with stable ischemic heart disease, who are being considered for revascularization of known coronary stenosis of unclear physiological significance.	I	B	31

[a]Class of recommendation
[b]Level of evidence

pharmacological stress CMR to gain prognostic information (page 33). It concludes: 1. "A normal stress CMR study with either vasodilator myocardial perfusion or inotropic stress cine imaging is associated with a low annual rate of cardiac death or myocardial infarction. 2. Detection of myocardial ischemia... and LGE imaging of infarction appear to provide complementary information. 3. An abnormal stress CMR with evidence of ischemia is associated with elevated likelihood of cardiac death or myocardial infarct". Another subchapter about "Future developments" (page 81) predicts increasing use of CMR in stable coronary artery disease in the future, being supported by upcoming technological developments, like image acquisition acceleration.

- 2014 AHA/ACC Guideline for the Management of Patients With Non–ST-Elevation Acute Coronary Syndromes [26]

This guideline deals with CMR in two scenarios. First, to determine early invasive versus ischemia-guided strategy in patients with NSTEMI, the guideline mentions that - among other factors – "noninvasive stress test findings, including magnetic resonance imaging, may aid in the identification of high-risk patients who could benefit from an invasive strategy" (page 28). Second, in patients presenting as NSTEMI but having angiographically normal coronary arteries, the guideline mentions that "Myocarditis may present with electrocardiographic and biomarker findings similar to ACS and can be distinguished by magnetic resonance imaging" (page 49). Furthermore, the recommendation to use CMR to assess the presence of stress (Takotsubo) cardiomyopathy is given (Table 11).

- 2014 AHA/ACC/HRS Guideline for the Management of Patients With Atrial Fibrillation [27]

CMR is mentioned in the text in the chapter "Mechanisms of atrial fibrillation and pathophysiology / Atrial structural abnormalities": "Late gadolinium-enhancement magnetic resonance imaging is used to image and quantitate atrial fibrosis noninvasively. Human studies show a strong correlation between regions of low voltage on electroanatomic mapping and areas of late enhancement on magnetic resonance imaging. Preliminary results suggest that the severity of atrial fibrosis correlates with the risk of stroke and decreased response to catheter ablation" (page 9–10).

Table 11 Recommendations for CMR in NSTEMI with angiographically normal coronary arteries

Stress (Takotsubo) cardiomyopathy	Class[a]	Level[b]	Page
Imaging with ventriculography, echocardiography, or magnetic resonance imaging should be performed to confirm or exclude the diagnosis of stress (Takotsubo) cardiomyopathy.	I	B	49

[a]Class of recommendation
[b]Level of evidence

- 2013 AHA/ACC/TOS Guideline for the Management of Overweight and Obesity in Adults [28]

CMR is not mentioned in this guideline.

- 2013 AHA/ACC Guideline on Lifestyle Management to Reduce Cardiovascular Risk [29]

CMR is not mentioned in this guideline.

- 2013 ACC/AHA Guideline on the Treatment of Blood Cholesterol to Reduce Atherosclerotic Cardiovascular Risk in Adults [30]

CMR is not mentioned in this guideline.

- 2013 ACC/AHA Guideline on the Assessment of Cardiovascular Risk [31]

CMR is not mentioned in this guideline.

- 2012 ACCF/AHA/HRS Focused Update Incorporated Into the ACCF/AHA/HRS 2008 Guidelines for Device-Based Therapy of Cardiac Rhythm Abnormalities [9]
- 2008 ACC/AHA/HRS Guidelines for Device-Based Therapy of Cardiac Rhythm Abnormalities [32]

In both issues, CMR is mentioned once in the text as a diagnostic tool to detect non-compaction of the left ventricle (page 36).

- 2011 ACCF/AHA Guideline for the Diagnosis and Treatment of Hypertrophic Cardiomyopathy [33]

This guideline includes CMR in several text passages as well as in specific recommendations for both diagnosis and risk stratification.

"The clinical diagnosis of HCM is conventionally made with cardiac imaging, at present most commonly with 2-dimensional echocardiography and increasingly with CMR" (page 10). "In terms of LV wall-thickness measurements, CMR is now used with increasing frequency, and the writing group presumes that data with this latter modality will increasingly emerge" (page 6). "Compared with other noninvasive cardiac imaging modalities, CMR provides superior spatial resolution with sharp contrast between blood and myocardium, as well as complete tomographic imaging of the entire LV myocardium and therefore the opportunity to more accurately characterize the presence, distribution, and extent of LV hypertrophy in HCM" (page 14). "There remain patients in whom the diagnosis of HCM is suspected but the echocardiogram is inconclusive, mostly because of

suboptimal imaging from poor acoustic windows or when hypertrophy is localized to regions of the LV myocardium not well visualized by echocardiography... (predominantly anterolateral wall... or confined to the apex)". (page 15). "Similarly, in the subgroup of patients with HCM who develop apical aneurysms, CMR can more readily detect the presence of an aneurysm" (page 15). Therefore, CMR is also mentioned as a diagnostic tool for HCM screening (page 11). Finally, other diseases may have overlapping phenotypes. CMR with LGE contributes to differentiate various forms of LV hypertrophy, like HCM, Anderson-Fabry disease or cardiac amyloidosis (page 15). Table 12 summarizes the specific recommendations for the use of CMR in HCM.

In addition to its diagnostic value, the use of CMR for risk stratification in HCM is also discussed in the guideline. "Patients with HCM with evidence of LGE on CMR imaging tend to have more markers of risk of sudden cardiac death, such as non-sustained VT, than patients without LGE" (page 15). It is a plausible and attractive concept that areas of LGE... could represent a substrate for the generation of malignant ventricular tachyarrhythmias in HCM and thus a marker for risk of SCD. Several studies have addressed this issue and have reported either trends in such a direction or significant associations between the presence of LGE ... and cardiac outcome events. "However, there is insufficient evidence at this time to support a significant association between the extent of LGE and outcome. ... Nonetheless, the present cross-data would support a potential role of ... LGE as an arbitrator to consider in clinical decision making for primary prevention ICDs in patients in whom high-risk status for sudden cardiac death remains uncertain after assessment of conventional risk factors" (page 15). This assessment is reflected in a specific recommendation (Table 12).

Finally, as HCM is regarded as a complex disease entity, the writing committee emphasizes establishing clinical excellence centers, including access to CMR imaging (page 8).

- 2011 ACCF/AHA Guideline for Coronary Artery Bypass Graft Surgery [34]

CMR is not mentioned in this guideline.

- 2011 AHA/ACCF Secondary Prevention and Risk Reduction Therapy for Patients With Coronary and Other Atherosclerotic Vascular Disease: 2011 Update [13]
- 2006 AHA/ACC Guidelines for Secondary Prevention for Patients With Coronary and Other Atherosclerotic Vascular Disease: 2006 Update [14]

CMR is not mentioned in these guideline updates.

Table 12 Recommendations for CMR in HCM

	Class[a]	Level[b]	Page
CMR for the diagnosis of HCM			
CMR imaging is indicated in patients with suspected HCM when echocardiography is inconclusive for diagnosis.	I	B	14
CMR imaging is indicated in patients with known HCM when additional information that may have an impact on management or decision making regarding invasive management, such as magnitude and distribution of hypertrophy or anatomy of the mitral valve apparatus or papillary muscles, is not adequately defined with echocardiography.	I	B	14
CMR imaging is reasonable in patients with HCM to define apical hypertrophy and/or aneurysm if echocardiography is inconclusive.	IIa	B	14
CMR imaging may be considered in patients with LV hypertrophy and the suspicion of alternative diagnoses to HCM, including cardiac amyloidosis, Fabry disease, and genetic phenocopies such as LAMP2 cardiomyopathy.	IIb	C	14
CMR for risk stratification in HCM			
In selected patients with known HCM, when SCD risk stratification is inconclusive after documentation of the conventional risk factors, CMR imaging with assessment of late gadolinium enhancement (LGE) may be considered in resolving clinical decision making.	IIb	C	14
The usefulness of the following potential SCD risk modifiers is unclear but might be considered in selected patients with HCM for whom risk remains borderline after documentation of conventional risk factors: CMR imaging with LGE.	IIb	C	27

[a]Class of recommendation
[b]Level of evidence

- 2011 ASA/ACCF/AHA/AANN/AANS/ACR/ASNR/ CNS/ SAIP/SCAI/SIR/SNIS/SVM/SVS Guideline on the Management of Patients With Extracranial Carotid and Vertebral Artery [20]

The guideline contains several specific recommendations for the use of MR angiography to assess both carotid and vertebral arteries (Table 13). In addition, the strength and limitations of MRA are described in detail. Among other aspects, the NASCET stenosis grade based on angiographic criteria corresponds well to sonography, CT angiography and MR angiography, although the latter may overestimate the severity of stenosis (page 17). It is also stated that patients with a high pretest probability of disease may be examined initially by MR angiography or CT angiography to more completely evaluate the

Table 13 Recommendations for MR in carotid and vertebral artery disease

	Class[a]	Level[b]	Page
Carotid artery			
In patients with acute, focal ischemic neurological symptoms corresponding to the territory supplied by the left or right internal carotid artery, magnetic resonance angiography (MRA) or computed tomography angiography (CTA) is indicated to detect carotid stenosis when sonography either cannot be obtained or yields equivocal or otherwise nondiagnostic results.	I	C	15
When an extracranial source of ischemia is not identified in patients with transient retinal or hemispheric neurological symptoms of suspected ischemic origin, CTA, MRA, or selective cerebral angiography can be useful to search for intracranial vascular disease.	IIa	C	15
When the results of initial noninvasive imaging are inconclusive, additional examination by use of another imaging method is reasonable. In candidates for revascularization, MRA or CTA can be useful when results of carotid duplex ultrasonography are equivocal or indeterminate.	IIa	C	15
When intervention for significant carotid stenosis detected by carotid duplex ultrasonography is planned, MRA, CTA, or catheter-based contrast angiography can be useful to evaluate the severity of stenosis and to identify intrathoracic or intracranial vascular lesions that are not adequately assessed by duplex ultrasonography.	IIa	C	15
MRA without contrast is reasonable to assess the extent of disease in patients with symptomatic carotid atherosclerosis and renal insufficiency or extensive vascular calcification.	IIa	C	15
When complete carotid arterial occlusion is suggested by duplex ultrasonography, MRA, or CTA in patients with retinal or hemispheric neurological symptoms of suspected ischemic origin, catheter-based contrast angiography may be considered to determine whether the arterial lumen is sufficiently patent to permit carotid revascularization.	IIb	C	15
Vertebral artery			
Noninvasive imaging by CTA or MRA for detection of vertebral artery disease should be part of the initial evaluation of patients with neurological symptoms referable to the posterior circulation and those with subclavian steal syndrome.	I	C	47
In patients whose symptoms suggest posterior cerebral or cerebellar ischemia, MRA or CTA is recommended rather than ultrasound imaging for evaluation of the vertebral arteries.	I	C	47
Contrast-enhanced CTA, MRA, and catheter-based contrast angiography are useful for diagnosis of cervical artery dissection.	I	C	52

[a]Class of recommendation
[b]Level of evidence

cerebral vessels distal to the aortic arch, because sono-graphic imaging alone does not provide assessment of intrathoracic or intracranial lesions beyond the limited range of the ultrasound probe (page 21). After carotid stenting, imaging by CT angiography or MR angiography may also be helpful for surveillance, particularly "when Doppler interrogation is difficult because of a superior anatomic location of the region of interest" (page 41).

- 2010 ACCF/AHA/AATS/ACR/ASA/SCA/SCAI/SIR/ STS/SVM Guidelines for the Diagnosis and Management of Patients With Thoracic Aortic Disease [21]

The guideline includes a chapter explaining the principles, strength and limitations of CMR to assess the thoracic aorta (page 17). CMR "has been shown to be very accurate in the diagnosis of thoracic aortic disease, with sensitivities and specificities that are equivalent to or may exceed those for CT and TEE" (page 17). "Advantages of CMR include the ability to identify anatomic variants of aortic dissection (intramural hematoma, penetrating aortic ulceration), assess branch artery involvement, and diagnose aortic valve pathology and left ventricular dysfunction without exposing the patient to either radiation or iodinated contrast" (page 17).

Throughout the text, the use of CMR in different clinical scenarios and pathologies is described and evaluated. CMR is an integral part of a number of diagnostic pathways illustrated in various figures, e.g., the aortic dissection pathway (figure 25 in the guideline, page 45) and the ascending aortic aneurysm pathway (figure 31 in the guideline, page 56). In addition, CMR is recommended for surveillance of stable and moderate thoracic aortic aneurysms (page 76), as well as for follow-up of aortic pathologies after repair or treatment (page 77, table 17 in the guideline). Finally, there are a number of specific recommendations on the use of CMR in patients with thoracic aortic disease (Table 14).

- 2010 ACCF/AHA Guideline for Assessment of Cardiovascular Risk in Asymptomatic Adults [18]

The use of CMR for the assessment of arterial stiffness by quantifying pulse wave velocity is mentioned. However, CMR "is more costly and therefore is typically not used for testing in asymptomatic persons" (page 23). CMR is described in detail as a method for "detection and quantification of atherosclerosis. ... Examination of plaque under different contrast weighting ... allows characterization of individual plaque components, including lipid-rich necrotic core, fibrous cap status,

Table 14 Recommendations for CMR in thoracic aortic disease

	Class[a]	Level[b]	Page
Recommendations for acute thoracic aortic disease			
Urgent and definitive imaging of the aorta using transesophageal echocardiogram, computed tomographic imaging, or magnetic resonance imaging is recommended to identify or exclude thoracic aortic dissection in patients at high risk for the disease by initial screening.	I	B	43
Recommendations for Takayasu arteritis and giant cell arteritis			
The initial evaluation of Takayasu arteritis or giant cell arteritis should include thoracic aorta and branch vessel computed tomographic imaging or magnetic resonance imaging to inves- tigate the possibility of aneurysm or occlusive disease in these vessels.	I	C	28
Recommendations for aortic arch aneurysms			
For patients with isolated aortic arch aneurysms less than 4.0 cm in diameter, it is reasonable to reimage using computed tomographic imaging or magnetic resonance imaging, at 12- month intervals, to detect enlargement of the aneurysm.	IIa	C	58
For patients with isolated aortic arch aneurysms 4.0 cm or greater in diameter, it is reasonable to reimage using computed tomographic imaging or magnetic resonance imaging, at 6-month intervals, to detect enlargement of the aneurysm.	IIa	C	58
Recommendations for chronic aortic diseases in pregnancy			
For imaging of pregnant women with aortic arch, descending, or abdominal aortic dilatation, magnetic resonance imaging (without gadolinium) is recommended over computed tomographic imaging to avoid exposing both the mother and fetus to ionizing radiation. Transesophageal echocardiogram is an option for imaging of the thoracic aorta.	I	C	64
Recommendations for surveillance of thoracic aortic disease or previously repaired patients			
Computed tomographic imaging or magnetic resonance imaging of the thoracic aorta is reasonable after a Type A or B aortic dissection or after prophylactic repair of the aortic root/ ascending aorta.	IIa	C	76
Computed tomographic imaging or magnetic resonance imaging of the aorta is reasonable at 1, 3, 6, and 12 months postdissection and, if stable, annually thereafter so that any threatening enlargement can be detected in a timely fashion.	IIa	C	76
If a thoracic aortic aneurysm is only moderate in size and remains relatively stable over time, magnetic resonance imaging instead of computed tomographic imaging is reasonable to minimize the patient's radiation exposure.	IIa	C	76

[a]Class of recommendation
[b]Level of evidence

hemorrhage, and calcification. ... It is recommended that additional large-scale multicenter trials be conducted to evaluate the possibility of using CMR in the detection of atherosclerosis in asymptomatic patients" (page 32). Yet, despite the potential of CMR for atherosclerotic plaque characterization, it is currently not recommended for screening asymptomatic subjects (Table 15).

- 2008 ACC/AHA Guidelines for the Management of Adults With Congenital Heart Disease (ACHD) [19]

In general, "cardiac MRI to assess ventricular anatomy and function, dimensions, myocardial perfusion, and ischemia in adults with unoperated or operated CHD is regarded as helpful" (page 29). CMR is also recommended as an integral part of regional ACHD centers (page 11, table 2 in the guideline). The guideline contains numerous text passages regarding the use of CMR in specific congenital heart diseases and clinical scenarios, such as ventricular septal defect (page 37), atrial septal defect (page 40), supravalvular aortic stenosis (page 51), and right ventricular outflow tract obstruction (page 56). To provide an example, the recommendations regarding aortic coarctation state that "MRI ... with 3-dimensional reconstruction identifies the precise location and anatomy of the coarctation and entire aorta, as well as collateral vessels. ... Magnetic resonance angiography may also be useful to quantify collateral flow." (page 53). In addition, a number of specific recommendations are made (Table 16).

- 2006 ACC/AHA/ESC Guidelines for Management of Patients With Ventricular Arrhythmias and the Prevention of Sudden Cardiac Death [35]

The guideline dedicates a paragraph to the strength of CMR "to evaluate both the structure and function of the beating heart. The excellent image resolution obtained with current techniques allows for the accurate quantification of chamber volumes, LV mass, and ventricular function. This is of particular value in patients with suspected arrhythmogenic RV cardiomyopathy (ARVC), in whom MRI provides excellent assessment of RV size, function, and regional wall motion and, importantly, may allow the detection of fatty infiltration within the RV myocardium. ... Cardiac MRI increasingly is being applied and validated for the detection of ischemia (adenosine stress perfusion and dobutamine stress wall motion studies) and the detection and quantification of

infarction/fibrosis, a substrate for VT." In addition, CMR is mentioned to detect cardiac involvement in sarcoidosis (page 41), "to be helpful in assessing extent of disease and predicting sudden cardiac death" (page 48), in hypertrophic cardiomyopathy, and "for the evaluation of patients with ventricular tachycardia arising from the RV in the absence of defined abnormalities on conventional testing particularly to exclude ARVC" (page 59). Finally, the guideline contains one specific recommendation for CMR for accurate assessment of LV and RV function and evaluation of structural changes (Table 17).

Discussion

This study demonstrates that CMR is mentioned in the majority of the AHA/ACC guidelines (66.7%) and that 50% of the AHA/ACC guidelines contain a total of 65 specific recommendations for when and how to use CMR. When analyzing the AHA/ACC guidelines in detail, some interesting aspects arise:

First, a look at the specific recommendations reveals that the indication category with the largest number of specific recommendations is vascular imaging. This is probably related to the fact that vascular imaging (MR angiography) is one of the most established CMR techniques. It is also worth noting that there is significant heterogeneity across the guidelines regarding whether a particular topic is only mentioned in the text, versus being included as a specific recommendation and assigned a class of recommendation and a level of evidence. Hence, to simply correlate the absolute number of specific recommendations with the importance of CMR across guideline documents may be flawed. Nevertheless, the large number of specific recommendations in the vascular disease category certainly underlines the well-defined role of CMR and MR angiography. This has also been reflected in the ESC guideline analysis, which showed in total 17 specific recommendations in the vascular category [3].

The category with the second highest number of recommendations is congenital heart disease. Patients with congenital heart disease are monitored and treated mostly in dedicated centers. The prevalence in CMR in AHA/ACC guidelines for congenital heart disease underscores the fact that CMR is commonly utilized in this population both in the preoperative state and during patient follow-up.

Regarding CMR myocardial stress testing, only eight specific recommendations exist. In relation to the

Table 15 Recommendations for CMR for assessment of cardiovascular risk in asymptomatic adults

Recommendation for imaging of plaque	Class[a]	Level[b]	Page
MRI for detection of vascular plaque is not recommended for cardiovascular risk assessment in asymptomatic adults.	III	C	32

[a]*Class of recommendation*
[b]*Level of evidence*

Table 16 Recommendations for CMR for management of adults with congenital heart disease

	Class[a]	Level[b]	Page
Recommendations for adults with congenital heart disease (ACHD)			
Diagnostic and interventional procedures, including imaging (ie, echocardiography, MRI, or CT, advanced cardiac catheterization, and electrophysiology procedures for adults with complex and moderate CHD should be performed in a regional ACHD center with appropriate experience in CHD and in a laboratory with appropriate personnel and equipment. Personnel performing such procedures should work as part of a team with expertise in the surgical and transcatheter management of patients with CHD.	I	C	12–13
Bicuspid aortic valve disease			
MRI/CT can be beneficial to add important information about the anatomy of the thoracic aorta.	IIa	C	45
MRI may be beneficial in quantifying aortic regurgitation when other data are ambiguous or borderline.	IIb	C	45
Supravalvular aortic stenosis			
TTE and/or TEE with Doppler and either MRI or CT should be performed to assess the anatomy of the LVOT, the ascending aorta, coronary artery anatomy and flow, and main and branch pulmonary artery anatomy and flow.	I	C	50
Aortic coarctation			
Every patient with coarctation (repaired or not) should have at least 1 cardiovascular MRI or CT scan for complete evaluation of the thoracic aorta and intracranial vessels.	I	B	52
Evaluation of the coarctation repair site by MRI/CT should be performed at intervals of 5 years or less, depending on the specific anatomic findings before and after repair.	I	C	53
Supravalvular, branch, and peripheral pulmonary stenosis			
Patients with suspected supravalvular, branch, or peripheral pulmonary stenosis should have baseline imaging with echocardiography-Doppler plus 1 of the following: MRI angiography, CT angiography, or contrast angiography.	I	C	61
Congenital coronary anomalies of ectopic arterial origin			
CT or MRA is useful as the initial screening method in centers with expertise in such imaging.	I	B	65
Coronary arteriovenous fistula			
If a continuous murmur is present, its origin should be defined either by echocardiography, MRI, CT angiography, or cardiac catheterization.	I	C	67
Congenital heart disease and pulmonary arterial hypertension			
The evaluation of all ACHD patients with suspected pulmonary arterial hypertension should include noninvasive assessment of cardiovascular anatomy and potential shunting, as detailed below: Diagnostic cardiovascular imaging via TTE, TEE, MRI, or CT as appropriate.	I	C	70
After repaired of tetralogy of Fallot			
Patients with tetralogy of Fallot should have echocardiographic examinations and/or MRIs performed by staff with expertise in ACHD.	I	C	73
Dextro-Transposition of the great arteries			
Additional imaging with TEE, CT, or MRI, as appropriate, should be performed in a regional ACHD center to evaluate the great arteries and veins, as well as ventricular function, in patients with prior atrial baffle repair of d-TGA.	I	B	80
Periodic MRI or CT can be considered appropriate to evaluate the anatomy and hemodynamics in more detail in patients with prior arterial switch operation.	IIa	C	80
Congenitally corrected transposition of the great arteries			
Echocardiography-Doppler study and/or MRI should be performed yearly or at least every other year by staff trained in imaging complex CHD.	I	C	87
The following diagnostic evaluations are recommended for patients with congenitally corrected transposition of the great arteries: ECG, chest x-ray, echocardiography-Doppler study, MRI, exercise testing.	I	C	87
In patients with prior repair of congenitally corrected transposition of the great arteries, echocardiography-Doppler study and/or MRI should be performed yearly or at least every other year by staff trained in imaging complex CHD.	I	C	89
After Fontan Procedure			
All patients with prior Fontan type of repair should have periodic echocardiographic and/or magnetic resonance examinations performed by staff with expertise in ACHD.	I	C	97

[a]Class of recommendation
[b]Level of evidence

Table 17 Recommendations for CMR for patients with ventricular arrhythmias and the prevention of sudden cardiac death

Recommendations for CMR for patients with ventricular arrhythmias and the prevention of sudden cardiac death	Class[a]	Level[b]	Page
MRI, cardiac computed tomography (CT), or radionuclide angiography can be useful in patients with ventricular arrhythmias when echocardiography does not provide accurate assessment of LV and RV function and/or evaluation of structural changes.	IIa	B	19

[a]Class of recommendation
[b]Level of evidence

number of guidelines dealing with coronary artery disease (guidelines for STEMI, NSTEMI and stable coronary artery disease), the evidence proving the diagnostic accuracy for CMR stress testing to detect coronary artery disease [2], and the dominance of coronary artery disease in clinical routine, this number suggests an underrepresentation of CMR stress testing. Conversely, CMR stress testing has a greater presence in the ESC guidelines where it is treated as equivalent with other modalities such as stress echocardiography and nuclear perfusion studies, ending up in a total of 28 specific recommendations [3]. With new data recently published, such as the CE-MARC 2 trial in 2016 that showed that CMR stress testing contributes to a lower rate of "unnecessary" invasive coronary angiographies [2], the role of CMR stress testing may increase in future editions of the AHA/ACC guidelines. The limited representation of CMR to assess viability to guide revascularization with only 3 specific recommendations can be interpreted in a similar sense.

Finally, there are only 6 specific recommendations regarding cardiomyopathies, all of which are part of the hypertrophic cardiomyopathy guidelines – a similar pattern as in the ESC guidelines [3]. In contrary, the evaluation of patients with known or suspected cardiomyopathy is the second largest indication group in clinical CMR in Europe, as expressed in the EuroCMR registry that included more than 27,000 patients [1]. This discrepancy may be attributed to the lack of a guideline covering cardiomyopathies in general. In case such a paper would be generated, there may be additional recommendations in favor of CMR, e.g., for assessment of arrhythmogenic ventricular cardiomyopathy, for risk stratification and differential diagnosis in dilated cardiomyopathy, for the diagnosis of non-compaction cardiomyopathy, and for diseases causing restrictive types of cardiomyopathies.

The use of CMR to assess myocarditis represents another discrepancy between representation in the AHA/ACC guidelines versus the level of evidence and clinical utilization in practice. Myocarditis is one of the most frequent indications for CMR in Europe [36] and the evidence for its diagnostic benefit is proven [37, 38]. In contrast, there is no single specific recommendation for CMR to assess myocarditis in the AHA/ACC guidelines. Only once in the context of differentiating acute coronary syndrome is CMR to assess myocarditis mentioned

[26]. This might be attributed to the lack of a focused guideline regarding inflammatory heart diseases. In this regard, the AHA/ACC guidelines resemble the ESC guidelines; only one ESC guideline (concerning patients with ventricular arrhythmias) contains a single specific recommendation to perform CMR for risk stratification in inflammatory heart disease [39].

When analyzing those guidelines that cover overlapping topics (e.g., ischemic heart disease), there exists considerable heterogeneity in how they deal with similar topics. For example, the 2014 guideline on stable coronary artery disease contains several specific recommendations for CMR stress testing. On the other hand, similar chapters in the guideline on NSTEMI or assessment of ventricular arrhythmias contain no specific recommendations for stress CMR. This may reflect the different publication dates, as the clinical evidence and utilization of stress CMR have continued to grow. In addition, a high degree of coordination is required to synchronize recommendations for indications that appear in multiple guidelines.

When looking at those guidelines that do not mention CMR at all, it seems understandable that the guidelines dealing with "supraventricular tachycardia", "overweight", "lifestyle management" and "blood cholesterol" would not include recommendations for CMR. In contrast it is rather surprising - based on the topic and the common indications for CMR - that the AHA/ACC guidelines dealing with "STEMI", "assessment of cardiovascular risk", "secondary prevention for patients with coronary vascular disease" and "CABG" do not mention CMR at all. In comparison, the ESC-STEMI guideline from 2012 contains 2 specific recommendations (for assessment of infarct size and resting LV function; for ischemia and viability).

Four AHA/ACC guidelines mention CMR in the text without including specific recommendations ("before noncardiac surgery", "atrial fibrillation", "percutanoues coronary intervention", "device therapy"). In future editions, some text passages may be accompanied by specific recommendations. On the other hand, the atrial fibrillation guideline from 2014 mentions late enhancement imaging of atrial fibrosis to predict therapeutic success [27]. Even though there is growing evidence for this application [40], its use within the CMR society is actually restricted to a small group. Thus, despite the intention to place CMR in the guidelines where the evidence supports this, modesty should also be part of the strategy to avoid the dilemma of creating non-accomplishable expectations.

Limitations of the study

This summary is not intended to provide a comparison of the various imaging modalities in the AHA/ACC guidelines, but is rather aimed at only describing the role of CMR. Its character is more descriptive than analytical, and its layout designed to allow the reader to easily locate CMR recommendations in the guidelines, rather than to serve as a scientific meta-analysis. Additional analyses, e.g., focusing on myocardial stress testing in all guidelines regarding all available methods, will be subject of future studies. Furthermore, there are guidelines, where every detail is represented in a specific recommendation, and others, where only general recommendations are made; this leads to significant heterogeneity in the number of recommendations included in different guidelines. Naturally, the composition of the writing groups influences the content of the guidelines, and therefore the representation of CMR. However, no systematic data are available regarding the inclusion of CMR experts in the writing groups and therefore this potential influencing factor cannot be evaluated. Another factor influencing the representation of CMR in the guidelines could be the length of time it takes to generate guideline documents. It can be a 5-year process from the time of conception to publication and thus some aspects may be out of date by the time of publication. Finally, a systematic and scientific comparison of the AHA/ACC and the ESC guidelines is difficult, as most of the corresponding guidelines were not published at the same time, and many topics are not covered by guidelines of both organizations. Hence, the comparative assessments that are included must be viewed with this limitation in mind.

Conclusions

CMR is represented in two thirds of the AHA/ACC guidelines, and these guidelines contain many recommendations in favor of the use of CMR in specific scenarios. In general, the representation of CMR is heterogeneous throughout the guidelines, with some topics (such as CMR in vascular disease and congenital heart disease) containing numerous recommendations for CMR, and others (such as those dealing with coronary artery disease) including few recommendations relative to the broad topic-related evidence. Although a direct comparison of the AHA/ACC to the ESC guidelines is difficult due to heterogeneous characteristics of both sets, CMR appears to be less represented in the AHA/ACC guidelines, in particular in coronary artery disease.

Abbreviations

ACC : American College of Cardiology; ACHD: Adults with congenital heart disease; AHA: American Heart Association; CMR : Cardiovascular magnetic resonance; CT: Computed tomography; EF: Ejection fraction; HCM: Hypertrophic cardiomyopathy; ICD: Implantable cardioverter defibrillator; LGE: Late gadolinium enhancement; LV: Left ventricle/left ventricular; LVOT: Left ventricular outflow tract; NSTEMI: Non-ST-elevation myocardial infarction; RV: Right ventricle/right ventricular; SCD: Sudden cardiac death; STEMI: ST-elevation myocardial infarction; TEE: Transesophageal echocardiography; TTE: Transthoracic echocardiography; VT: Ventricular tachycardia

Acknowledgements

We thank Orlando Simonetti, PhD, for carefully editing the manuscript, as well as Edyta Blaszczyk, MD, for assisting in preparing the manuscript.

Funding

There is no specific funding for the project underlying this manuscript.

Authors' contributions

FvKB was responsible for conception and design, acquisition of data, analysis and interpretation of data and drafted the manuscript. GP and JSM revised the manuscript critically for important intellectual content and gave final approval of the version to be published. All authors agree to be accountable for all aspects of the work in ensuring that questions related to the accuracy or integrity of any part of the work are appropriately investigated and resolved. All authors read and approved the final manuscript.

Consent for publication

Not applicable.

Competing interests

Jeanette Schulz-Menger is immediate past-president of the Society for Cardiovascular Magnetic Resonance. Florian von Knobelsdorff-Brenkenhoff is member of the executive committee of the working group CMR of the German Society for Cardiology.

Author details

[1]Department of Cardiology, Clinic Agatharied, Ludwig-Maximilians-University Munich, Norbert-Kerkel-Platz, 83734 Hausham, Germany. [2]Charité – Universitätsmedizin Berlin, corporate member of Freie Universität Berlin, Humboldt-Universität zu Berlin, and Berlin Institute of Health, DZHK (German Centre for Cardiovascular Research), partner site Berlin, Berlin, Germany. [3]Working Group Cardiovascular Magnetic Resonance, Experimental and Clinical Research Center, a joint cooperation between the Charité Medical Faculty and the Max-Delbrueck Center for Molecular Medicine and HELIOS Klinikum Berlin Buch, Department of Cardiology and Nephrology, Berlin, Germany.

References

1. Bruder O, Wagner A, Lombardi M, Schwitter J, van Rossum A, Pilz G, et al. European cardiovascular magnetic resonance (EuroCMR) registry–multi national results from 57 centers in 15 countries. J Cardiovasc Magn Reson. 2013;15:9.
2. Greenwood JP, Ripley DP, Berry C, McCann GP, Plein S, Bucciarelli-Ducci C, et al. Effect of care guided by cardiovascular magnetic resonance, myocardial perfusion Scintigraphy, or NICE guidelines on subsequent unnecessary angiography rates: the CE-MARC 2 randomized clinical trial. JAMA. 2016;316:1051–60.
3. von Knobelsdorff-Brenkenhoff F, Schulz-Menger J. Role of cardiovascular magnetic resonance in the guidelines of the European Society of Cardiology. J Cardiovasc Magn Reson. 2016;18:6.
4. Gerhard-Herman MD, Gornik HL, Barrett C, Barshes NR, Corriere MA, Drachman DE, et al. 2016 AHA/ACC guideline on the Management of Patients with Lower

Extremity Peripheral Artery Disease: executive summary: a report of the American College of Cardiology/American Heart Association task force on clinical practice guidelines. J Am Coll Cardiol. 2017;69:1465–508.

5. Yancy CW, Jessup M, Bozkurt B, Butler J, Casey DE, Jr., Colvin MM et al. 2017 ACC/AHA/HFSA Focused Update of the 2013 ACCF/AHA Guideline for the Management of Heart Failure: A Report of the American College of Cardiology/American Heart Association Task Force on Clinical Practice Guidelines and the Heart Failure Society of America. J Am Coll Cardiol. 2017;70:776-803.

6. Yancy CW, Jessup M, Bozkurt B, Butler J, Casey DE Jr, Colvin MM, et al. 2016 ACC/AHA/HFSA focused update on new pharmacological therapy for heart failure: an update of the 2013 ACCF/AHA guideline for the Management of Heart Failure: a report of the American College of Cardiology/American Heart Association task force on clinical practice guidelines and the Heart Failure Society of America. J Am Coll Cardiol. 2016;68:1476–88.

7. Nishimura RA, Otto CM, Bonow RO, Carabello BA, Erwin JP, 3rd, Fleisher LA et al. 2017 AHA/ACC Focused Update of the 2014 AHA/ACC Guideline for the Management of Patients With Valvular Heart Disease: A Report of the American College of Cardiology/American Heart Association Task Force on Clinical Practice Guidelines. J Am Coll Cardiol. 2017;70:252-289.

8. Fihn SD, Blankenship JC, Alexander KP, Bittl JA, Byrne JG, Fletcher BJ, et al. 2014 ACC/AHA/AATS/PCNA/SCAI/STS focused update of the guideline for the diagnosis and management of patients with stable ischemic heart disease: a report of the American College of Cardiology/American Heart Association task force on practice guidelines, and the American Association for Thoracic Surgery, preventive cardiovascular nurses association, Society for Cardiovascular Angiography and Interventions, and Society of Thoracic Surgeons. J Am Coll Cardiol. 2014;64:1929–49.

9. Epstein AE, DiMarco JP, Ellenbogen KA, Estes NA 3rd, Freedman RA, Gettes LS, et al. 2012 ACCF/AHA/HRS focused update incorporated into the ACCF/AHA/HRS 2008 guidelines for device-based therapy of cardiac rhythm abnormalities: a report of the American College of Cardiology Foundation/American Heart Association task force on practice guidelines and the Heart Rhythm Society. J Am Coll Cardiol. 2013;61:e6–75.

10. Levine GN, Bates ER, Blankenship JC, Bailey SR, Bittl JA, Cercek B, et al. 2015 ACC/AHA/SCAI focused update on primary Percutaneous coronary intervention for patients with ST-elevation myocardial infarction: an update of the 2011 ACCF/AHA/SCAI guideline for Percutaneous coronary intervention and the 2013 ACCF/AHA guideline for the management of ST-elevation myocardial infarction. J Am Coll Cardiol. 2016;67:1235–50.

11. American College of Emergency P, Society for Cardiovascular A, Interventions, O'Gara PT, Kushner FG, Ascheim DD, et al. 2013 ACCF/AHA guideline for the management of ST-elevation myocardial infarction: a report of the American College of Cardiology Foundation/American Heart Association task force on practice guidelines. J Am Coll Cardiol. 2013;61:e78–140.

12. Levine GN, Bates ER, Blankenship JC, Bailey SR, Bittl JA, Cercek B, et al. 2011 ACCF/AHA/SCAI guideline for Percutaneous coronary intervention. A report of the American College of Cardiology Foundation/American Heart Association task force on practice guidelines and the Society for Cardiovascular Angiography and Interventions. J Am Coll Cardiol. 2011;58:e44–122.

13. Smith SC Jr, Benjamin EJ, Bonow RO, Braun LT, Creager MA, Franklin BA, et al. AHA/ACCF secondary prevention and risk reduction therapy for patients with coronary and other atherosclerotic vascular disease: 2011 update: a guideline from the American Heart Association and American College of Cardiology Foundation endorsed by the world heart federation and the preventive cardiovascular nurses association. J Am Coll Cardiol. 2011;58:2432–46.

14. Aha, Acc, National Heart L, Blood I, Smith SC Jr, Allen J, et al. AHA/ACC guidelines for secondary prevention for patients with coronary and other atherosclerotic vascular disease: 2006 update endorsed by the National Heart, Lung, and Blood Institute. J Am Coll Cardiol. 2006;47:2130–9.

15. Fleisher LA, Fleischmann KE, Auerbach AD, Barnason SA, Beckman JA, Bozkurt B, et al. 2014 ACC/AHA guideline on perioperative cardiovascular evaluation and management of patients undergoing noncardiac surgery: a report of the American College of Cardiology/American Heart Association task force on practice guidelines. J Am Coll Cardiol. 2014;64:e77–137.

16. Fleisher LA, Beckman JA, Brown KA, Calkins H, Chaikof EL, Fleischmann KE, et al. ACC/AHA 2007 guidelines on Perioperative cardiovascular evaluation and Care for Noncardiac Surgery: executive summary: a report of the American College of Cardiology/American Heart Association task force on practice guidelines (writing committee to revise the 2002 guidelines on Perioperative cardiovascular evaluation for noncardiac surgery) developed in collaboration with the American Society of Echocardiography, American Society of Nuclear Cardiology, Heart Rhythm Society, Society of Cardiovascular Anesthesiologists, Society for Cardiovascular Angiography and Interventions, Society for Vascular Medicine and Biology, and society for vascular surgery. J Am Coll Cardiol. 2007;50:1707–32.

17. Fihn SD, Gardin JM, Abrams J, Berra K, Blankenship JC, Dallas AP, et al. 2012 ACCF/AHA/ACP/AATS/PCNA/SCAI/STS guideline for the diagnosis and management of patients with stable ischemic heart disease: a report of the American College of Cardiology Foundation/American Heart Association task force on practice guidelines, and the American College of Physicians, American Association for Thoracic Surgery, preventive cardiovascular nurses association, Society for Cardiovascular Angiography and Interventions, and Society of Thoracic Surgeons. J Am Coll Cardiol. 2012;60:e44–e164.

18. Greenland P, Alpert JS, Beller GA, Benjamin EJ, Budoff MJ, Fayad ZA, et al. 2010 ACCF/AHA guideline for assessment of cardiovascular risk in asymptomatic adults: a report of the American College of Cardiology Foundation/American Heart Association task force on practice guidelines. J Am Coll Cardiol. 2010;56:e50–103.

19. Warnes CA, Williams RG, Bashore TM, Child JS, Connolly HM, Dearani JA, et al. ACC/AHA 2008 guidelines for the management of adults with congenital heart disease: a report of the American College of Cardiology/American Heart Association task force on practice guidelines (writing committee to develop guidelines on the Management of Adults with Congenital Heart Disease). Developed in collaboration with the American Society of Echocardiography, Heart Rhythm Society, International Society for Adult Congenital Heart Disease, Society for Cardiovascular Angiography and Interventions, and Society of Thoracic Surgeons. J Am Coll Cardiol. 2008;52:e143–263.

20. Brott TG, Halperin JL, Abbara S, Bacharach JM, Barr JD, Bush RL, et al. 2011 ASA/ACCF/AHA/AANN/AANS/ACR/ASNR/CNS/SAIP/SCAI/SIR/SNIS/SVM/SVS guideline on the management of patients with extracranial carotid and vertebral artery disease: executive summary: a report of the American College of Cardiology Foundation/American Heart Association task force on practice guidelines, and the American Stroke Association, American Association of Neuroscience Nurses, American Association of Neurological Surgeons, American College of Radiology, American Society of Neuroradiology, Congress of Neurological Surgeons, Society of Atherosclerosis Imaging and Prevention, Society for Cardiovascular Angiography and Interventions, Society of Interventional Radiology, society of NeuroInterventional surgery, Society for Vascular Medicine, and Society for Vascular Surgery. J Am Coll Cardiol. 2011;57:1002–44.

21. Hiratzka LF, Bakris GL, Beckman JA, Bersin RM, Carr VF, Casey DE Jr, et al. 2010 ACCF/AHA/AATS/ACR/ASA/SCA/SCAI/SIR/STS/SVM guidelines for the diagnosis and management of patients with thoracic aortic disease. A report of the American College of Cardiology Foundation/American Heart Association task force on practice guidelines, American Association for Thoracic Surgery, American College of Radiology,American Stroke Association, Society of Cardiovascular Anesthesiologists, Society for Cardiovascular Angiography and Interventions, Society of Interventional Radiology, Society of Thoracic Surgeons,and Society for Vascular Medicine. J Am Coll Cardiol. 2010;55:e27–e129.

22. Yancy CW, Jessup M, Bozkurt B, Butler J, Casey DE Jr, Drazner MH, et al. 2013 ACCF/AHA guideline for the management of heart failure: a report of the American College of Cardiology Foundation/American Heart Association task force on practice guidelines. J Am Coll Cardiol. 2013;62:e147–239.

23. Nishimura RA, Otto CM, Bonow RO, Carabello BA, Erwin JP 3rd, Guyton RA, et al. 2014 AHA/ACC guideline for the management of patients with valvular heart disease: executive summary: a report of the American College of Cardiology/American Heart Association task force on practice guidelines. J Am Coll Cardiol. 2014;63:2438–88.

24. Shen WK, Sheldon RS, Benditt DG, Cohen MI, Forman DE, Goldberger ZD et al. 2017 ACC/AHA/HRS Guideline for the Evaluation and Management of Patients With Syncope: A Report of the American College of Cardiology/American Heart Association Task Force on Clinical Practice Guidelines, and the Heart Rhythm Society. J Am Coll Cardiol. 2017.

25. Page RL, Joglar JA, Caldwell MA, Calkins H, Conti JB, Deal BJ, et al. 2015 ACC/AHA/HRS guideline for the Management of Adult Patients with Supraventricular Tachycardia: a report of the American College of Cardiology/American Heart Association task force on clinical practice guidelines and the Heart Rhythm Society. J Am Coll Cardiol. 2016;67:e27–e115.

26. Amsterdam EA, Wenger NK, Brindis RG, Casey DE Jr, Ganiats TG, Holmes DR Jr, et al. 2014 AHA/ACC guideline for the Management of Patients with

non-ST-elevation acute coronary syndromes: a report of the American College of Cardiology/American Heart Association task force on practice guidelines. J Am Coll Cardiol. 2014;64:e139–228.

27. January CT, Wann LS, Alpert JS, Calkins H, Cigarroa JE, Cleveland JC Jr, et al. 2014 AHA/ACC/HRS guideline for the management of patients with atrial fibrillation: a report of the American College of Cardiology/American Heart Association task force on practice guidelines and the Heart Rhythm Society. J Am Coll Cardiol. 2014;64:e1–76.

28. Jensen MD, Ryan DH, Apovian CM, Ard JD, Comuzzie AG, Donato KA, et al. 2013 AHA/ACC/TOS guideline for the management of overweight and obesity in adults: a report of the American College of Cardiology/American Heart Association task force on practice guidelines and the Obesity Society. J Am Coll Cardiol. 2014;63:2985–3023.

29. Eckel RH, Jakicic JM, Ard JD, de Jesus JM, Houston Miller N, Hubbard VS, et al. 2013 AHA/ACC guideline on lifestyle management to reduce cardiovascular risk: a report of the American College of Cardiology/American Heart Association task force on practice guidelines. J Am Coll Cardiol. 2014;63:2960–84.

30. Stone NJ, Robinson JG, Lichtenstein AH, Bairey Merz CN, Blum CB, Eckel RH, et al. 2013 ACC/AHA guideline on the treatment of blood cholesterol to reduce atherosclerotic cardiovascular risk in adults: a report of the American College of Cardiology/American Heart Association task force on practice guidelines. J Am Coll Cardiol. 2014;63:2889–934.

31. Goff DC Jr, Lloyd-Jones DM, Bennett G, Coady S, D'Agostino RB Sr, Gibbons R, et al. 2013 ACC/AHA guideline on the assessment of cardiovascular risk: a report of the American College of Cardiology/American Heart Association task force on practice guidelines. J Am Coll Cardiol. 2014;63:2935–59.

32. Epstein AE, JP DM, Ellenbogen KA, Estes NA 3rd, Freedman RA, Gettes LS, et al. ACC/AHA/HRS 2008 guidelines for device-based therapy of cardiac rhythm abnormalities: a report of the American College of Cardiology/American Heart Association task force on practice guidelines (writing committee to revise the ACC/AHA/NASPE 2002 guideline update for implantation of cardiac pacemakers and Antiarrhythmia devices) developed in collaboration with the American Association for Thoracic Surgery and Society of Thoracic Surgeons. J Am Coll Cardiol. 2008;51:e1–62.

33. Gersh BJ, Maron BJ, Bonow RO, Dearani JA, Fifer MA, Link MS, et al. 2011 ACCF/AHA guideline for the diagnosis and treatment of hypertrophic Cardiomyopathy: a report of the American College of Cardiology Foundation/American Heart Association task force on practice guidelines. Developed in collaboration with the American Association for Thoracic Surgery, American Society of Echocardiography, American Society of Nuclear Cardiology, Heart Failure Society of America, Heart Rhythm Society, Society for Cardiovascular Angiography and Interventions, and Society of Thoracic Surgeons. J Am Coll Cardiol. 2011, 58:e212–60.

34. Hillis LD, Smith PK, Anderson JL, Bittl JA, Bridges CR, Byrne JG et al. 2011 ACCF/AHA Guideline for Coronary Artery Bypass Graft Surgery. A report of the American College of Cardiology Foundation/American Heart Association Task Force on Practice Guidelines. Developed in collaboration with the American Association for Thoracic Surgery, Society of Cardiovascular Anesthesiologists, and Society of Thoracic Surgeons. J Am Coll Cardiol. 2011;58:e123-e210.

35. European Heart Rhythm A, Heart Rhythm S, Zipes DP, Camm AJ, Borggrefe M, Buxton AE, et al. ACC/AHA/ESC 2006 guidelines for management of patients with ventricular arrhythmias and the prevention of sudden cardiac death: a report of the American College of Cardiology/American Heart Association task force and the European Society of Cardiology Committee for practice guidelines (writing committee to develop guidelines for Management of Patients with Ventricular Arrhythmias and the prevention of sudden cardiac death). J Am Coll Cardiol. 2006;48:e247–346.

36. von Knobelsdorff-Brenkenhoff F, Bublak A, El-Mahmoud S, Wassmuth R, Opitz C, Schulz-Menger J. Single-centre survey of the application of cardiovascular magnetic resonance in clinical routine. Eur Heart J Cardiovasc Imaging. 2013;14:62–8.

37. Friedrich MG, Sechtem U, Schulz-Menger J, Holmvang G, Alakija P, Cooper LT, et al. Cardiovascular magnetic resonance in myocarditis: a JACC white paper. J Am Coll Cardiol. 2009;53:1475–87.

38. von Knobelsdorff-Brenkenhoff F, Schuler J, Doganguzel S, Dieringer MA, Rudolph A, Greiser A et al. Detection and Monitoring of Acute Myocarditis Applying Quantitative Cardiovascular Magnetic Resonance. Circ Cardiovasc Imaging. 2017;10.

39. Authors/Task Force M, Priori SG, Blomstrom-Lundqvist C, Mazzanti A, Blom N, Borggrefe M et al. 2015 ESC Guidelines for the management of patients with ventricular arrhythmias and the prevention of sudden cardiac death: The Task Force for the Management of Patients with Ventricular Arrhythmias and the Prevention of Sudden Cardiac Death of the European Society of Cardiology (ESC)Endorsed by: Association for European Paediatric and Congenital Cardiology (AEPC). Eur Heart J. 2015;36:2793-867.

40. Marrouche NF, Wilber D, Hindricks G, Jais P, Akoum N, Marchlinski F, et al. Association of atrial tissue fibrosis identified by delayed enhancement MRI and atrial fibrillation catheter ablation: the DECAAF study. JAMA. 2014;311:498–506.

9

Diagnostic performance of semi-quantitative and quantitative stress CMR perfusion analysis

R. van Dijk[1,3], M. van Assen[1], R. Vliegenthart[1,2], G. H. de Bock[4], P. van der Harst[3] and M. Oudkerk[1*]

Abstract

Background: Stress cardiovascular magnetic resonance (CMR) perfusion imaging is a promising modality for the evaluation of coronary artery disease (CAD) due to high spatial resolution and absence of radiation. Semi-quantitative and quantitative analysis of CMR perfusion are based on signal-intensity curves produced during the first-pass of gadolinium contrast. Multiple semi-quantitative and quantitative parameters have been introduced. Diagnostic performance of these parameters varies extensively among studies and standardized protocols are lacking. This study aims to determine the diagnostic accuracy of semi- quantitative and quantitative CMR perfusion parameters, compared to multiple reference standards.

Method: Pubmed, WebOfScience, and Embase were systematically searched using predefined criteria (3272 articles). A check for duplicates was performed (1967 articles). Eligibility and relevance of the articles was determined by two reviewers using pre-defined criteria. The primary data extraction was performed independently by two researchers with the use of a predefined template. Differences in extracted data were resolved by discussion between the two researchers. The quality of the included studies was assessed using the 'Quality Assessment of Diagnostic Accuracy Studies Tool' (QUADAS-2). True positives, false positives, true negatives, and false negatives were subtracted/calculated from the articles. The principal summary measures used to assess diagnostic accuracy were sensitivity, specificity, andarea under the receiver operating curve (AUC). Data was pooled according to analysis territory, reference standard and perfusion parameter.

Results: Twenty-two articles were eligible based on the predefined study eligibility criteria. The pooled diagnostic accuracy for segment-, territory- and patient-based analyses showed good diagnostic performance with sensitivity of 0. 88, 0.82, and 0.83, specificity of 0.72, 0.83, and 0.76 and AUC of 0.90, 0.84, and 0.87, respectively. In per territory analysis our results show similar diagnostic accuracy comparing anatomical (AUC 0.86(0.83–0.89)) and functional reference standards (AUC 0.88(0.84–0.90)). Only the per territory analysis sensitivity did not show significant heterogeneity. None of the groups showed signs of publication bias.

Conclusions: The clinical value of semi-quantitative and quantitative CMR perfusion analysis remains uncertain due to extensive inter-study heterogeneity and large differences in CMR perfusion acquisition protocols, reference standards, and methods of assessment of myocardial perfusion parameters. For wide spread implementation, standardization of CMR perfusion techniques is essential.

Keywords: Magnetic resonance imaging, Coronary artery disease, Myocardial perfusion imaging

* Correspondence: m.oudkerk@umcg.nl
[1]Center for Medical Imaging, University Medical Center Groningen, University of Groningen, Hanzeplein 1 EB 45, Groningen, The Netherlands
Full list of author information is available at the end of the article

Background

In recent years it has become apparent that information on the functional consequence of a stenosis in the coronary arteries is essential in prognostication and treatment of patients with coronary artery disease (CAD) [1–3]. Invasive coronary angiography is the current gold standard for the assessment of CAD according to the ESC guidelines [4, 5]. Fractional flow reserve (FFR) measurements are used to assess the functional significance by determining the pressure drop over an epicardial stenosis [6]. The disadvantage of invasive coronary angiography is that it is an invasive procedure, exposing patients to procedural risks and radiation [7–11]. In addition, in up to 60% of the patients undergoing invasive angiography, no significant stenosis is present suggesting that the pre-selection of patients for invasive coronary angiography can be improved [12].

A variety of noninvasive imaging modalities exists which show potential to be used in the (functional) assessment of patients suspected of CAD. These modalities include positron emission tomography (PET), cardiovascular magnetic resonance (CMR), computed tomography (CT), and single-photon emission computed tomography (SPECT). The different myocardial perfusion imaging (MPI) modalities all show a high diagnostic accuracy with an area under the curve (AUC) of 0.95 (0.91–0.99) for CMR perfusion imaging in general compared to 0.93 for PET, 0.93 for CT, and 0.82 for SPECT, respectively [13]. A disadvantage of MPI performed with either PET, SPECT or CT is the radiation exposure during the examination [11, 14].

MPI by stress CMR perfusion combines a high spatial resolution with the absence of radiation. These features make CMR perfusion an interesting modality for routine clinical assessment of CAD. The diagnostic accuracy of CMR perfusion imaging has been assessed in multiple studies and recent meta-analyses have provided extensive overviews of available evidence [13, 15–18], however these meta-analyses do not discriminate between qualitative and quantitative assessment. Currently, the visual assessment of perfusion defects is used in clinical practice [19].Visual assessment however, is subjective and highly dependent on expertise. However, analysis of the signal-intensity curves (SI-curves) that can be acquired during the first wash-in of the paramagnetic contrast agent gadolinium have potential to provide quantitative information on myocardial perfusion. These SI-curves to evaluate the myocardial blood flow (MBF) can be evaluated by semi-quantitative or quantitative methods [20]. The semi-quantitative method is based on the maximal upslope of the tissue attenuation curve (TAC) [21]. The quantitative method is based on model dependent deconvolution using the SI-curves. A variety of tracer kinetic models are used providing a MBF value related to the physiological MBF [22]. There are various proposed models for model dependent deconvolution with varying complexity. Both the semi-quantitative and quantitative parameters can be analyzed relatively as a ratio between values during stress and rest MPI or as absolute values. Although a large number of studies have been performed, meta-analysis of CMR perfusion available to date did not evaluate the diagnostic performance of these semi-quantitative and quantitative analysis of the SI-curves acquired during the first-pass perfusion.

Therefore, the aim of this meta-analysis was to assess the diagnostic accuracy of semi-quantitative or quantitative CMR perfusion imaging analysis based on SI time (SI-curves) as compared to either anatomical(quantitative coronary angiography (QCA)) or functional reference standards (invasive coronary angiography +/– FFR) in patients with suspected or known CAD.

Methods

Protocol and registration

This meta-analysis was performed in concordance with the Preferred Reporting Items for Systematic Reviews and Meta-analyses (PRISMA) statement and was registered at PROSPERO (http://www.crd.york.ac.uk/PROS-PERO/display_record.asp?ID=CRD42016040176) under registration number: 42016040176.

Eligibility criteria

To produce an extensive overview of the diagnostic accuracy of both semi-quantitative and quantitative CMR perfusion analysis, the following criteria to determine eligibility where used: study domain – patients with known or suspected CAD. Index test – quantitative or semi-quantitative CMR perfusion. Reference standard – invasive coronary angiography +/– FFR and QCA. Study results – diagnostic accuracy of index test compared to reference standard. Study design – observational. Overlap in study population between studies was corrected for by only including the study with the highest number of patients. Studies evaluating visual CMR perfusion outcome measures not based on time intensity curves, evaluation on a segmental basis, animal studies, phantom studies, and dose ranging studies were excluded from both the qualitative and quantitative analysis. Furthermore, reviews and overview documents were excluded from the quantitative analysis.

Search strategy

The following search strategy was used in Pubmed: ("Myocardial Ischemia"[Mesh] OR myocardial OR cardiac OR "coronary artery") AND ("Magnetic Resonance Imaging"[Mesh] OR Magnetic Resonance[tiab] OR mri[tiab] OR MRP[tiab]) AND ("Perfusion Imaging"[Mesh] OR perfusion[tiab]) AND (Quantification*[tiab] OR quantitative[-tiab] OR deconvolut*[tiab] OR myocardial perfusion reserve[tiab] OR mpr[tiab] OR semiquantitative [tiab] OR semiquantitative [tiab] OR semiquantitative OR MPRI

[tiab] OR myocardial blood flow [tiab] OR MBF [tiab] OR contrast enhancement ratio [tiab] OR left ventricular up-slope [tiab] OR upslope integral [tiab] OR CER [tiab] OR SLP [tiab] OR INT [tiab]). Additionally, Embase and Web of Science were searched using adjusted search strategy to fit the search matrix of the source.

Study selection
The search strategy was set-up in collaboration with the local Medical Library (Central Medical Library University Medical Center Groningen). One researcher (RvD) executed the search and gathered the results in Mendeley (version 1.16.1). A check for duplicates was performed with both the built in 'check for duplicates' function as well as manually (RvD). Screening for study eligibility and relevance of the articles retrieved by the search strategy was performed individually by two reviewers (RvD and MvA) using the pre-defined study eligibility criteria. Studies were categorized as includable, possibly includable, non-includable by screening the titles and abstracts. Inter-reviewer categorization was compared and in case of disagreement discussed to obtain consensus.

Data collection process
The primary data extraction was performed independently by both researchers (RvD and MvA) with the use of a predefined template. Data extraction was cross checked and discussed to achieve consensus. In case of missing or unclear data the corresponding authors were contacted ($n = 12$), in absence of a response the studies were excluded.

Data items
The following patient characteristics were collected: age, gender, prevalence of CAD, and coronary artery disease risk factors. Data on study design was collected, including: prospective/retrospective set up, number of patients enrolled, number of patients excluded, scanner type and manufacturer, stressor agent and dose, contrast agent, perfusion sequence, cardiac segmentation method, reference standard, outcome measures with reported sensitivity, specificity, negative predictive value, positive predictive. The number of true positives (TP), false positives (FP), true negatives (TN), and false negatives (FN) were derived directly from the article or calculated from the sensitivity and specificity reported in the articles. All the figures and tables in this article are original for this article.

Quality assessment
Two reviewers (RvD and MvA) independently evaluated the study quality of the included studies using the 'Quality Assessment of Diagnostic Accuracy Studies Tool' (QUADAS-2) [23]. Risk of bias was assessed across all

studies and within each individual study using RevMan software (version 5.3.5, Cochrane collaboration).

Statistical analysis
The principal summary measures used to assess diagnostic accuracy were sensitivity, specificity, Diagnostic Odds Ratio (DOR), and AUC. In case studies performed multiple semi-quantitative or quantitative analyses we chose the maximal upslope parameter as a representative measure for semi-quantitative analysis and absolute MBF for quantitative analysis. Furthermore, transmural ratios were used when studies reported sub-endocardial, sub-epicardial, and transmural outcomes. When multiple tracer kinetic models were used for quantitative analysis, the Fermi model was selected. When both a semi-quantitative and a quantitative outcome, or both 1.5 T as well as 3.0 T were used, both outcomes were taken into account for the analysis.

The primary data synthesis was based on bivariate mixed-effects binary regression modeling. Sensitivity, specificity, and heterogeneity (using the Q-statistic and I^2 index) were calculated and displayed in forest plots. Significant heterogeneity was defined as Q-statistic $p < 0.10$ and/or $I^2 > 50\%$. Separate subgroup forest plots were evaluated when >5 studies were available.

The Deeks' funnel test was used to test for publication bias, with a value <0.05 indicative of publication bias or systematic difference between results of larger and smaller studies. The DORs were used to calculate the summary receiver operating curves (sROC). Based on the ROC curves the AUC was calculated. Data analysis was performed with STATA (version 13.0; STATA corporation, Lakeway Drive, College Station, Texas, USA).

Results
The systematic search in Pubmed, WebOfScience, and Embase identified 3272 articles. After the removal of duplicates, 1967 articles were screened based on title and abstract. The resulting 137 articles were assessed in full text for eligibility. Of these, 23 articles were deemed eligible based on the predefined study eligibility criteria including a total of patients, with mean age ranging from 57 to 67 years. The PRISMA flowchart is shown in Fig. 1. The final analysis included 22 articles due to exclusion of one study using dobutamine as a stressor agent in which an inadequate heart rate response for diagnosis was achieved in most age groups.

Studies were performed at 1.5 T in 20 (91%) studies and at 3 T in 6 (27%) studies (Bernhardt et al. used both 1.5 T as well as 3.0 T). The stressor agent used was either adenosine or dipyridamole in 18 (82%) and 6 (27%), studies, respectively. Segment based outcome data was available in 4 (18%) of all studies, territory based outcome data was available in 13 (59%) and patient based outcome data in

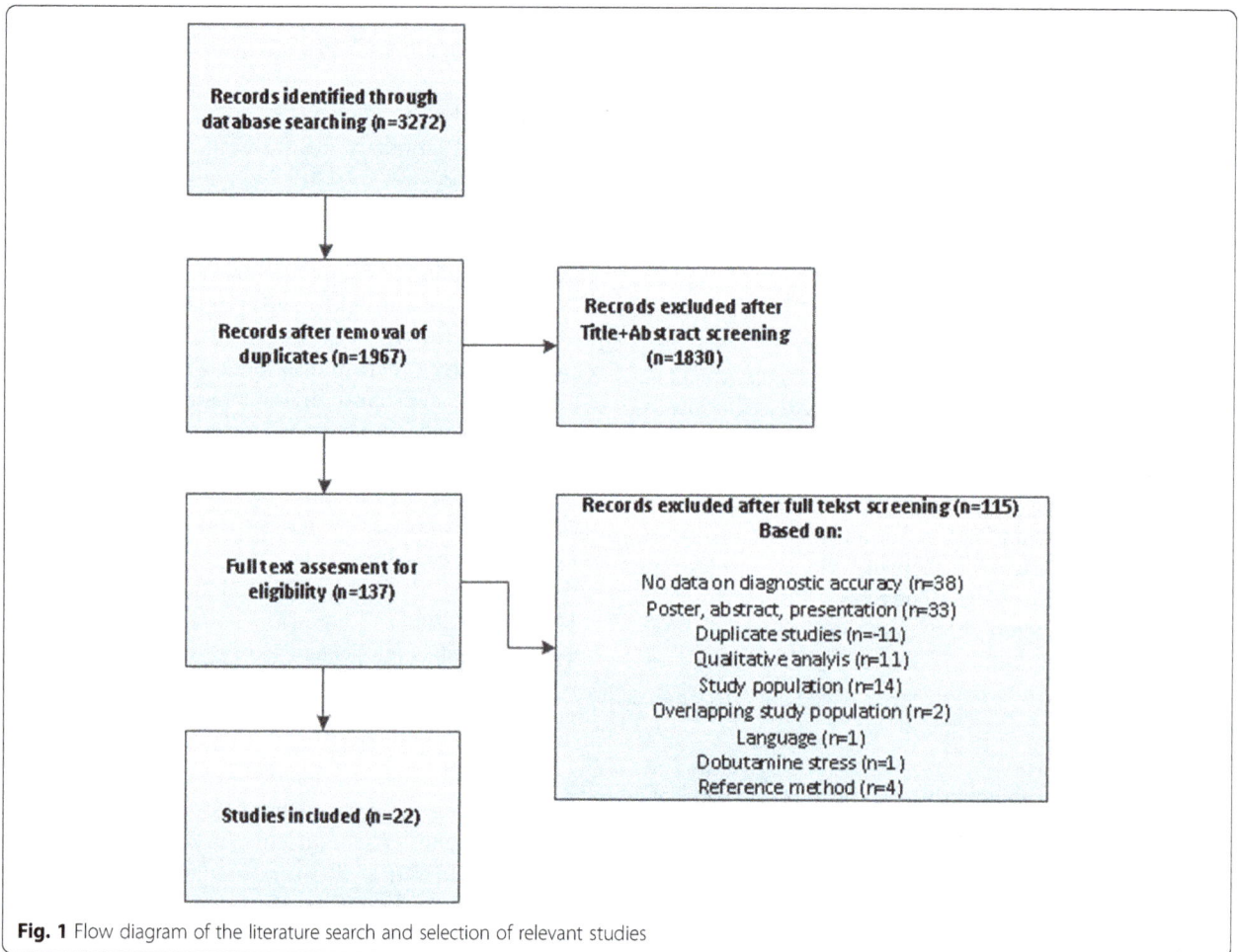

Fig. 1 Flow diagram of the literature search and selection of relevant studies

11 (50%) studies included (Bertschinger et al. and Papanastasiou et al. reported both territory and patient based data). Perfusion analysis was performed semi-quantitative in 16 (73%) studies and quantitative in 10 (45%) (Huber et al. and Mordini et al. reported data on both semi-quantitative and quantitative analysis). The reference standard was anatomical in 15 (68%) studies and functional in 11 (50%). See Tables 1, 2 and 3.

Diagnostic performance

Four studies with per segment-based analysis could be included, all using an anatomical reference method (QCA). Segment-based pooled sensitivity, specificity, and DOR were 0.88 (95% CI, 0.82–0.93), 0.72 (95%CI, 0.56–0.84), and 19 (95% CI, 9–40), respectively. ROC curve analysis showed an AUC of 0.90 (95% CI, 0.87–0.92). See Table 4 and Figs. 2 and 3.

Eleven studies were included analyzing the perfusion data on a per territory basis with Huber et al. [24] reporting on both semi-quantitative and quantitative analysis, including twelve study outcomes in the final per territory analysis. Territory-based pooled sensitivity, specificity, and DOR were 0.82 (95% CI, 0.77–0.86), 0.83

(95% CI, 0.74–0.90), and 21 (95% CI, 10–45), respectively. ROC curve analysis showed an AUC of 0.84 (95% CI, 0.81–0.87). See Table 4 and Figs. 4 and 5. Quantitative analysis (n = 6) on a per territory base yielded a sensitivity, specificity, and DOR of 0.77 (95% CI, 0.62–0.87), 0.86 (95% CI, 0.72–0.94), and 21 (95% CI, 6–8) with an AUC of 0.88 (95% CI, 0.85–0.91), while semi-quantitative analysis (n = 6) yielded a sensitivity and specificity of 0.77 (95% CI, 0.60–0.88) and 0.84 (95% CI, 0.76–0.89) with an AUC of 0.87 (95% CI, 0.84–0.90). Using a functional reference (n = 7) standard yielded a sensitivity, specificity, and DOR of 0.77 (95% CI, 0.63–0.86), 0.85 (95% CI, 0.73–0.92), and 18 (95% CI, 6–59) with an AUC of 0.88 (95% CI, 0.84–0.90), while the use of an anatomical reference (n = 5) showed sensitivity, specificity, and DOR of 0.85 (95% CI 0.78–0.90), 0.83 (95% CI, 0.72–0.91), and 28 (95% CI, 13–63) with an AUC of 0.86 (95% CI, 0.83–0.89).

Eight studies were included analyzing the CMR perfusion data on a per patient basis, of which Mordini et al. [20] reported on both semi-quantitative and quantitative outcome and Bernhardt et al. [25] performed analysis at both 1.5 T and 3.0 T, in the end including ten study outcomes in the final per patient analysis. Six had

Table 1 Overview of patient demographics for all included studies

Study	No. Patients	Male	Age[a]	HT (%)	DM (%)	smoking	Hypercholesterolemia (%)	History of PCI/ CABG (5)	prevalence of CAD %	Previous MI (%)
Al-Saadi 2000 [27]	34	32	59+/−11	NS	NS	NS	NS	NS	100	NS
Bertschinger 2001 [28]	14	NS	NS	NS	NS	NS	NS	NS	93	NS
Ibrahim 2002 [29]	25	19	63+/−13	NS	28	NS	68	56	100	12
Nagel 2003 [30]	84	73	63+/−8	0	0	21	NS	NS	51	0
Giang 2004 [31]	29	25	58+/−8	45	14	34	59	52	66	38
Plein 2005 [32]	92	68	58+/−11	30	8	35	54	NS	64	19
Rieber 2006 [33]	43	38	66+/−8	86	23	35	NS	28	67	19
Positano 2006 [34]	32	20	65+/−10	NS	NS	NS	NS	NS	50	NS
Costa 2007 [35]	37	16	65+/−11	80	23	20	57	NS	97	NS
Pignitore 2008 [36]	125	51 / 14	62+/−7 / 60+/−5	73 / 78	27 / 26	51 / 59	70 / 66	NS	71	NS
KrittayaPhong 2009 [37]	66	38	61+/−12	62	27	8	62	Exclusion criterium	58	Exclusion criterium
Kirschbaum 2011 [38]	40	27	62+/−7	49	15	29	41	NS	34	NS
Lockie 2011 [39]	42	33	57+/−10	NS	19	21	Exclusion criterium	19	NS	Exclusion criterium
Bernhardt 2012 [25]	34	26	62+/−11	80	15	47	53	NS	62	NS
Huber 2012 [24]	23	27	67+/−12	36	23	85	29	NS	55	19
Motwani 2012 [40]	40	27	64+/−8	NS	NS	NS	NS	NS	53	NS
Chiribiri 2013 [41]	30	22	59+/−11	NS	27	27	NS	NS	80	NS
Mordini 2014 [20]	67	45	60+/−11	60	16	42	75	25	34	25
Motwani 2014 [42]	35	26	62+/−8	51	17	40	54	9	57	9
Yun 2015 [43]	58	17	60+/−11	59	26	28	48	10	31	16
Pan 2015 [44]	71	57	60+/−6	8	31	61	62	9	55	NS
Papanastasiou 2016 [45]	24	20	63 ± 7	13	3	6	NS	4	67	7

[a]Age either mean+/−SD or mean(range). *HT* hypertension, *DM* diabetes mellitus, *PCI* percutaneous coronary intervention, *CABG* coronary artery bypass graft, *CAD* Coronary Artery Disease, *MI* myocardial infarct

an anatomical reference standard and 4 a functional reference standard. Patient based sensitivity, specificity, and DOR were 0.83 (95% CI, 0.75–0.88), 0.76 (95% CI, 0.65–0.85), and 15 (95%CI 6–36). ROC curve analysis showed an AUC of 0.87 (95% CI, 0.84–0.90). See Table 4 and Figs. 6 and 7.

Diagnostic accuracy in patients with decreased left ventricular ejection fraction or multi-vessel disease

The study of Krittayaphong et al. reported on the diagnostic accuracy of MPRI in patients with decreased left ventricular ejection fraction (LVEF). They report a decreased sensitivity, specificity and diagnostic accuracy in the subgroup of patients with decreased LVEF (sensitivity 88.9%, specificity 58.3% and diagnostic accuracy 71.5) as compared to patients with normal LVEF (sensitivity 89.7%, specificity 93.8% and diagnostic accuracy 91.1). Mordini et al. report that all their patients with multivessel disease (*n* = 7) were correctly identified with quantitative perfusion analysis. Giang et al. present a similar sensitivity and specificity whether patients with three vessel disease were included or not across all tested doses (e.g. 94/71% sensitivity/specificity when patients with three vessel disease included at dose 3 compared to a 91%/71% sensitivity/specificity when patients with three vessel disease excluded).

Table 2 Overview of the study specific acquisition protocol

Study	Scanner	Protocol	Stressor agent	Contrast agent	Contrast dosage	Perfusion sequence
Al-Saadi 2000 [27]	1.5 T, Philips	Rest/stress	Dipyridamole	Gadopentate (Magnevist)	0.025 mmol/kg	T1-weighted inversion recovery single-shot turbo gradient echo
Bertschinger 2001 [28]	1.5 T, G.E.	Stress only	Dipyridamole	Gadodiamide (Omniscan)	NS	interleaved gradient-echo EPI
Ibrahim 2002 [29]	1.5 T, Phillips	Rest/stress	Adenosine	Gadopentate (Magnevist)	0.05 mmol/l	A fast hybrid, gated-imaging sequence consisting of three short-axis slices was used
Nagel 2003 [30]	1.5 T, Philips	Rest/stress	Adenosine	Diethylenetriaminepentaacetic acid-gadolinium	0.025 mmol/kg	single shot segmented k-space turbo-gradient-echo/echo-planar-imaging (EPI)-hybrid
Giang 2004 [31]	1.5 T, G.E.	Stress only	Adenosine	Gadopentate (Magnevist)	0.05 mmol/kg	hybrid echo planar
Plein 2005 [32]	1.5 T, Philips	Rest/stress	Adenosine	Gadopentate (Magnevist)	0.05 mmol/kg	dynamic segmented k-space gradient-echo combined with SENSE
Rieber 2006 [33]	1.5 T, Siemens	Stress/rest	Adenosine	Gadodiamide (Omniscan)	0.05 mmol/kg	T1-weighted saturation recovery turbo flash
Positano 2006 [34]	1.5 G.E.	Rest/stress	Dipyridamole	Gadodiamide (Omniscan)	0.1 mmol/kg	fast gradient-echo train
Costa 2007 [35]	1.5 Siemens	Stress/rest	Adenosine	Gadolinium (Magnevist)	0.1 mmol/kg	single-shot gradient-echo
Pignitore 2008 [36]	1.5 G.E.	Rest/stress	Dipyridamole	Gadodiamide (Omniscan)	0.1 mmol/kg	fast gradient-echo train
KrittayaPhong 2009 [37]	1.5 T, Phillips	Stress/rest	adenosine	Gadopentate (Magnevist)	0.05 mmol/l	ECG-triggered, T1 weighted, inversion receovery single shot turbo gradient echo sequence
Kirschbaum 2011 [38]	1.5 T, GE Medical Systems	Rest/stress	adenosine	Gadopentate (Magnevist)	0.05 mmol/kg	steady state free-precession technique
Lockie 2011 [39]	3.0 T, Philips	Stress/rest	Adenosine	Gadopentate (Magnevist)	0.05 mmol/kg	saturation recovery gradient echo method
Bernhardt 2012 [25]	1.5 T/ 3.0 T, Philips	Stress/rest	Adenosine	Gadoterate meglumine (Dotarem)	0.075 mmol/kg	steady state free-precession technique
Huber 2012 [24]	1.5 T, Siemens	NS	Adenosine	Gadopentate (Magnevist)	0.05 mmol/kg	saturation turboFlash
Motwani 2012 [40]	3.0 Phillips	Stress/rest	Adenosine	Gadopentate (Magnevist)	0.05 mmol/kg	Saturation-recovery gradient echo
Chiribiri 2013 [41]	3.0 T, Philips	Stress/rest	Adenosine	Gadopentate (Magnevist)	0.05 mmol/kg	saturation-recovery gradient echo
Mordini 2014 [20]	1.5 T, Siemens	Stress/rest	Dipyridamole	Gadopentate (Magnevist)	0.005 mmol/kg followed by 0.1 mmol/kg	saturation recovery hybrid echo-planar
Motwani 2014 [42]	3.0 T, Philips	Stress/rest	Adenosine	Gadobutrol (Gadovist)	0.075 mmol/kg	3D spoiled turbo gradient-echo
Yun 2015 [43]	3.0 T, Philips	Stress/rest	Dipyridamole	Gadobenate Dimeglumine (Multihance)	0.05 mmol/kg	saturation recovery gradient-echo T1-weighted
Pan 2015 [44]	3.0 T, Siemens	Stress/rest	Adenosine	Gadobutrol (Gadovist)	0.075 mmol/kg	T1-weighted saturation recovery turbo flash
Papanastasiou 2016 [45]	3.0 T, Siemens	Stress/rest	Adenosine	Gadobutrol (Gadovist)	0.05 mmol/kg	Turbo-fast low saturation recovery single-shot gradient echo

Study quality assessment and publication bias

The overall methodological quality of the studies was good See Figs. 10 and 11. The per territory analysis pooled sensitivity, per territory anatomical reference standard sensitivity and per territory semi-quantitative specificity did not show significant heterogeneity See Figs. 2, 4, 6 and Table 4. The Deeks' Funnel plots did not indicate publication bias or systematic difference between results of larger and smaller studies See Figs. 8 and 9.

Table 3 Overview of study specific cardiac segmentation method, data interpretation, reference standard, cut-off values for significant stenosis and semi-quantitative and/or quantitative analysis

Study	Segmentation	Data interpretation	Reference standard	Cut-off values	Outcome variables
Al-Saadi 2000 [27]	6 segments (mid ventricular)	Territory	QCA	≥75% DS	Semi-quantitative
Bertschinger 2001 [28]	4 × 8 segments	Patient/ Territory	QCA	≥50% stenosis	Semi-quantitative
Ibrahim 2002 [29]	3 short axis slices 18 segments per slice/polar maps subdivided into 6 segments	Territory	QCA	>75% DS	Semi-quantitative
Nagel 2003 [30]	5 short axis slices 6 segments per slice	Patient	Visual ICA	≥75% DS	Quantitative
Giang 2004 [31]	3 × 8 segments good quality score	Patient	QCA	≥50% DS	Semi-quantitative
Plein 2005 [32]	16 segments (AHA)	Patient	Visual ICA	>70% DS	Quantitative
Rieber 2006 [33]	16 segments (AHA)	Territory	QCA + FFR	>50% DS on QCA and FFR ≤0.75	Semi-quantitative
Positano 2006 [34]	3 short axis slices 16 segments	Segment	QCA	≥75% DS	Semi-quantitative
Costa 2007 [35]	3 short axis 8 segments per slice	Segment	QCA	>70% DS	Quantitaive
Pignitore 2008 [36]	3 short axis slices 16 segments	Segment	QCA	≥50% DS	Semi-quantitative
KrittayaPhong 2009 [37]	16 segments (AHA)	Patient	Visual ICA	≥50%	Semi-quantitative
Kirschbaum 2011 [38]	16 segments (AHA)	Patient	ICA with CFR	CFR < 2.0	Semi-quantitative
Lockie 2011 [39]	16 segments (AHA)	Territory	FFR	<0.75	Quantitative
Bernhardt 2012 [25]	16 segments (AHA)	Patient	FFR	≤0.80	Semi-quantitative
Huber 2012 [24]	18 segments (6 per slice)	Territory	QCA + FFR	>75% DS on QCA or 51 - 75% DS on QCA + FFR <0.75	Semi-quantitative/ Quantitative
Motwani 2012 [40]	1 midventricular slice 6 segments	Segment	QCA	>70% DS	Quantitative
Chiribiri 2013 [41]	16 segments (AHA)	Territory	FFR	<0.80	Quantitative
Mordini 2014 [20]	3 short axis slices 12 segments per slice	Patient	QCA	>70% DS	Semi-quantitative/ Quantitative
Motwani 2014 [42]	Whole heart	Territory	QCA	≥75% DS	Quantitative
Yun 2015 [43]	16 segments (AHA)	Territory	QCA	>70% DS	Semi-quantitative
Pan 2015 [44]	16 segments (AHA) (mean of 2 lowest value assigned to coronary territories)	Territory	FFR	≤0.75	Quantitative
Papanastasiou 2016 [45]	16 segments (AHA)	Patient/ Territory	ICA + FFR	≥70% DS on ICA or FFR <0.80 and luminal stenosis ≥50%	Quantitative

Discussion

Summary of evidence

The pooled diagnostic accuracy for segment-, territory- and patient-based analyses showed good diagnostic performance. The diagnostic accuracy of CMR perfusion analysis has been assessed in previous meta-analyses [13, 15–18].

However, this meta-analysis is the first focusing on the semi-quantitative and quantitative analysis of the SI-curves. The diagnostic accuracy of CMR perfusion (pooled for visual, semi-quantitative, and quantitative analysis) reported in the earlier meta-analyses range from AUC 0.90 to 0.94 [13, 15–18]. When comparing our results, the SI-curve based

Table 4 Pooled diagnostic accuracy of semi-quantitative and quantitative CMR perfusion analysis on segmental, territory, and per patient basis (bold) and subgroup analysis of anatomical/functional reference standard or semi-quantitative/quantitative analysis (unbold)

	No. Studies	No. S/T/P	Sensitivity	Q-statistics p-value[a]	I[2b]	Specificity	Q-statistics p-value[a]	I[2b]	PLR	NLR	DOR	AUC
Per Segment	4	3838	**0.88 (0.82–0.93)**	**0.00**	**82.04**	**0.72 (0.56–0.84)**	**0.00**	**96.23**	**3.1 (1.0–5.10)**	**0.16 (0.10–0.26)**	**19 (9–40)**	**0.90 (0.870.92)**
Per territory	12	1058	**0.82 (0.77–0.86)**	**0.49**	**0.00**	**0.83 (0.74–0.90)**	**0.00**	**90.68**	**5.0 (3.1–7.9)**	**0.22 (0.17–0.29)**	**23 (12–44)**	**0.84 (0.81–0.87)**
Anatomical reference	5	370	0.85 (0.78–0.90)	0.49	0.00	0.83 (0.72–0.91)	0.00	78.11	5.1 (2.9–9.2)	0.18 (0.12–0.27)	28 (13–63)	0.86 (0.83–0.89)
Functional reference	7	688	0.77 (0.63–0.86)	0.00	86.70	0.85 (0.73–0.92)	0.00	93.19	5.1 (2.5–10.3)	0.28 (0.16–0.48)	18 (6–59)	0.88 (0.84–0.90)
Semi-quantitative	6	343	0.77 (0.60–0.88)	0.00	86.96	0.84 (0.76–0.89)	0.30	17.10	4.7 (2.9–7.8)	0.28 (0.15–0.53)	17 (6–50)	0.87 (0.84–0.90)
Quantitative	6	729	0.77 (0.62–0.87)	0.00	89.39	0.86 (0.72–0.94)	0.00	94.92	5.5 (2.4–12.6)	0.27 (0.14–0.49)	21 (6–8)	0.88 (0.85–0.91)
Per patient	10	566	**0.83 (0.75–0.88)**	**0.01**	**60.71**	**0.76 (0.65–0.85)**	**0.00**	**66.27**	**3.5 (2.2–5.5)**	**0.23 (0.14–0.36)**	**15 (6–36)**	**0.87 (0.84–0.90)**

[a]Q statistic p-value <0.10 and/or [b]I[2] > 50% is considered to indicate heterogeneity. Subgroup analysis was performed when ≥5 studies were available

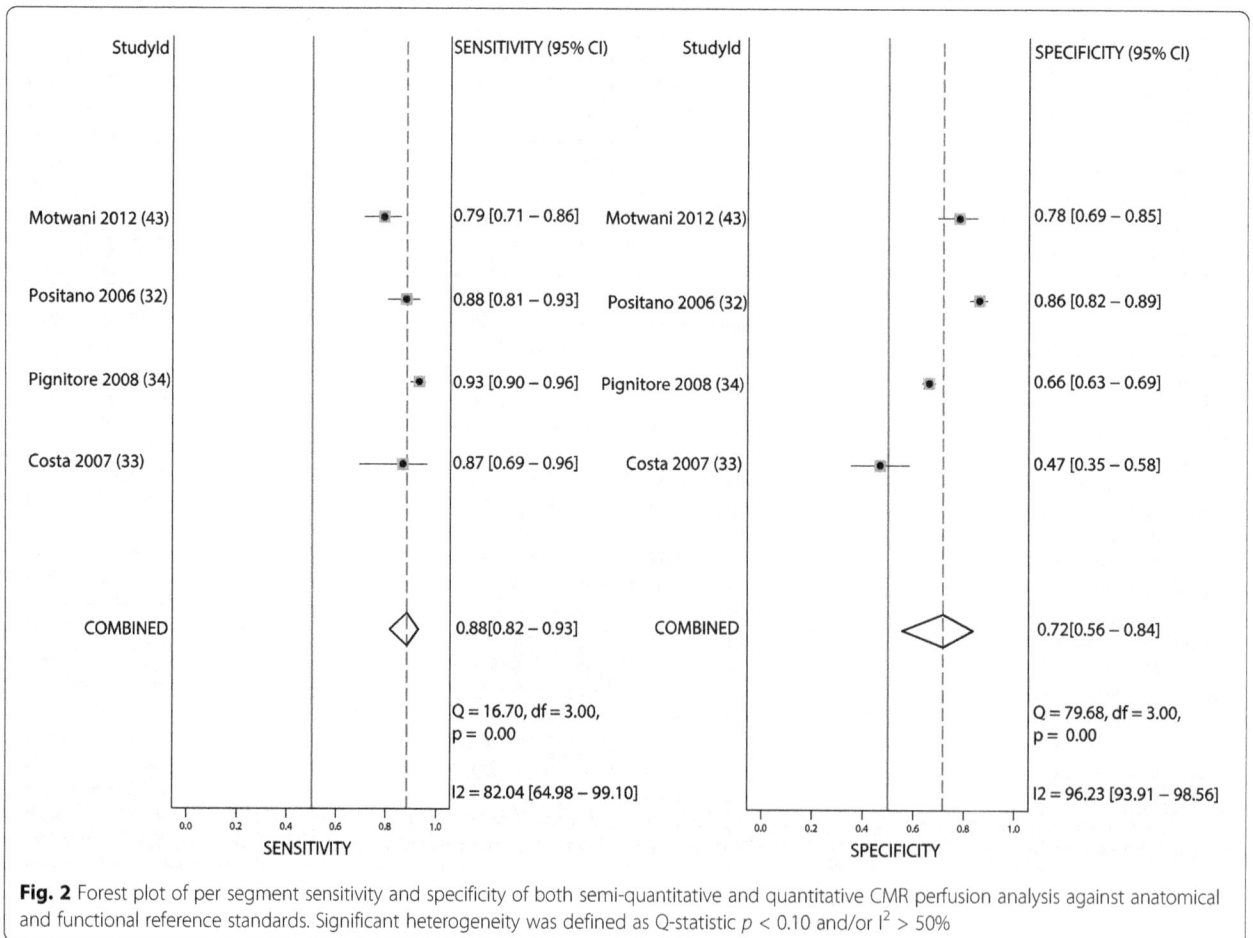

Fig. 2 Forest plot of per segment sensitivity and specificity of both semi-quantitative and quantitative CMR perfusion analysis against anatomical and functional reference standards. Significant heterogeneity was defined as Q-statistic p < 0.10 and/or I[2] > 50%

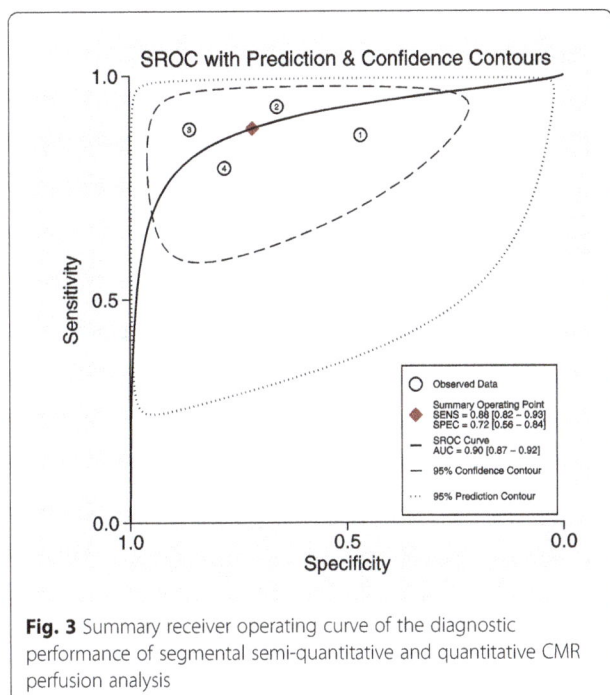

Fig. 3 Summary receiver operating curve of the diagnostic performance of segmental semi-quantitative and quantitative CMR perfusion analysis

analysis of CMR perfusion does not lead to an increase in the diagnostic accuracy as compared to the combined diagnostic accuracy of CMR perfusion as reported in these previous papers. Visual analysis of CMR perfusion does not yield lower diagnostic accuracy. This is possibly due to the fact that visual observations are made upon fewer and less complex assumptions than both the semi-quantitative and quantitative analysis methods that are used. Both semi-quantitative and quantitative perfusion analysis are based on SI-curves and calculate a derivative of myocardial blood flow based on certain assumptions. The models used for quantitative analysis are mathematical representations of a physiological process and rely on assumptions made about the dynamic of contrast and blood plasma and pre-existing knowledge about the physiologic process and model dynamics. In these models it is assumed that there is no diffusion of contrast medium into the intracellular space. Unfortunately, only in a few specific contrast agents this is the case. Different models are used for CMR perfusion analysis, with different degrees of complexity, and the optimal model is yet to be determined. The complexity of this modeling process, the many assumptions made and thereby the selection of a suitable model makes model-dependent perfusion analysis highly susceptible to error and with inconsistent results as a consequence. The use of different models with varying results could add to the heterogeneity in the quantitative analysis group. Semi-quantitative analysis, although in theory inferior to quantitative analysis, is a relatively simple method to estimate perfusion. The low complexity of these methods make it a robust method,

allowing for less variation among research groups. As visual CMR perfusion analysis is relatively simple as compared to either semi-quantitative and/or quantitative CMR perfusion analysis, it is possible that this method is less susceptible to methodological errors (causing false conclusions). However, the methods used for assessing semi-quantitative CMR perfusion also vary within studies. The large variation in both semi-quantitative and quantitative CMR perfusion post processing techniques make it challenging to make an accurate comparison due to extensive inter-study heterogeneity. We compared the diagnostic accuracy of semi-quantitative and quantitative CMR perfusion analysis on a per territory basis and observed that the diagnostic accuracy slightly decreased using quantitative analysis (AUC of 0.87(0.83–0.89) compared to 0.81(0.78–0.85)). This is possibly due to the fact that quantitative analysis is based on multiple assumptions.

If the noninvasive MPI techniques are to be used as a gatekeeper for further diagnosis and treatment it is important to select a modality in which the amount of false negative results is low to assure that patients with significant disease are not missed. This requires the sensitivity of the gatekeeper test to be high. We were also performed subgroup analyses in the per territory group, based on the reference standards used. The anatomical reference standards merely depict the presence or absence of epicardial coronary stenosis (visual invasive coronary angiography, QCA), whereas the functional reference standards contained functional information on either pressure drop across the stenosis (FFR).

Our results show similar diagnostic accuracy when anatomical reference standards were used (0.85(0.82–0.88)) as compared to the diagnostic accuracy of SI-curve analysis with the use of functional reference standards (0.82(0.79–0.86)) in the per territory analysis.

For the anatomical reference standard, a DS >50, >70% or >75% were generally used as the cut-off value for significant CAD in both QCA and visual angiographic assessment. For the functional reference standard, a FFR of either <0.75 or <0.8 were used to indicate significant CAD. The accuracy of the anatomical reference standards as well as the currently used gold standard for functional reference of invasive coronary angiography +/− FFR for determining flow limiting CAD are debatable. Furthermore, pooling of the different threshold also increases heterogeneity in this meta-analysis. Previous research has shown that the anatomical presence of a stenosis, with cut-off values of either >50% DS or >70% DS have a poor correlation with FFR [1]. The use of the functional FFR measurement to guide therapy has proven to be superior as compared to anatomical assessment alone [2]. The FFR measurement is based on the measurement of a pressure drop across an epicardial vessel pre- and post-stenosis and a value of either <0.75

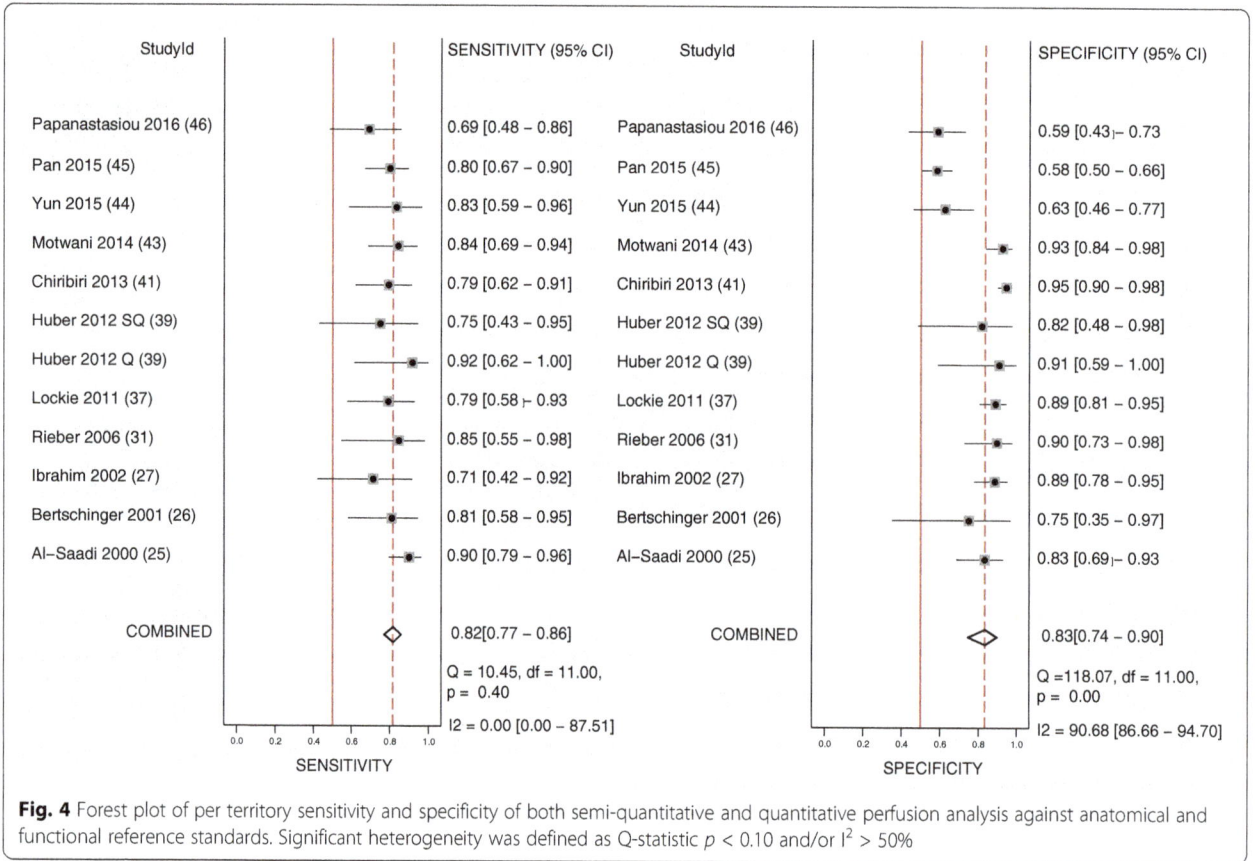

Fig. 4 Forest plot of per territory sensitivity and specificity of both semi-quantitative and quantitative perfusion analysis against anatomical and functional reference standards. Significant heterogeneity was defined as Q-statistic $p < 0.10$ and/or $I^2 > 50\%$

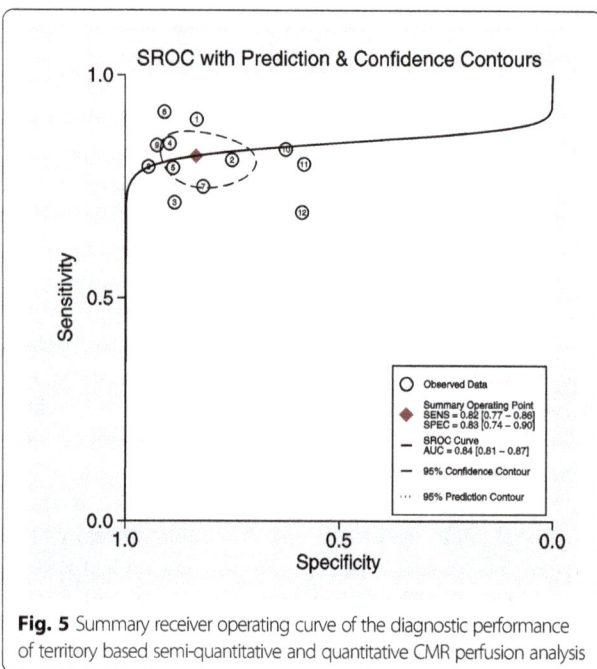

Fig. 5 Summary receiver operating curve of the diagnostic performance of territory based semi-quantitative and quantitative CMR perfusion analysis

or a more liberal cut-off of <0.8 is used to indicate a functionally significant epicardial stenosis. However, what both the anatomical reference standard and the functional FFR measurement ignore microvasculature perfusion defects and the assumptions of a linear relationship between increasing stenosis or decreasing pressure with decreasing flow is made. To better understand the myocardial perfusion, van de Hoef et al. aimed to determine the relationship between invasively measured FFR and coronary flow reserve. The results of this study indicate a non-linear relationship between FFR (pressure drop information) and coronary flow reserve (flow information). The authors conclude that the disagreement between FFR and coronary flow reserve is caused by the involvement of the microvasculature and this indicates that the functional FFR measurement is not an accurate representation of myocardial perfusion [26]. We believe that there is a trend towards a better understanding of the complex process of myocardial perfusion and that the currently used reference standard as of yet fail to accurately represent myocardial perfusion. The need for a well validated and robust measurement technique for measuring myocardial perfusion is necessary and this technique might be used in the

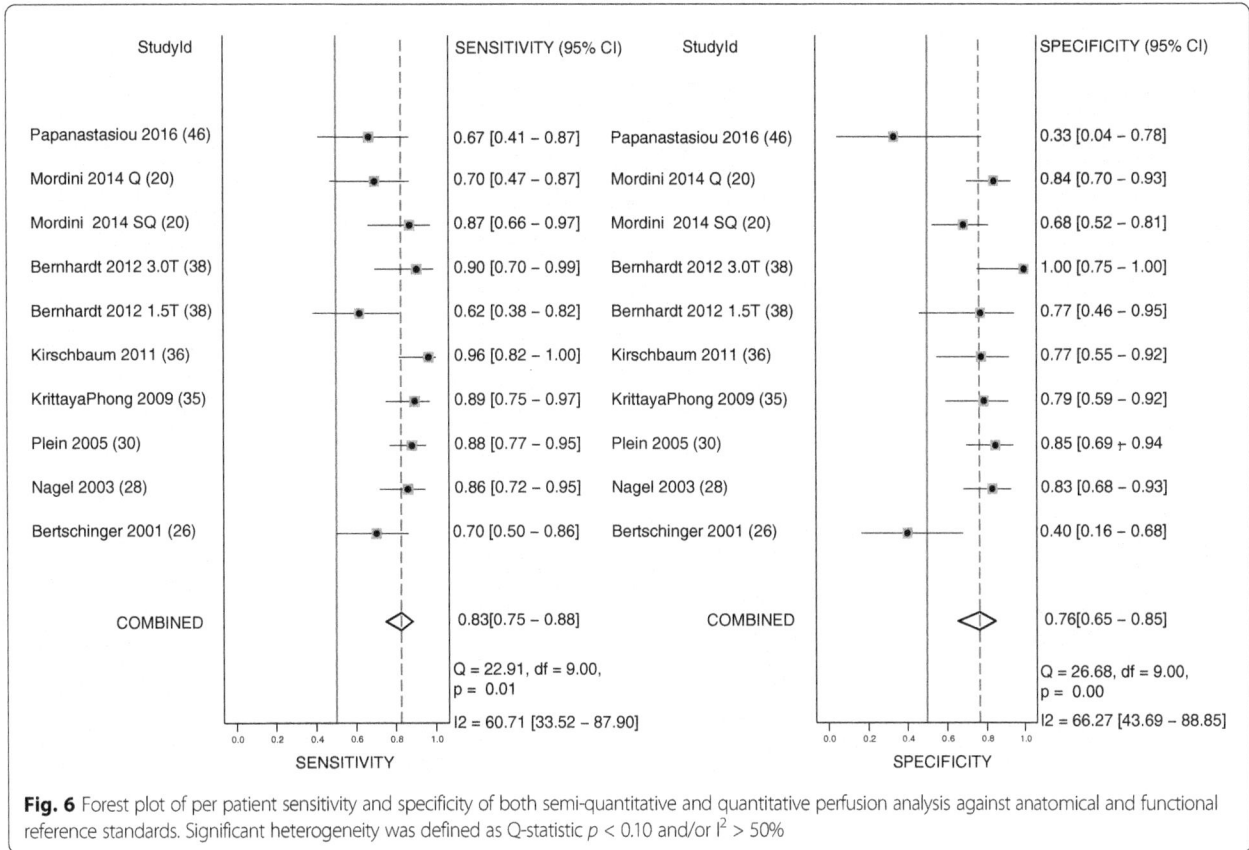

Fig. 6 Forest plot of per patient sensitivity and specificity of both semi-quantitative and quantitative perfusion analysis against anatomical and functional reference standards. Significant heterogeneity was defined as Q-statistic p < 0.10 and/or I² > 50%

future as the gold standard. The inability of both the anatomical and functional reference standards to accurately represent myocardial blood flow might have influenced the results and so the results of this meta-analysis should be interpreted with caution.

Further research is necessary to determine the ideal golden standard for myocardial perfusion. We emphasize that it might be beneficial to first critically review phantom or ex-vivo research regarding the determination of myocardial perfusion in search for the measurement which represents true myocardial blood flow as accurately as possible.

In our meta-analysis we found an extensive variation in study population, CMR protocols, post processing techniques, and reference standards used. The lack of standardized CMR perfusion protocols or post processing techniques might have influenced our estimates of a lower diagnostic accuracy than expected of semi-quantitative and quantitative CMR perfusion analysis as compared to visual assessment. The extensive heterogeneity between the study protocols should be taken into account in the interpretation of these results. Standardization of the analysis protocols is needed to make more generalizable recommendations.

Future research should focus on the construction of a quantitative model that accurately depicts physiological myocardial blood flow. The different quantitative models should be compared and validated within a well-structured standardized CMR perfusion protocol preferably against a well validated perfusion method to determine which of the models accurately describes the perfusion process. Specific cut-off values to distinguish between normal and ischemic myocardium should be determined, and CMR protocols should be calibrated between the different CMR scanners. Visual CMR perfusion analysis alone is already highly accurate in the assessment of significant CAD and might also benefit from standardization of CMR protocols. The included studies reported results per segment, vessel territory or per patient. In this study we chose to include all three groups and report the results separately. However, it should be noted that a per segment based analysis holds more anatomical value since CAD often involves only specific coronary branches and not an entire vessel, affecting an entire vessel territory. This could have resulted in a lower diagnostic accuracy for the territory based results. The per territory analysis however, has a high clinical value since intervention more likely target the main coronary vessels instead of the secondary branches.

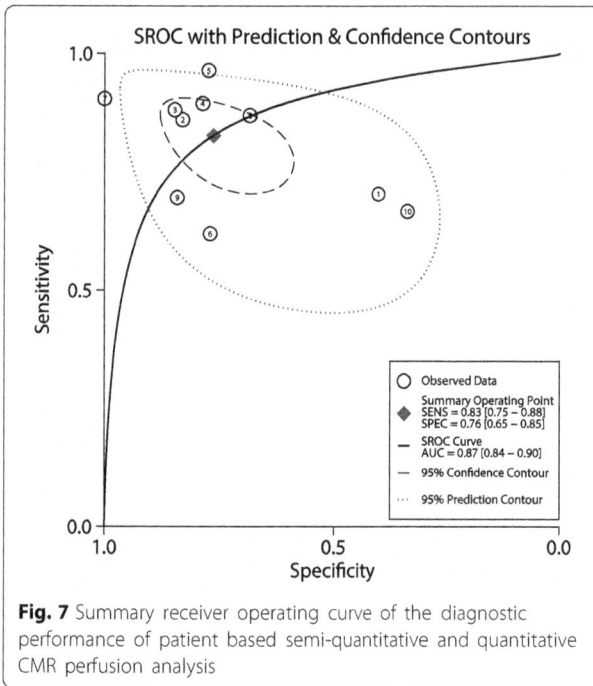

Fig. 7 Summary receiver operating curve of the diagnostic performance of patient based semi-quantitative and quantitative CMR perfusion analysis

Limitations

The main limitations for this meta-analysis is the small number of studies available regarding either segment, territory or patient based semi-quantitative or quantitative analysis of SI-curves in the assessment of myocardial perfusion using CMR and the wide variety of CMR protocols used in these studies. This resulted in a high degree of heterogeneity and possible bias making inter-study comparison difficult. Furthermore, there was an overrepresentation of male patients in the included studies. This limitation makes the findings less generalizable for women. We also decided not to include visual CMR perfusion analysis as the diagnostic accuracy of this assessment has been assessed in previous meta-analyses and our aim was to explore the diagnostic accuracy of SI-curve based assessment.

Another limitation regarding this meta-analysis are the wide variety of reference standards used. We decided to pool all reference standards used to provide a more complete overview of the evidence regarding SI-curve analysis during CMR perfusion. For our subgroup analysis we decided to group reference standards on either providing anatomical or functional information and observed a difference in diagnostic accuracy when using either anatomical or functional reference standards.

We conclude that the reference standard used has an influence on the diagnostic accuracy of SI-curve CMR-perfusion analysis and discussed the unclear

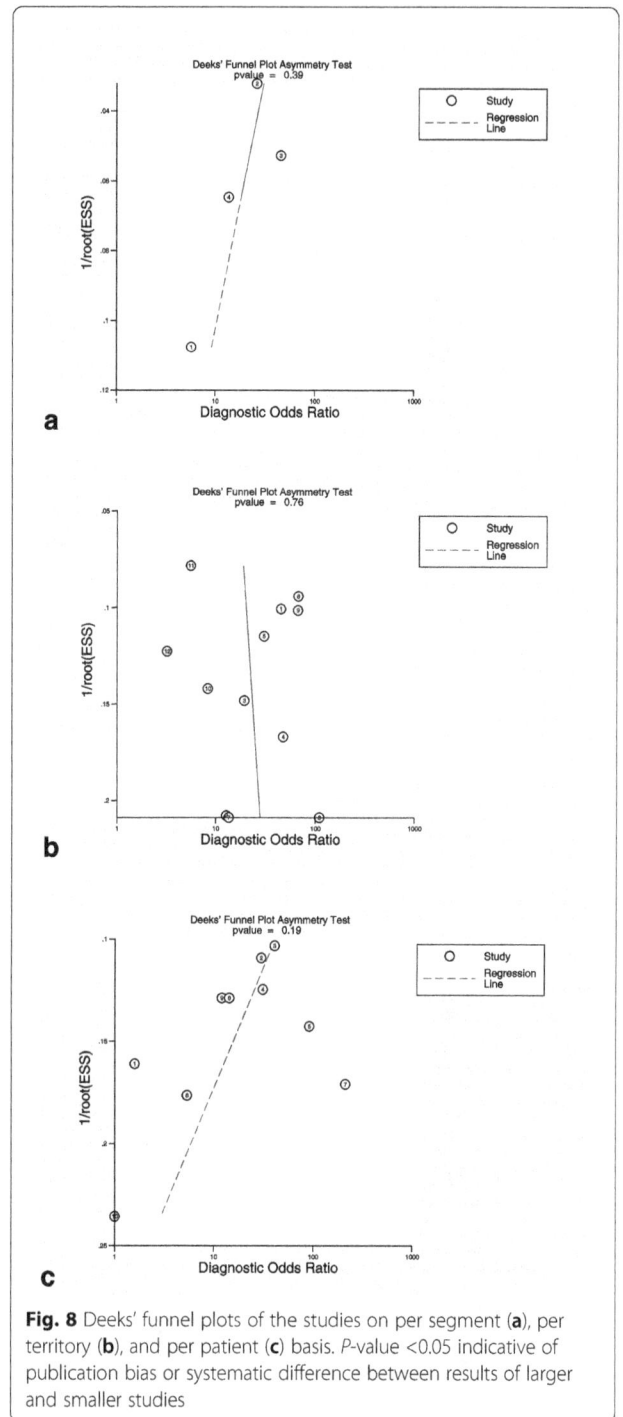

Fig. 8 Deeks' funnel plots of the studies on per segment (**a**), per territory (**b**), and per patient (**c**) basis. *P*-value <0.05 indicative of publication bias or systematic difference between results of larger and smaller studies

relationship of both currently used anatomical and functional reference standards with myocardial flow and perfusion.

Conclusions

This meta-analysis provides an overview of 23 original studies reporting on the diagnostic accuracy of semi-

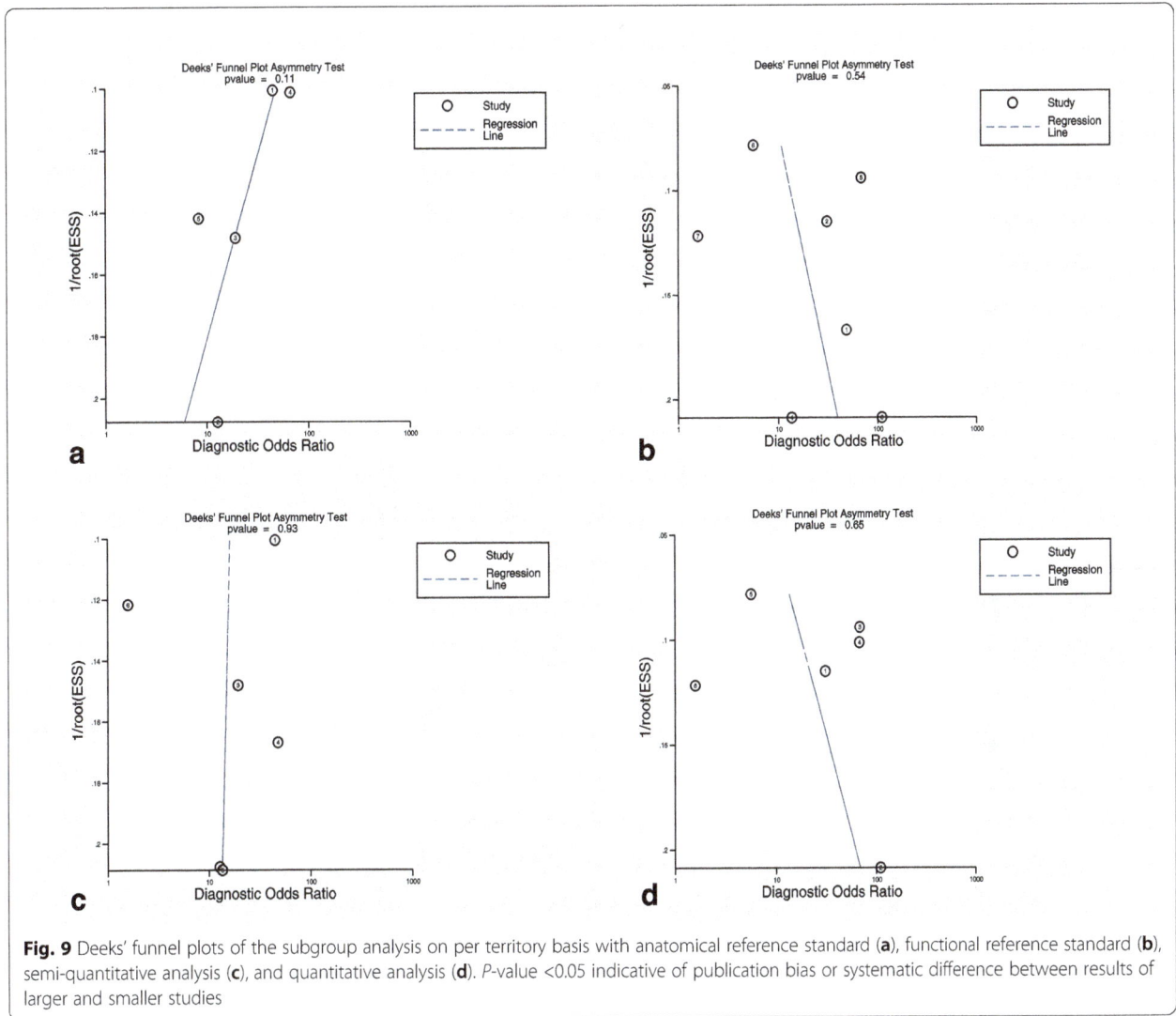

Fig. 9 Deeks' funnel plots of the subgroup analysis on per territory basis with anatomical reference standard (**a**), functional reference standard (**b**), semi-quantitative analysis (**c**), and quantitative analysis (**d**). *P*-value <0.05 indicative of publication bias or systematic difference between results of larger and smaller studies

quantitative or quantitative analysis of stress CMR perfusion on a per segment, per territory or per patient basis for the assessment of significant CAD. Based on our results we conclude that due to a high degree of inter-study heterogeneity the real value of signal intensity curve based analyses of stress CMR perfusion still remains unclear. Semi-quantitative analysis showed a higher diagnostic accuracy for per territory analysis in this meta-analysis, possibly because it is less complex and less susceptible to false assumptions during the calculation. However, quantitative analysis still shows the potential to be used for absolute quantification of myocardial blood flow and further studies should be performed to determine the quantitative model that best represent true myocardial blood flow. The

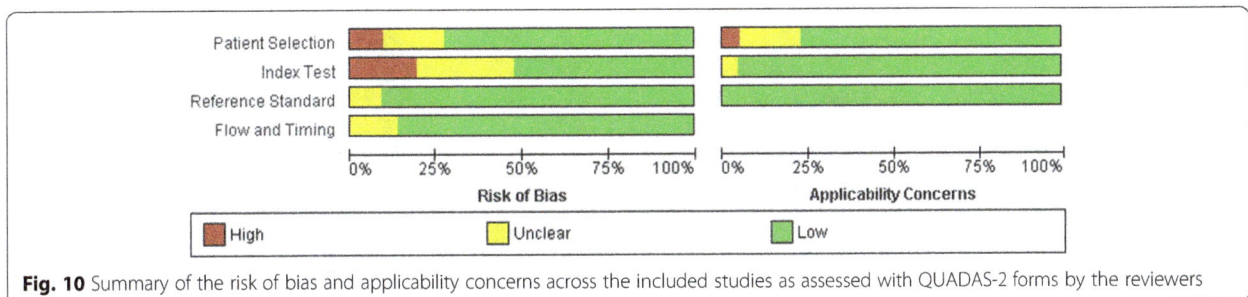

Fig. 10 Summary of the risk of bias and applicability concerns across the included studies as assessed with QUADAS-2 forms by the reviewers

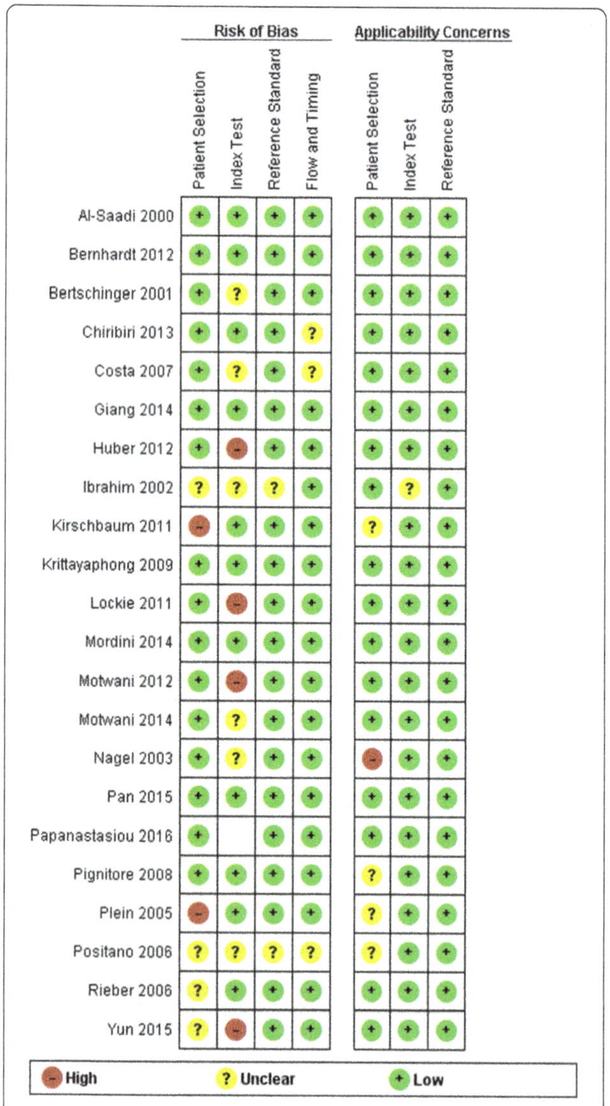

98   Handbook of Cardiovascular Magnetic Resonance Imaging

Fig. 11 Risk of bias and applicability concerns assessment with an overview of the reviewers judgment about each separate domain for each included study

standardization and validation of semi-quantitative or quantitative stress CMR perfusion is necessary before it can be safely implemented in clinical practice.

Abbreviations

AUC: Area under the curve; CAD: Coronary artery disease; CMR: Cardiovascular magnetic resonance; CT: Computed tomography; DOR: Diagnostic odds ratio; FFR: Fractional flow reserve; FN: False negative; FP: False positive; LVEF: Left ventricular ejection fraction; MBF: Myocardial blood flow; MPI: Myocardial perfusion imaging; PET: Positron emission tomography; QCA: Quantitative coronary angiography; SI: Signal intensity; SPECT: Single-photon emission computed tomography; sROC: Summary receiver operating curve; TAC: Tissue attenuation curve; TN: True negative; TP: True positive

Acknowledgements
N/A.

Funding
No funding.

Authors' contributions
RvD and MvA equally contributed to this manuscript. RvD and MvA were responsible for the data acquisition and writing the manuscript. GHdB, RvD and MvA were responsible for the statistical method behind the analysis. GHdB, RV, PvdH and MO were major contributors in interpretation of the data and in revising the manuscript. All authors read and approved the final manuscript.

Competing interests
The authors declare that they have no competing interests.

Author details
[1]Center for Medical Imaging, University Medical Center Groningen, University of Groningen, Hanzeplein 1 EB 45, Groningen, The Netherlands. [2]Department of Radiology, University Medical Center Groningen, University of Groningen, Groningen, The Netherlands. [3]Department of Cardiology, University Medical Center Groningen, University of Groningen, Groningen, The Netherlands. [4]Department of Epidemiology, University Medical Center Groningen, University of Groningen, Groningen, The Netherlands.

References

1. Christou MAC, Siontis GCM, Katritsis DG, Ioannidis JPA. Meta-analysis of fractional flow reserve versus quantitative coronary angiography and noninvasive imaging for evaluation of myocardial ischemia. Am J Cardiol. 2007;99(4):450–6.
2. Tonino PAL, Fearon WF, De Bruyne B, Oldroyd KG, Leesar MA, Ver Lee PN, et al. Angiographic versus functional severity of coronary artery Stenoses in the FAME study. Fractional flow reserve versus angiography in multivessel evaluation. J Am Coll Cardiol. 2010;55(25):2816–21.
3. Hamon MM, Fau G, Née G, Ehtisham J, Morello R, Hamon MM, et al. Meta-analysis of the diagnostic performance of stress perfusion cardiovascular magnetic resonance for detection of coronary artery disease. J Cardiovasc Magn Reson. 2010;56(3):29.
4. Montalescot G, Sechtem U, Achenbach S, Andreotti F, Arden C, Budaj A, et al. 2013 ESC guidelines on the management of stable coronary artery disease. Eur Heart J. 2013;34(38):2949–3003.
5. Fihn SD, Blankenship JC, Alexander KP, Bittl JA, Byrne JG, Fletcher BJ, et al. 2014 ACC/AHA/AATS/PCNA/SCAI/STS focused update of the guideline for the diagnosis and Management of Patients with Stable Ischemic Heart Disease: A Report of the American College of Cardiology /American Heart Association Task Force on Practice Cardiovascul. Circulation. 2014;130:1749–67.
6. Pijls NHJ, De Bruyne B, Peels K, Van Der Voort PH, Bonnier HJRM, Bartunek J, Koolen JJ, et al. Measurement of fractional flow reserve to assess the functional severity of coronary-artery Stenoses. N Engl J Med. 1996;334(26):1703–8.
7. Jolly SS, Yusuf S, Cairns J, Niemel K, Xavier D, Widimsky P, et al. Radial versus femoral access for coronary angiography and intervention in patients with acute coronary syndromes (RIVAL): a randomised, parallel group, multicentre trial. Lancet. 2011;377(9775):1409–20.
8. Arora N, Matheny ME, Sepke C, Resnic FS. A propensity analysis of the risk of vascular complications after cardiac catheterization procedures with the use of vascular closure devices. Am Heart J. 2007;153(4):606–11.
9. Noto TJ, Johnson L, Krone R. Cardiac catheterization 1990: a report of the Registryt of the Society for Cardiac Angiography and Intervention s(SCA&!). Catheter Cardiovasc Diagn. 1991;24:75–83.
10. Bokhari S, Raina A, Rosenweig EB, Schulze PC, Bokhari J, Einstein AJ, et al. PET imaging may provide a novel biomarker and understanding of right ventricular dysfunction in patients with idiopathic pulmonary arterial hypertension. Circ Cardiovasc Imaging. 2011;4(6):641–7.
11. Einstein AJ. Radiation risk from coronary artery disease imaging: how do different diagnostic tests compare? Heart. 2008;94(12):1519–21.
12. Patel MR, Peterson ED, Dai D, Brennan JM, Redberg RF, Anderson HV, et al. Low diagnostic yield of elective coronary angiography. N Engl J Med. 2010; 362(10):886–95.

13. Takx RAP, Blomberg BA, Aidi HE, Habets J, de Jong PA, Nagel E, et al. Diagnostic accuracy of stress myocardial perfusion imaging compared to invasive coronary angiography with fractional flow reserve meta-analysis. Circ Cardiovasc Imaging. 2015;8(1):e002666.

14. Einstein AJ. Effects of radiation exposure from cardiac Imaging : how good are the data? J Am Coll Cardiol. 2012;59(6):553–65.

15. Nandalur KR, Dwamena BA, Choudhri AF, Nandalur MR, Carlos RC. Diagnostic performance of stress cardiac magnetic resonance imaging in the detection of coronary artery disease: a meta-analysis. J Am Coll Cardiol. 2007;50(14):1343–53.

16. Hamlin SA, Henry TS, Little BP, Lerakis S, Stillman AE. Mapping the future of cardiac MR imaging: case-based review of T1 and T2 mapping techniques. Radiographics. 2014;34(6):1594–611.

17. Desai RR, Jha S. Diagnostic performance of cardiac stress perfusion mri in the detection of coronary artery disease using fractional flow reserve as the reference standard: a meta-analysis. Am J Roentgenol. 2013; 201(2):245–52.

18. Li M, Zhou T, Yang L, Peng Z, Ding J, Sun G, et al. Diagnostic accuracy of myocardial magnetic resonance perfusion to diagnose ischemic Stenosis with fractional flow reserve as reference. JACC Cardiovasc Imaging. 2014; 7(11):1098–105.

19. Ebersberger U, Makowski MR, Schoepf UJ, Platz U, Schmidtler F, Rose J, et al. Magnetic resonance myocardial perfusion imaging at 3.0 Tesla for the identification of myocardial ischaemia: comparison with coronary catheter angiography and fractional flow reserve measurements. Eur Heart J Cardiovasc Imaging. 2013;14(12):1174–80.

20. Mordini FE, Haddad T, Hsu L-YY, Kellman P, Lowrey TB, Aletras AH, et al. Diagnostic accuracy of stress perfusion CMR in comparison with quantitative coronary angiography: fully quantitative, semiquantitative, and qualitative assessment. JACC Cardiovasc Imaging. 2014;7(1):14–22.

21. Handayani A, Sijens PE, Lubbers DD, Triadyaksa P, Oudkerk M, van Ooijen PMA, et al. Influence of the choice of software package on the outcome of semiquantitative MR myocardial perfusion analysis. Radiology. 2013;266(3):759–65.

22. Handayani A, Triadyaksa P, Dijkstra H, Pelgrim GJ, van Ooijen PM, Prakken NH, et al. Intermodel agreement of myocardial blood flow estimation from stress-rest myocardial perfusion magnetic resonance imaging in patients with coronary artery disease. Investig Radiol. 2015; 50(4):275–82.

23. Whiting PF, Rutjes AWS, Westwood ME, Mallet S, Deeks JJ, Reitsma JB, et al. Research and reporting methods accuracy studies. Ann Intern Med. 2011; 155(4):529–36.

24. Huber A, Sourbron S, Klauss V, Schaefer J, Bauner KU, Schweyer M, et al. Magnetic resonance perfusion of the myocardium: semiquantitative and quantitative evaluation in comparison with coronary angiography and fractional flow reserve. Investig Radiol. 2012;47(6):332–8.

25. Bernhardt P, Walcher T, Rottbauer W, Wöhrle J, Wohrle J, Wöhrle J. Quantification of myocardial perfusion reserve at 1.5 and 3.0 tesla: a comparison to fractional flow reserve. Int J Cardiovasc Imaging. 2012; 28(8):2049–56.

26. Van De Hoef TP, Van Lavieren MA, Damman P, Delewi R, Piek MA, Chamuleau SAJ, et al. Physiological basis and long-term clinical outcome of discordance between fractional flow reserve and coronary flow velocity reserve in coronary stenoses of intermediate severity. Circ Cardiovasc Interv. 2014;7(3):301–11.

27. Al-Saadi N, Nagel E, Gross M, Bornstedt A, Schnackenburg B, Klein C, et al. Noninvasive detection of myocardial ischemia from perfusion reserve based on cardiovascular magnetic resonance. Circulation. 2000; 101(12):1379–83.

28. Bertschinger KM, Nanz D, Buechi M, Luescher TF, Marincek B, von Schulthess GK, et al. Magnetic resonance myocardial first-pass perfusion imaging: parameter optimization for signal response and cardiac coverage. J Magn Reson Imaging. 2001;14(5):556–62.

29. Ibrahim T, Nekolla SG, Schreiber K, Odaka K, Volz S, Mehilli J, et al. Assessment of coronary flow reserve: comparison between contrast-enhanced magnetic resonance imaging and positron emission tomography. J Am Coll Cardiol. 2002;39(5):864–70.

30. Nagel E, Klein C, Paetsch I, Hettwer S, Schnackenburg B, Wegscheider K, et al. Magnetic resonance perfusion measurements for the noninvasive detection of coronary artery disease. Circulation. 2003;108(4):432–7.

31. Giang TH, Nanz D, Coulden R, Friedrich M, Graves M, Al-Saadi N, et al. Detection of coronary artery disease by magnetic resonance myocardial perfusion imaging with various contrast medium doses: first European multi-centre experience. Eur Heart J. 2004;25(18):1657–65.

32. Plein S, Radjenovic A, Ridgway JP, Barmby D, Greenwood JP, Ball SG, et al. Coronary artery disease: myocardial perfusion MR imaging with sensitivity encoding versus conventional angiography. Radiology. 2005; 235(2):423–30.

33. Rieber J, Huber A, Erhard I, Mueller S, Schweyer M, Koenig A, et al. Cardiac magnetic resonance perfusion imaging for the functional assessment of coronary artery disease: a comparison with coronary angiography and fractional flow reserve. Eur Heart J. 2006;27(12):1465–71.

34. Positano V, Pingitore A, Scattini B, Santarelli MF, De Marchi D, Favilli B, et al. Myocardial perfusion by first pass contrast magnetic resonance: a robust method for quantitative regional assessment of perfusion reserve index. Heart. 2006;92(5):689–90.

35. Costa MA, Shoemaker S, Futamatsu H, Klassen C, Angiolillo DJ, Nguyen M, et al. Quantitative magnetic resonance perfusion imaging detects anatomic and physiologic coronary artery disease as measured by coronary angiography and fractional flow reserve. J Am Coll Cardiol. 2007;50(6):514–22.

36. Pingitore A, Lombardi M, Scattini B, De Marchi D, Aquaro GD, Positano V, et al. Head to head comparison between perfusion and function during accelerated high-dose dipyridamole magnetic resonance stress for the detection of coronary artery disease. Am J Cardiol. 2008;101(1):8–14.

37. Krittayaphong R, Boonyasirinant T, Saiviroonporn P, Nakyen S, Thanapiboonpol P, Yindeengam A, et al. Myocardial perfusion cardiac magnetic resonance for the diagnosis of coronary artery disease: do we need rest images? Int J Cardiovasc Imaging. 2009;25(Suppl 1):139–48.

38. Kirschbaum SW, Nieman K, Springeling T, Weustink AC, Ramcharitar S, van Mieghem C, et al. Non-invasive diagnostic workup of patients with suspected stable angina by combined computed tomography coronary angiography and magnetic resonance perfusion imaging. Circ J. 2011;75(7):1678–84.

39. Lockie T, Ishida M, Perera D, Chiribiri A, De Silva K, Kozerke S, et al. High-resolution magnetic resonance myocardial perfusion imaging at 3.0-Tesla to detect hemodynamically significant coronary stenoses as determined by fractional flow reserve. J Am Coll Cardiol. 2011;57(1):70–5.

40. Motwani M, Fairbairn TA, Larghat A, Mather AN, Biglands JD, Radjenovic A, et al. Systolic versus diastolic acquisition in myocardial perfusion MR imaging. Radiology. 2012;262(3):816–23.

41. Chiribiri A, Hautvast GLTF, Lockie T, Schuster A, Bigalke B, Olivotti L, et al. Assessment of coronary artery stenosis severity and location: quantitative analysis of transmural perfusion gradients by high-resolution MRI versus FFR. JACC Cardiovasc Imaging. 2013;6(5):600–9.

42. Motwani M, Kidambi A, Sourbron S, Fairbairn TA, Uddin A, Kozerke S, et al. Quantitative three-dimensional cardiovascular magnetic resonance myocardial perfusion imaging in systole and diastole. J Cardiovasc Magn Reson. 2014;16:19.

43. Yun C-H, Tsai J-P, Tsai C-T, Mok GSP, Sun J-Y, Hung C-L, et al. Qualitative and semi-quantitative evaluation of myocardium perfusion with 3 T stress cardiac MRI. BMC Cardiovasc Disord. 2015;15(1):164.

44. Pan J, Huang S, Lu Z, Li J, Wan Q, Zhang J, et al. Comparison of myocardial Transmural perfusion gradient by magnetic resonance imaging to fractional flow Reserve in Patients with Suspected Coronary Artery Disease. Am J Cardiol. 2015;115(10):1333–40.

10

3D whole-heart phase sensitive inversion recovery CMR for simultaneous black-blood late gadolinium enhancement and bright-blood coronary CMR angiography

Giulia Ginami[1]*[iD], Radhouene Neji[1,2], Imran Rashid[1], Amedeo Chiribiri[1], Tevfik F. Ismail[1], René M. Botnar[1,3] and Claudia Prieto[1,3]

Abstract

Background: Phase sensitive inversion recovery (PSIR) applied to late gadolinium enhancement (LGE) imaging is widely used in clinical practice. However, conventional 2D PSIR LGE sequences provide sub-optimal contrast between scar tissue and blood pool, rendering the detection of subendocardial infarcts and scar segmentation challenging. Furthermore, the acquisition of a low flip angle reference image doubles the acquisition time without providing any additional diagnostic information. The purpose of this study was to develop and test a novel 3D whole-heart PSIR-like framework, named *BOOST*, enabling simultaneous black-blood LGE assessment and bright-blood visualization of cardiac anatomy.

Methods: The proposed approach alternates the acquisition of a 3D volume preceded by a T_2-prepared Inversion Recovery (T_2Prep-IR) module (magnitude image) with the acquisition of a T_2-prepared 3D volume (reference image). The two volumes (T_2Prep-IR BOOST and bright-blood T_2Prep BOOST) are combined in a PSIR-like reconstruction to obtain a complementary 3D black-blood volume for LGE assessment (PSIR BOOST). The black-blood PSIR BOOST and the bright-blood T_2Prep BOOST datasets were compared to conventional clinical sequences for scar detection and coronary CMR angiography (CMRA) in 18 patients with a spectrum of cardiovascular disease (CVD).

Results: Datasets from 12 patients were quantitatively analysed. The black-blood PSIR BOOST dataset provided statistically improved contrast to noise ratio (CNR) between blood and scar when compared to a clinical 2D PSIR sequence (15.8 ± 3.3 and 4.1 ± 5.6, respectively). Overall agreement in LGE depiction was found between 3D black-blood PSIR BOOST and clinical 2D PSIR acquisitions, with 11/12 PSIR BOOST datasets considered diagnostic. The bright-blood T_2Prep BOOST dataset provided high quality depiction of the proximal coronary segments, with improvement of visual score when compared to a clinical CMRA sequence. Acquisition time of BOOST (~10 min), providing information on both LGE uptake and heart anatomy, was comparable to that of a clinical single CMRA sequence.

Conclusions: The feasibility of BOOST for simultaneous black-blood LGE assessment and bright-blood coronary angiography was successfully tested in patients with cardiovascular disease. The framework enables free-breathing multi-contrast whole-heart acquisitions with 100% scan efficiency and predictable scan time. Complementary information on 3D LGE and heart anatomy are obtained reducing examination time.

Keywords: Whole-heart, Black-blood, Bright-blood, Late gadolinium enhancement (LGE), Coronary MR angiography

* Correspondence: giulia.ginami@kcl.ac.uk
Dr. Debiao Li served as a guest editor for this manuscript.
[1]School of Biomedical Engineering and Imaging Sciences, King's College London, St Thomas' Hospital (Lambeth Wing), Westminster Bridge Rd, London SE1 7EH, UK
Full list of author information is available at the end of the article

Background

Late gadolinium enhancement (LGE) cardiovascular magnetic resonance (CMR) imaging has become the gold standard for the assessment of myocardial viability in different cardiac pathologies, including myocardial infarction [1, 2] and myocarditis [3–5]. In addition, LGE imaging provides pre-interventional assessment of arrhythmogenic substrate in patients undergoing electrophysiology procedures as well as visualization of lesions after ablation [6–8], and is gaining importance in the characterization of fibrosis in non-ischemic cardiomyopathies [9–12]. LGE imaging is typically performed 10–20 min after the administration of a gadolinium (Gd)-based contrast agent using T_1-weighted inversion recovery (IR) sequences [1, 13–15]. The inversion time (TI) is normally set to null the signal from the healthy myocardium, thus enhancing the contrast to noise ratio (CNR) between viable and diseased myocardial tissue. IR sequences, however, are prone to reduced scar to blood and scar to remote myocardium contrast when a sub-optimal TI is selected. Phase-sensitive IR (PSIR) LGE acquisitions have been introduced to provide intrinsic robustness with respect to the TI selection [16]. Conventional PSIR sequences are based on the acquisition of an IR-prepared image (referred to as "magnitude image"), interleaved with a proton density image (referred to as "reference image") that is acquired at a low flip-angle, which are then combined as described in [16]. Although PSIR normally achieves excellent contrast between viable myocardium and scar tissue, the contrast between blood pool and LGE uptake is often suboptimal. This leads to difficulties in delineating sub-endocardial infarcts that are adjacent to the blood pool. Furthermore, unclear borders between scar tissue and blood affect the accuracy of scar segmentation that is crucial for infarct size and transmurality measurements as well as for the planning of electrophysiology procedures [17, 18]. Black-blood PSIR LGE has been introduced [19] to improve the contrast between the blood pool and scar tissue by exploiting an inversion pulse in combination with a T_2 preparation (T_2Prep) module (T_2Prep-IR) [19–21]. However, a limitation of all PSIR frameworks is that the acquisition efficiency is intrinsically sub-optimal as the low flip-angle reference image has limited diagnostic value. Furthermore, most of the LGE PSIR implementations are limited to 2D acquisitions that are performed during a breath-hold to minimize respiratory motion artefacts. Recently, free-breathing whole-heart PSIR acquisitions have been introduced [22, 23] and integrated with diaphragmatic navigator gating [24]. The use of diaphragmatic navigator gating, however, leads to reduced scan efficiency and unpredictable acquisition times that can make the selection of the correct TI challenging. In addition, residual imaging artefacts may be observed as a result of the combination of the inversion pulse with the diaphragmatic navigator [25]. In order to overcome these drawbacks, we propose the extension of a 3D whole-heart Bright-blood and black-blOOd phase SensiTive inversion recovery (BOOST) sequence [26] – that has been recently introduced for non-contrast enhanced visualization of coronary lumen and thrombus – to black-blood LGE imaging. The proposed post-contrast BOOST sequence exploits a T_2Prep-IR module for the acquisition of the magnitude image, enabling black-blood LGE PSIR reconstruction. Furthermore, the acquisition of the reference image is designed to provide a complementary and fully co-registered bright-blood dataset for the visualization of the heart anatomy, the great vessels, and the coronary lumen. The entire framework has been integrated with image-based navigation [27] to achieve 100% scan efficiency and predictable scan time. In this study, the feasibility of BOOST for post-contrast simultaneous black-blood LGE imaging and bright-blood heart anatomy, great vessels, and coronary lumen visualization was tested in a cohort of cardiovascular patients at the end of a clinical CMR examination.

Methods

Framework implementation

An electrocardiogram -triggered free-breathing 3D whole-heart balanced steady-state free precession (bSSFP) prototype sequence was implemented as described in [26] and as illustrated in Fig. 1. The sequence alternates the acquisition of a T_2-prepared IR volume in odd heartbeats (T_2Prep-IR BOOST, magnitude image) and a T_2-prepared volume in even heartbeats (bright-blood T_2Prep BOOST, reference image). Both acquisitions are performed with a Cartesian trajectory with spiral profile order [28] and with a high flip-angle of 90 degrees. A 2D low-resolution image-based navigator (iNAV) [27] is acquired at each heartbeat to estimate translational respiratory motion along the superior-inferior (SI) and right-left (RL) directions and to enable beat-to-beat motion correction with 100% scan efficiency and predictable scan time. Prior to data acquisition, a rectangular region of interest (ROI) is selected covering the whole heart along the RL direction and covering the base and the mid part of the heart along the SI direction. RL and SI translational motion is then estimated using a template-matching algorithm [29] and motion compensation is performed by modulating the k-space data with a linear shift before image reconstruction [27]. Motion estimation is performed for the T_2Prep-IR BOOST and T_2Prep BOOST datasets independently. For each dataset, respiratory motion correction is performed at the end-expiratory level [30].

The motion corrected T_2Prep-IR BOOST and T_2Prep BOOST volumes are then rigidly co-registered and combined in a PSIR-like reconstruction as described in [16] to obtain a complimentary PSIR BOOST black-blood

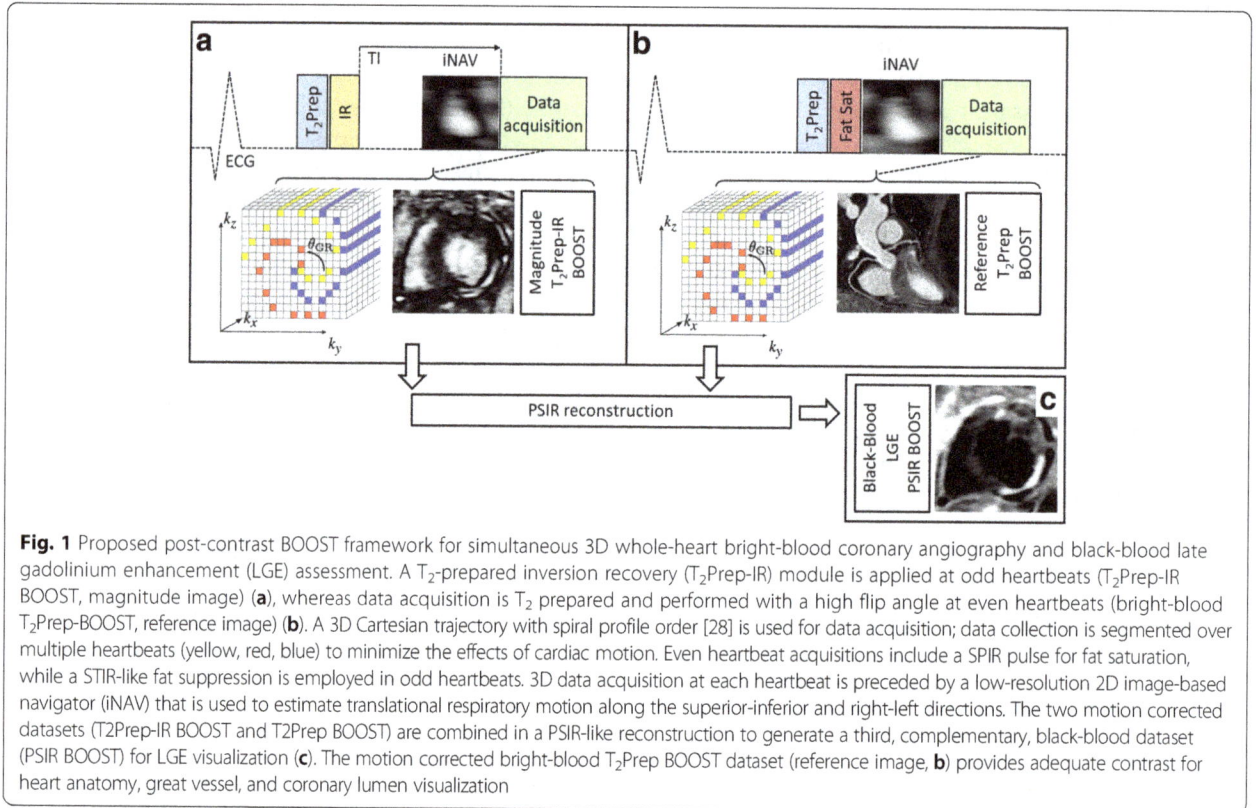

Fig. 1 Proposed post-contrast BOOST framework for simultaneous 3D whole-heart bright-blood coronary angiography and black-blood late gadolinium enhancement (LGE) assessment. A T_2-prepared inversion recovery (T_2Prep-IR) module is applied at odd heartbeats (T_2Prep-IR BOOST, magnitude image) (**a**), whereas data acquisition is T_2 prepared and performed with a high flip angle at even heartbeats (bright-blood T_2Prep-BOOST, reference image) (**b**). A 3D Cartesian trajectory with spiral profile order [28] is used for data acquisition; data collection is segmented over multiple heartbeats (yellow, red, blue) to minimize the effects of cardiac motion. Even heartbeat acquisitions include a SPIR pulse for fat saturation, while a STIR-like fat suppression is employed in odd heartbeats. 3D data acquisition at each heartbeat is preceded by a low-resolution 2D image-based navigator (iNAV) that is used to estimate translational respiratory motion along the superior-inferior and right-left directions. The two motion corrected datasets (T2Prep-IR BOOST and T2Prep BOOST) are combined in a PSIR-like reconstruction to generate a third, complementary, black-blood dataset (PSIR BOOST) for LGE visualization (**c**). The motion corrected bright-blood T_2Prep BOOST dataset (reference image, **b**) provides adequate contrast for heart anatomy, great vessel, and coronary lumen visualization

volume. The PSIR-like reconstruction is performed using the T_2Prep BOOST dataset as reference image. As the T_2Prep BOOST is designed for coronary lumen visualization, it exhibits high tissue contrast. Thus, voxel-by-voxel intensity normalization of the resulting PSIR BOOST volume by the reference image is not performed in order to preserve adequate contrast in the resulting black-blood LGE volume.

All acquisitions reported in this study were performed on a 1.5 T CMR system (Magnetom Aera, Siemens Healthineers, Erlangen, Germany) using an 18-channel chest-coil and a 32-channel spine coil. The study was approved by the National Research Ethics Service (15/NS/0030) and written informed consent was obtained from each participant according to institutional guidelines. Motion estimation and correction, image reconstruction, and PSIR-like computation were implemented using the scanner software (Syngo MR E11A, Siemens Healthineers).

Sequence simulations

The longitudinal magnetization behavior of healthy viable myocardium, scar and blood was investigated via simulations for the proposed post-contrast BOOST sequence. This was compared against the corresponding simulations for previously published LGE PSIR and bright-blood coronary angiography

post-contrast sequences. Sequence simulations were performed in Matlab R2016a (The MathWorks, Inc., Natick, Massachusetts, USA).

Three different CMR sequences were simulated using the extended phase graphs (EPG) formalism [31]: 1) the BOOST sequence as illustrated in Fig. 1; 2) a conventional PSIR sequence for LGE assessment as described in [16]; 3) a dedicated T_2-prepared bright-blood sequence for coronary CMRA [32]. The simulated tissue parameters were set as follows: healthy viable myocardium $T_1 = 550$ ms, $T_2 = 45$ ms; scar $T_1 = 300$ ms, $T_2 = 45$ ms; and post-contrast blood $T_1 = 450$ ms, $T_2 = 200$ ms. The T_1 and T_2 values of the tissues of interest were set to match those of the standardized phantom [33] used in this study, as described in the following paragraphs, and to approximate the properties of tissues about 15 min after gadolinium contrast injection [33, 34]. Accordingly, imaging parameters were set to match those of the performed phantom acquisitions. For both the BOOST and the conventional PSIR sequences, the TI was set to null the signal from healthy viable myocardium at odd heartbeats (corresponding to TI = 150 ms for the BOOST sequence and to TI = 350 ms for the conventional PSIR sequence). T_2Prep duration was set to 40 ms for odd and even heartbeats of the BOOST sequence, and for the CMRA sequence. A flip-angle of 90 degrees was simulated for both the acquisition of the magnitude and the bright-blood reference image in the BOOST sequence as well as for the acquisition of the magnitude image in the conventional PSIR sequence. A flip-angle of 8 degrees was simulated for the reference image of the conventional PSIR sequence. For the CMRA sequence, a 90 degrees flip angle was simulated for each heartbeat. For all three sequences (BOOST, conventional PSIR, and CMRA), and for each individual heartbeat, a data acquisition duration equal to 120 ms was simulated, corresponding to 33 k-space lines. To minimize signal oscillations during acquisition, and to generate the iNAVs at each individual heartbeat, 14 bSSFP linear ramp-up pulses were simulated prior to imaging data acquisition. The heart-rate was simulated at 60 beats per minute with a total of 50 heartbeats (of which 2 were dummy heartbeats).

For all the simulated sequences, expected magnetization M_z/M_0 as well as absolute signal differences between the tissues of interest were computed. All the absolute signal differences (that are preserved in the final PSIR reconstruction) were computed at the beginning of the data acquisition using centric k-space ordering.

Phantom experiments
Data acquisition
A standardized T_1 and T_2 phantom, with different vials resembling T_1 and T_2 values of the most relevant cardiac compartments [33], was used for data acquisition. Healthy myocardium, scar, and post-contrast blood T_1 and T_2 values were identical to the simulated ones. Data acquisition was performed using the BOOST sequence, the conventional PSIR sequence, and the dedicated CMRA acquisition. T_2Prep durations, TIs, heart rate, number of k-space lines acquired per heartbeat and flip angle values were kept identical to those used in the simulations. Additional imaging parameters included: transverse orientation, Field of view (FOV) = 320x320x60 mm^3, in-plane spatial resolution = 1 mm^2, slice thickness = 2 mm, echo-time (TE) / repetition time (TR) = 1.56/3.6 ms, pixel bandwidth 977 Hz/pixel. The PSIR BOOST reconstruction was performed with and without intensity normalization for comparison purposes.

Data analysis
Signal to noise ratio (SNR) and CNR were quantified for the three sequences (BOOST, conventional PSIR, and dedicated CMRA). SNR of blood (SNR_{blood}), healthy viable myocardium (SNR_{myo}) and scar (SNR_{scar}) were calculated for the odd heartbeats of BOOST and conventional PSIR, together with CNR between blood and healthy myocardium ($CNR_{blood-myo}$), scar and blood ($CNR_{scar-blood}$), and scar and healthy viable myocardium ($CNR_{scar-myo}$). SNR_{blood} and $CNR_{blood-myo}$ were quantified for even heartbeats for both the BOOST and the conventional PSIR sequence as well as for the dedicated CMRA

acquisition. For the PSIR images obtained from the BOOST sequence (with and without intensity normalization) and the conventional PSIR sequence, $CNR_{blood-myo}$, $CNR_{scar-blood}$, and $CNR_{scar-myo}$ were quantified after the removal of low spatial frequency signal components as described in [16, 35].

In-vivo experiments
Data acquisition
Eighteen patients (52.7 ± 13.2 years, 9 males) who were referred for a clinical CMR examination were recruited for this study. In 16 out of 18 (89%) patients, a conventional 2D multi-slice and multi breath-hold bSSFP Cartesian PSIR sequence [16] was acquired in different orientations (four chamber view, three chamber view, short-axis view) starting 10 min after gadobutrol (0.2 mmol/kg) administration (Gadovist, Bayer, Berlin, Germany). Relevant imaging parameters for this acquisition include: FOV = 292 × 152 mm^2, slice thickness = 8 mm, in plane spatial resolution = 1.4 mm^2, 10 slices acquired for the short axis view, TE/TR = 1.26/2.9 ms, pixel bandwidth = 775 Hz/pixel, flip angle = 45 degrees, ECG triggering to the most quiescent diastolic period. The TI (typically ranging from 200 ms – 300 ms) was selected with a dedicated TI scout scan and was set to null the signal from the healthy viable myocardium. In 7 out of 18 (39%) subjects, a conventional free-breathing navigator-gated bright-blood whole-heart T_2-prepared bSSFP (CMRA) Cartesian sequence was acquired after the breath-hold 2D PSIR sequences. For this acquisition, imaging parameters were set as follows: sagittal orientation, subject-specific FOV = 410x307x160–192 mm^3, in plane spatial resolution = 1.4 mm^2, slice thickness = 1.4 mm, TE/TR = 1.56/3.6 ms, pixel bandwidth = 575 Hz/pixel, flip angle = 90 degrees, T_2Prep duration = 40 ms, 2× GRAPPA parallel imaging acceleration [36] with 24 calibration lines. Respiratory motion was compensated using diaphragmatic navigator gating and tracking (tracking factor equal to 0.6 [37]), with an acceptance window placed in end-expiration and with an amplitude equal to ±3.5 mm.

At the end of the clinical examination, the proposed ECG-triggered BOOST sequence was acquired under free-breathing and using the following imaging parameters: coronal orientation, in-plane spatial resolution = 1 mm^2, slice thickness = 4 mm (interpolated to 2 mm during image reconstruction), subject-specific FOV = 320x320x80–130 mm^3, TE/TR = 1.56/3.6 ms, pixel bandwidth 977 Hz/pixel. For both the magnitude image T_2Prep-IR BOOST and the reference image T_2Prep BOOST, the flip angle was set to 90 degrees and the T_2Prep duration was equal to 40 ms. The subject-specific TI (typically ranging in the interval 100–180 ms) was selected to null the signal from viable healthy myocardium by acquiring a dedicated 2D BOOST TI scout scan during a breath-hold; such scout scan consisted of a magnetization-prepared cine sequence where a T_2Prep-IR module is applied right after the R-wave at odd heartbeats, whereas T_2-preparation solely is performed at the beginning of the cardiac cycle in even heartbeats. Cine frames belonging to the odd heartbeats were visually inspected to determine the optimized TI. In odd heartbeats, fat signal was suppressed for the effect of the inversion pulse (STIR-like approach) [38], while spectral pre-saturation (SPIR) [39] was used to suppress signal from epicardial fat at even heartbeats (Fig. 1). Images obtained in patients for whom BOOST data acquisition did not start later than 40 min after contrast injection were considered for further quantitative and qualitative data analyses. This temporal restriction was set to avoid a too pronounced washout of the contrast agent.

Quantitative data analysis

Quantitative data analysis was performed for the images acquired with the clinical 2D PSIR sequence, and for the 3D black-blood LGE and bright-blood CMRA datasets obtained with BOOST (PSIR BOOST and T_2Prep BOOST, respectively). ROIs were manually drawn in blood, healthy viable myocardium and scar tissue (when present) at matching anatomical locations for both the clinical 2D PSIR and the 3D whole-heart PSIR BOOST images. Background noise was computed from a ROI with uniform signal positioned at the level of the liver, following the removal of low spatial frequency signal components as performed for the phantom images [16, 35]. $CNR_{blood-myo}$, $CNR_{scar-blood}$ and $CNR_{scar-myo}$ were quantified for both the clinical 2D PSIR and the 3D whole-heart PSIR BOOST images. CNR values were quantified in the subjects for whom both the 2D PSIR and BOOST sequences were acquired, and compared using a paired 2-tailed Student t-test. $P = 0.05$ was set as the threshold to determine statistical significance. Acquisition times of all the acquired sequences (2D PSIR acquisition – including pauses between breath-holds –, clinical whole-heart CMRA, and BOOST) were recorded. In addition, scan efficiency was recorded for the clinical CMRA acquisition with diaphragmatic navigator gating.

Qualitative data analysis

All the datasets (3D black-blood PSIR BOOST, 3D bright-blood T_2Prep BOOST, conventional 3D CMRA acquisition, and clinical 2D PSIR) were anonymized and stored in a randomized order. Qualitative grading of the anonymized images was performed by two experienced cardiologists (T.F.I. and I.R., *SCMR III* certification) blinded to clinical data. For all the LGE images (black-blood 3D PSIR BOOST and 2D clinical PSIR), presence and location of LGE were assessed. Furthermore, images were graded in terms of diagnostic quality on consensus

basis using a 4-point scale system where *1* indicates a fully diagnostic dataset without the presence of artefacts, *2* indicates a diagnostic dataset with only minor artefacts present, *3* indicates a diagnostic dataset with significant artefacts, and *4* indicates an artefacts-rendering images non-diagnostic dataset. Subjective scores for LGE visualization were compared with a paired Wilcoxon signed-rank test to assess statistical differences; $P < 0.05$ was considered statistically significant. Statistical analyses were performed considering the cases for whom both the clinical 2D PSIR and the BOOST sequences were acquired. For all acquired bright-blood datasets (conventional 3D CMRA and T_2Prep BOOST), the ability to identify the origin and the proximal course of the coronary arteries was graded for four relevant coronary segments: left main (LM), left anterior descending coronary artery (LAD), left circumflex coronary artery (LCX), and right coronary artery (RCA). Grading was performed on consensus basis using a 4-point scale system as that used for the grading of LGE datasets.

Results

All data acquisitions and reconstructions were carried out successfully and all quantified endpoints are reported hereafter.

Sequence simulations

All simulated pulse sequences (proposed post-contrast BOOST sequence, conventional PSIR sequence [16], and dedicated post-contrast CMRA acquisition [32]) and the resulting steady state magnetization behavior for blood, myocardium and scar tissues are reported in Fig. 2. For the T_2Prep-IR BOOST sequence (odd heartbeats) the expected magnetization M_z/M_0 of the healthy viable myocardium, blood and scar varied within the intervals 0.000–0.059, –0.158 – 0.003, and 0.108–0.116, respectively, during imaging data acquisition. This resulted in an absolute signal difference between myocardium and scar of +0.108 and of +0.266 between blood and scar. For the conventional PSIR sequence, and in correspondence to the acquisition of the magnitude image, the expected magnetization M_z/M_0 of the healthy viable myocardium varied within the interval – 0.002 – 0.058, whereas the expected magnetization M_z/M_0 of blood and scar varied within the intervals 0.056–0.146 and 0.207–0.144, respectively. This resulted in an absolute signal difference between healthy myocardium and scar amounting to +0.208, and of +0.151 between blood and scar. For the conventional PSIR sequence, the reference image at even heartbeats (low flip-angle) exhibited high values of expected magnetization M_z/M_0, varying in the intervals 0.807–0.858, 0.877–0.919 and 0.951–0.967, for healthy viable myocardium, blood, and scar tissue, respectively. Conversely, even heartbeats of the BOOST

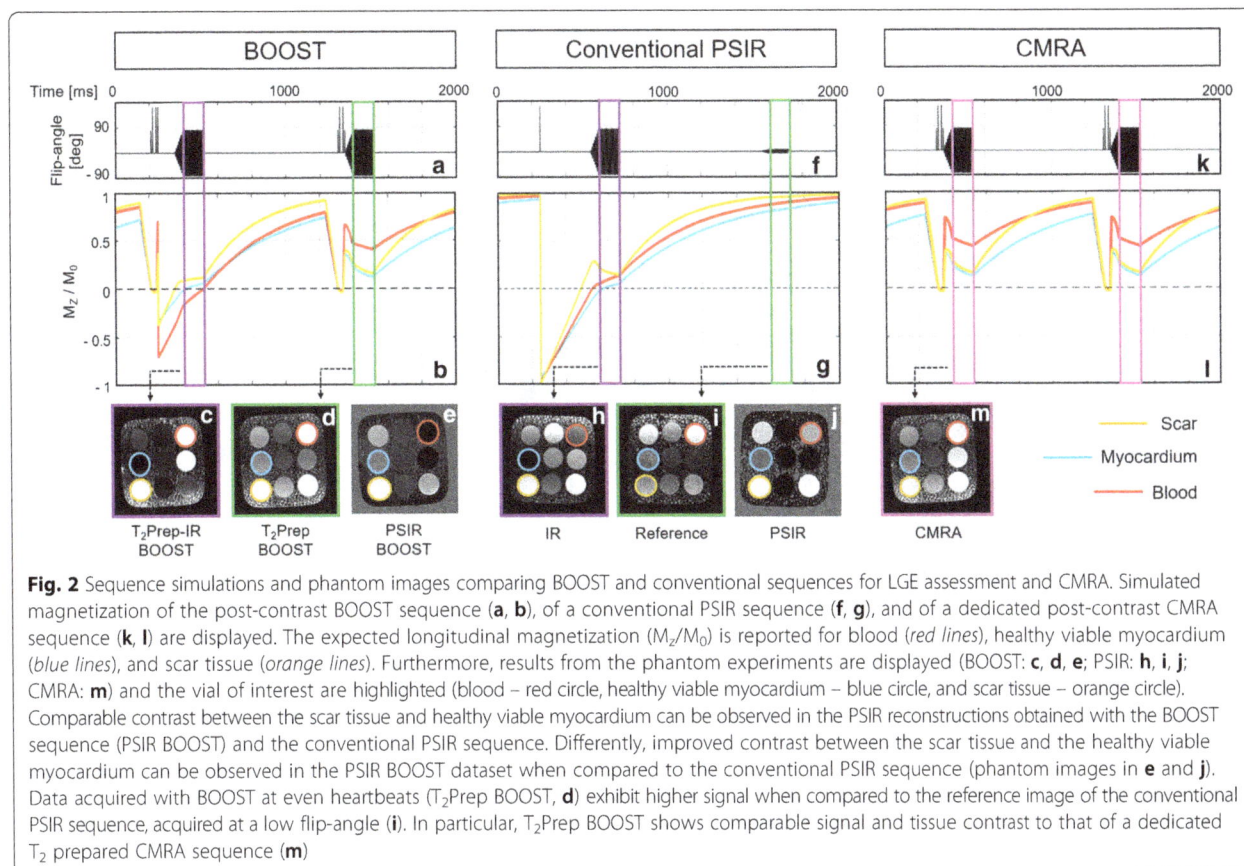

Fig. 2 Sequence simulations and phantom images comparing BOOST and conventional sequences for LGE assessment and CMRA. Simulated magnetization of the post-contrast BOOST sequence (**a**, **b**), of a conventional PSIR sequence (**f**, **g**), and of a dedicated post-contrast CMRA sequence (**k**, **l**) are displayed. The expected longitudinal magnetization (M_z/M_0) is reported for blood (*red lines*), healthy viable myocardium (*blue lines*), and scar tissue (*orange lines*). Furthermore, results from the phantom experiments are displayed (BOOST: **c**, **d**, **e**; PSIR: **h**, **i**, **j**; CMRA: **m**) and the vial of interest are highlighted (blood – red circle, healthy viable myocardium – blue circle, and scar tissue – orange circle). Comparable contrast between the scar tissue and healthy viable myocardium can be observed in the PSIR reconstructions obtained with the BOOST sequence (PSIR BOOST) and the conventional PSIR sequence. Differently, improved contrast between the scar tissue and the healthy viable myocardium can be observed in the PSIR BOOST dataset when compared to the conventional PSIR sequence (phantom images in **e** and **j**). Data acquired with BOOST at even heartbeats (T$_2$Prep BOOST, **d**) exhibit higher signal when compared to the reference image of the conventional PSIR sequence, acquired at a low flip-angle (**i**). In particular, T$_2$Prep BOOST shows comparable signal and tissue contrast to that of a dedicated T$_2$ prepared CMRA sequence (**m**)

sequence (T$_2$Prep BOOST) exhibited reduced expected magnetization M_z/M_0 for the tissues of interest, since data acquisition is performed with higher flip-angle and is preceded by a T$_2$Prep. Specifically, the expected magnetization M_z/M_0 of healthy viable myocardium, blood and scar varied within the intervals 0.230–0.123, 0.490–0.420 and 0.267–0.167, respectively. This resulted in a blood/myocardium ratio of 2.13, which is adequate for anatomy and coronary lumen visualization. Similarly, for the conventional post-contrast CMRA sequence, the expected magnetization M_z/M_0 of healthy viable myocardium, blood and scar varied within the intervals 0.220–0.100, 0.498–0.438, and 0.267–0.161, respectively, leading to a blood/myocardium ratio equal to 2.26.

Phantom experiments

Phantom images obtained with the proposed post-contrast BOOST sequence, the conventional PSIR sequence [16], and the dedicated post-contrast CMRA acquisition are shown in Fig. 2. ROIs corresponding to post-contrast blood, healthy viable myocardium, and scar are indicated by red, blue and yellow circles, respectively. All the endpoints that were quantified for the phantom acquisitions are summarized in the Additional file 1. The T$_2$Prep-IR BOOST phantom dataset showed strong signal from both blood and scar tissue, while providing suppression of the signal belonging

to the vial mimicking the viable myocardium. The magnitude image of the conventional PSIR acquisition showed effective suppression of signal from the viable myocardium, and high signal from the vial mimicking the scar. The reference image T$_2$Prep BOOST, designed for the visualization of the heart anatomy, great vessels, and coronary lumen, showed SNR$_{blood}$ and CNR$_{blood-myo}$ comparable to those provided by the dedicated CMRA acquisition. Conversely, the reference image of the conventional PSIR acquisition (acquired at a low flip angle) showed reduced SNR$_{blood}$ and CNR$_{blood-myo}$. The PSIR reconstructions obtained using the BOOST sequence with and without normalization are displayed in Fig. 3. Reduced tissue contrast is observed for the PSIR reconstruction with intensity normalization. Conversely, tissue contrast was restored in the PSIR reconstruction without intensity normalization. The PSIR BOOST phantom dataset (obtained without intensity normalization) showed effective blood signal suppression, leading to improved CNR$_{scar-blood}$ when compared to the more conventional PSIR sequence.

In-vivo experiments

Quantitative and qualitative data analysis was performed for 12 of 18 patients for whom BOOST data acquisition started less than 40 min after contrast agent injection. The average time after injection for the BOOST datasets

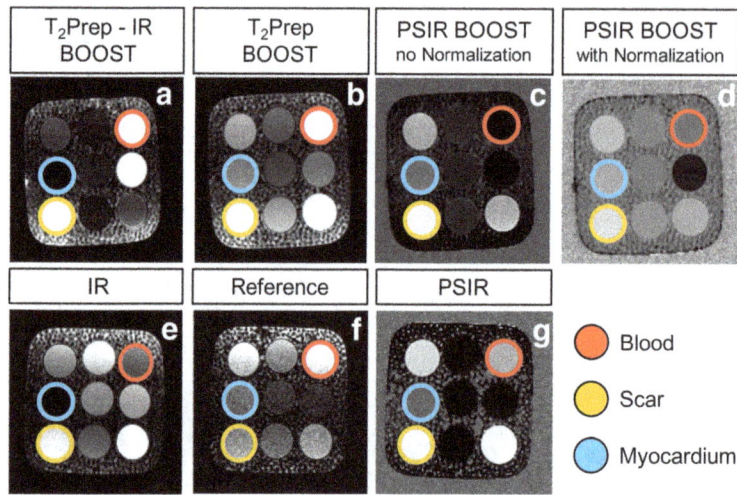

Fig. 3 Phantom images obtained with the BOOST and the conventional PSIR sequence. Imaging data were acquired by nulling the signal from the healthy viable myocardium (*blue vial*) in the magnitude images (**a**, **e**). Differently from **f**, the T$_2$Prep BOOST dataset, acquired at a high flip-angle, exhibits both high signal from the blood (*red vial*) and pronounced contrast between blood and healthy viable myocardium (**b**). The PSIR reconstruction obtained with BOOST and using intensity normalization (**d**) shows reduced tissue contrast, which is restored once intensity normalization is not applied (**c**). Furthermore, such restored contrast between the scar tissue (*orange vial*) and the healthy viable myocardium is comparable to that of the PSIR reconstruction in (**g**), while improved contrast between scar and blood can be appreciated

was 27:47 ± 3:35 min. Among those patients, the acquisition of the clinical 2D PSIR sequence and of the clinical 3D whole-heart CMRA with diaphragmatic navigator was performed in 10 and 6 cases, respectively. Clinical, imaging, and demographic characteristics are summarized in Table 1. Acquisition times were 7:48 ± 4:03 min for the clinical 2D PSIR sequence (including pauses between breath-holds), 13:06 ± 3:05 min for the conventional CMRA acquisition with diaphragmatic navigator (with an average scan efficiency of ~ 47%), and 12:07 ± 1:56 min for data acquisition with BOOST that provides both black-blood LGE and bright-blood anatomical images. For the BOOST sequence, image-based navigation enabled data acquisition with 100% scan efficiency (i.e., none of the acquired data was discarded during image reconstruction) and predictable scan time. Furthermore, translational motion correction led to effective respiratory motion correction for both the bright-blood T$_2$Prep and the black-blood PSIR BOOST datasets in most cases, as shown in Fig. 4 for two representative patients.

Quantitative data analysis

The endpoints quantified for the conventional 2D PSIR sequence amounted to CNR$_{\text{blood-myo}}$ = 15.2 ± 8.1, CNR$_{\text{blood-scar}}$ = 4.1 ± 5.6 and CNR$_{\text{scar-myo}}$ = 12.3 ± 9.3. The black-blood PSIR BOOST datasets presented effective nulling of the blood signal, leading to significantly improved CNR$_{\text{blood-scar}}$ (equal to 15.8 ± 3.3, $P < 0.025$) and significantly reduced CNR$_{\text{blood-myo}}$ (4.2 ± 3.6, $P < 0.001$) when compared to the clinical 2D PSIR sequence (Fig. 5).

Quantified CNR$_{\text{scar-myo}}$ was equal to 13.02 ± 4.56 (P = NS in comparison to the clinical 2D PSIR sequence).

Qualitative data analysis

Eleven of 12 3D PSIR BOOST datasets were considered diagnostic, with an average grade of 1.75 ± 1.21; specifically, 8/12 cases were graded *1*, one single case was graded *2*, two cases – where incomplete blood suppression was observed – were graded *3*, and one single case was graded *4* due to the presence of residual motion and pronounced artefacts originating from the rigid translation of the chest wall and arms. Complete correspondence between clinical 2D PSIR acquisitions and 3D PSIR BOOST datasets was found in 8/10 cases in terms of LGE findings and location of the LGE uptake. In two individual cases (Patient 08 and Patient 10) LGE was not visible in the 3D PSIR BOOST dataset. Both datasets were graded *1*, meaning no residual artefacts were visible and optimal blood signal suppression was achieved. In these two cases, however, BOOST data acquisition started 39:57 min and 39:32 min after contrast injection, following a conventional 3D CMRA acquisition (duration 17:04 min and 11:31 min) that was performed between the 2D clinical PSIR and the 3D BOOST sequences. This particularly pronounced delay between the two LGE acquisitions, together with the absence of residual artefacts and the achievement of adequate blood signal suppression in the PSIR BOOST datasets, suggests that contrast agent washout prevented adequate scar depiction. Clinical 2D PSIR images were graded 1 for all the 10 patients where the sequence was acquired. No

Table 1 Summary of patients' data used for quantitative analysis

	Gender	Age (years)	Heartbeats per minute	Clinical Condition	LGE findings	3D whole heart CMRA
Patient 01	F	25	85	Atrial fibrillation	No	Yes
Patient 02	F	30	70	Atrial fibrillation (previous myocarditis)	No	No
Patient 03	F	48	70	Eosinophilic Granulomatous Polyangitis (Churg-Strauss syndrome)	No	No
Patient 04	M	50	80	Myocarditis	Yes Diffuse mid-wall	No
Patient 05	M	67	55	Myocardial infarction	Yes Transmural	No
Patient 06	M	56	65	Advanced Hypertensive heart disease	No (no 2D PSIR)	Yes
Patient 07	M	66	70	Myocardial infarction	Yes Transmural and subendocardial	No
Patient 08	M	62	80	Myocardial infarction	Yes Mid-wall	Yes
Patient 09	M	59	45	Myocardial infarction	Yes Subendocardial	Yes
Patient 10	F	30	75	Myocardial infarction	Yes Subendocardial	Yes
Patient 11	F	74	80	Myocardial infarction	Yes Transmural	No
Patient 12	M	52	75	Suspected myocardial infarction	No (no 2D PSIR)	Yes

Furthermore, the presence of LGE findings is stated ("no 2D PSIR" pertains the cases where 2D PSIR acquisition was not performed and presence of LGE uptake was assessed with BOOST only). In addition, it is indicated whether the acquisition of the conventional, 3D whole-heart CMRA sequence was performed or not

statistically significant difference was found in terms of visual grading (P = NS) when comparing the 3D PSIR BOOST datasets and the clinical 2D PSIR counterpart (average grade of BOOST in these 10 patients: 1.80 ± 1.31). In terms of coronary conspicuity, image quality scores evaluated by consensus grading were 1.50 ± 1.22 (LM), 2.00 ± 1.54 (LAD), 2.50 ± 1.64 (LCX) and 2.83 ± 1.16 (RCA) for the conventional CMRA with diaphragmatic navigator (6 patients, Table 1). A trend of improvement in terms of coronary delineation was quantified with BOOST in the same 6 patients; for those subjects, LM and LAD were graded 1 in all cases. For LCX and RCA, average grades were equal to 1.50 ± 1.22 and 1.50 ± 0.83, respectively. A visual comparison between T_2Prep BOOST datasets and conventional CMRA is shown in Fig. 6. Overall visual grading obtained with T_2Prep BOOST (considering the entire cohort of 12 patients, which includes cases where the acquisition of the conventional CMRA was not performed) was 1.07 ± 0.27 for the LM, 1.07 ± 0.27 for the LAD, 1.07 ± 0.27 for the LCX, and 1.53 ± 0.77 for the RCA.

Fusion of a bright-blood T_2Prep BOOST with a black-blood PSIR BOOST datasets (obtained with the Horos software, V1.1.7) is illustrated in Fig. 7 to demonstrate the location and transmurality of the infarct obtained from the black-blood PSIR dataset.

Discussion

In this study, we extended the use of a novel PSIR-like framework, referred to as BOOST, to post-contrast applications for simultaneous 1) black-blood LGE assessment and 2) bright-blood heart anatomy, great vessels, and coronary lumen visualization. With the BOOST framework, the acquisition of the magnitude image (T_2Prep-IR BOOST) is based on a T_2Prep-IR module for optimal contrast between the blood pool and scar tissue after PSIR computation (black-blood PSIR BOOST). Furthermore, the acquisition of the reference image (bright-blood T_2Prep BOOST) is performed with a high flip-angle and it is preceded by a T_2Prep module. This ensures adequate signal and tissue contrast for the visualization of heart anatomy, great vessels, and the coronary lumen. In contrast to previously published approaches providing a single bright-blood dataset for the simultaneous visualization of LGE and proximal coronary arteries [40], our framework generates two separate yet co-registered 3D volumes, each one being specifically designed and optimized for the visualization of the coronary lumen (bright-blood T_2Prep BOOST) and myocardial scar (black-blood PSIR BOOST).

Sequence simulations and phantom acquisitions showed that the proposed post-contrast PSIR BOOST dataset achieves improved scar-blood contrast when compared to

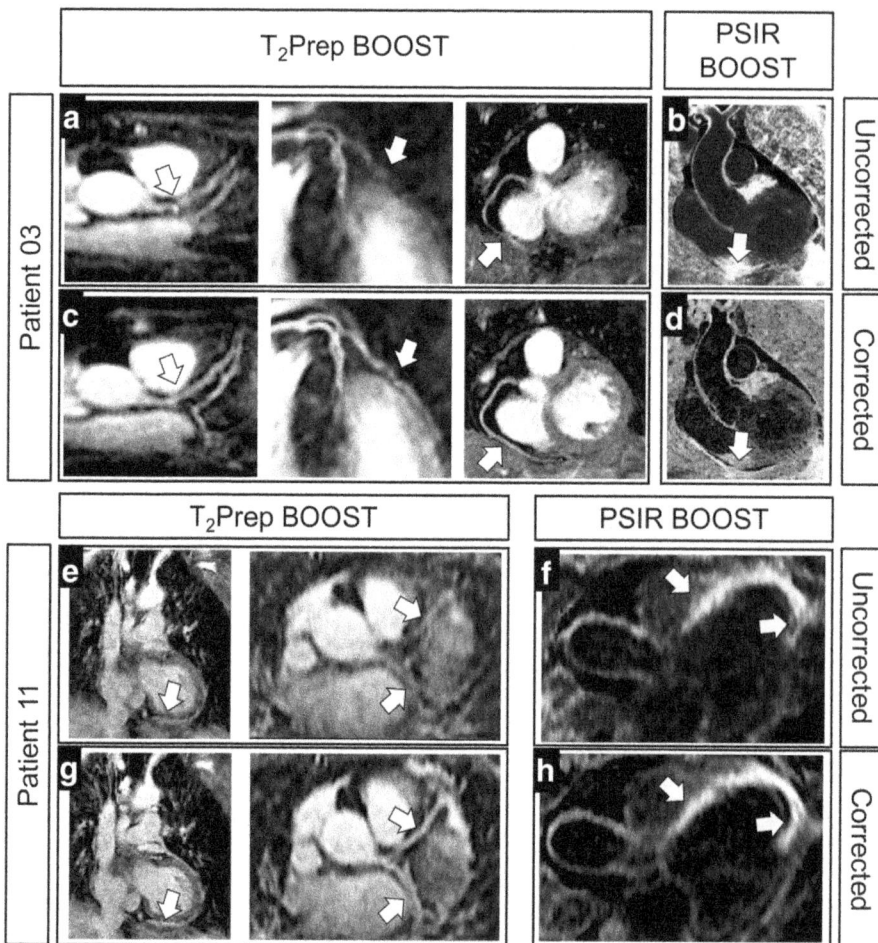

Fig. 4 Improvement in BOOST image quality after translational motion correction in two representative patients. The use of translational motion correction along the SI and RL directions reduces blurring artefacts and improves coronary vessel sharpness in the bright-blood T$_2$Prep BOOST datasets (arrows in **a**, **c**, **e**, and **g**). Motion compensation recovers also small details as showed in the zoomed images. Furthermore, improved image sharpness can be observed on the black-blood PSIR-like reconstructions (arrows in **b**, **d**, **f**, and **h**), where a sharper delineation of the LGE uptake can be appreciated following motion correction (**f** versus **h**)

a more conventional PSIR sequence for LGE imaging [16]; this was confirmed by in vivo measurements in patients. While the PSIR BOOST volume provided adequate LGE depiction in most of the patients with positive findings, phantom experiments indicate higher CNR$_{scar-myo}$ in the T$_2$Prep-IR BOOST datasets, where precise viable myocardial nulling is achieved; this can be qualitatively appreciated in vivo as shown in Fig. 5. As such, referring to the T$_2$Prep-IR BOOST dataset for the detection of subtle, non-ischemic, fibrosis patterns might be preferable; this aspect, however, needs further investigation and will be analyzed in future studies. Furthermore, sequence simulations show that the bright-blood T$_2$Prep BOOST dataset provides SNR$_{blood}$ and CNR$_{blood-myo}$ similar to those of a dedicated T$_2$-prepared post-contrast CMRA acquisition. In vivo acquisitions showed that respiratory motion corrected bright-blood T$_2$Prep BOOST datasets allowed visualization of the origin and the proximal course of the

coronary arteries (LM, LAD, LCX, and RCA) with high diagnostic quality. A trend of improvement was observed in comparison to the conventional CMRA; respiratory motion compensation performed with diaphragmatic navigator gating assumes a fixed linear correlation between the respiratory motion of the liver and that of the heart. The fixed correlation factor of 0.6 [37] that was used in this study might have been inexact for some of the subjects, thus leading to sub-optimal motion compensation. Conversely, with the use of image-based navigation, respiratory motion information can be directly extracted from the heart itself, thus avoiding the risk of imprecise approximations. In addition, with image-based navigation, it is possible to correct for movements along both SI and RL directions [27]. These aspects may have been a contributing factor of the improved coronary delineation that was obtained with BOOST. Furthermore, and as predicted by sequence simulations, the black-blood PSIR BOOST

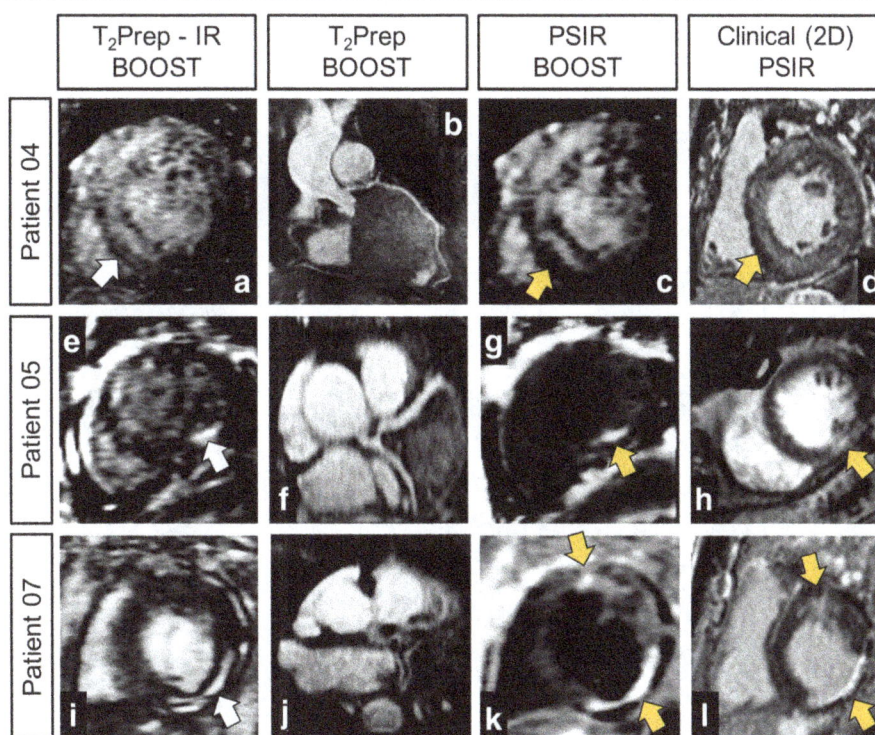

Fig. 5 Comparison between the proposed 3D whole-heart BOOST framework and the clinical 2D PSIR acquisition. Images in **a**, **e**, and **i** show the LGE uptake as depicted in the T$_2$Prep-IR BOOST datasets (*white arrows*), where signal from the blood pool is present and the viable myocardium is suppressed. Reformats in **b**, **f**, and **j** show the coronary reformats obtained from the 3D whole-heart bright-blood T$_2$Prep BOOST dataset. Complementary 3D black-blood LGE images obtained with BOOST are shown in **c**, **g**, and **k**. All the images from the T$_2$Prep-IR BOOST and the PSIR BOOST datasets were reformatted to match the orientation of the clinical 2D PSIR acquisitions (**d**, **h**, and **l**). The LGE uptake identified in both the T$_2$Prep-IR BOOST and PSIR BOOST datasets matches that of the clinical 2D PSIR acquisition. Furthermore, improved contrast between the scar tissue and the blood pool can be appreciated in the 3D PSIR BOOST datasets when compared to the 2D PSIR acquisition (**g**, **k** versus **h**, **l**, *orange arrows*). LGE uptake appears more shallow and blood pool signal is not entirely suppressed in Patient 04 with myocarditis (**c**, **d**, *orange arrows*), due to a longer TI

reconstruction provided visualization of LGE with diagnostic quality in most cases and significantly improved CNR$_{\text{scar-blood}}$ was quantified in comparison to clinical 2D PSIR acquisitions [16].

The PSIR reconstruction performed with the proposed framework exactly follows that described in [16], with the exception of the intensity normalization step that is conventionally performed at the end of the PSIR pipeline. In contrast to previously published post-contrast PSIR sequences [16], the reference image (T$_2$Prep BOOST) acquired in our approach exhibits high tissue contrast, thus preventing the application of surface coil intensity normalization. In fact, the presence of high tissue contrast in the reference image significantly alters the resulting contrast of the normalized PSIR reconstruction (Fig. 3). The use of surface coil intensity normalization is typically exploited to compensate for large variations in the intensity of the image caused by rapid fall-off of the surface-coil fields, thus improving the local tissue contrast. This was shown to be particularly beneficial for the visualization of subendocardial

infarcts, given the fact that the contrast between scar tissue and blood is particularly reduced in conventional PSIR acquisitions [16]. With this new sequence configuration, however, intrinsically enhanced contrast between blood and scar tissue is provided using a T$_2$Prep-IR module for the acquisition of the magnitude image; in addition, the use of pre-scan based normalization readily available on commercial scanners can be exploited to compensate for variations in signal intensity. This might alleviate the need for surface coil intensity normalization, however further validation may be needed to corroborate this point.

The integration of the framework with image-based navigation enabled data acquisition during free-breathing with 100% scan efficiency and predictable scan time. The acquisition time for BOOST (approximately 12 min) was similar to that of a conventional CMRA acquisition with diaphragmatic navigator (approximately 13 min), considering an average scan efficiency of 50% and 2× parallel imaging acceleration. The BOOST framework, however, provides both a bright- and black-

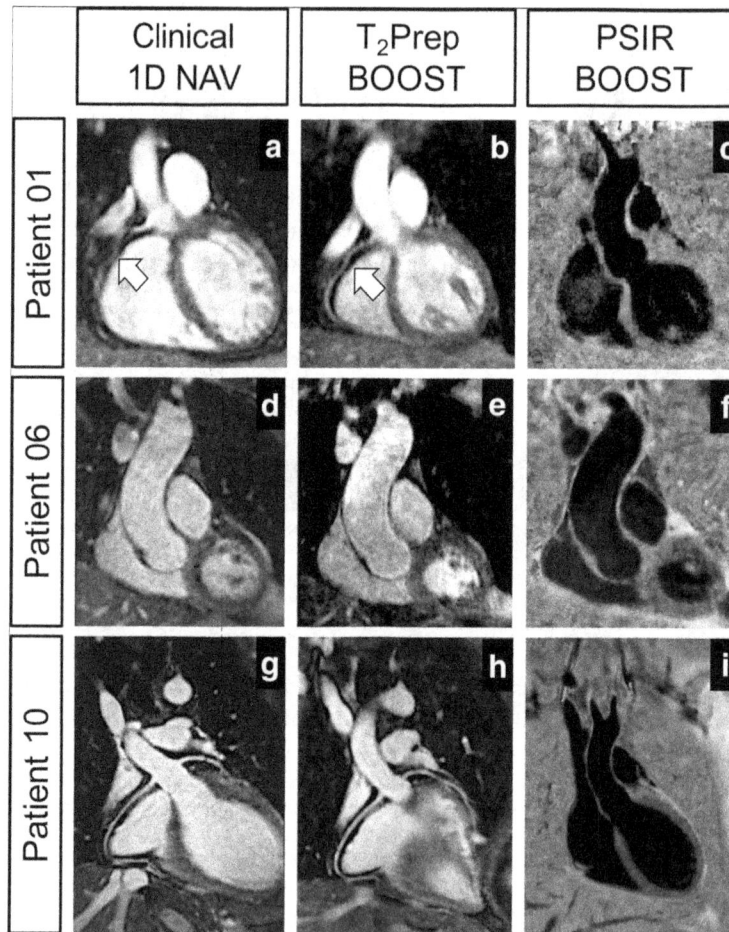

Fig. 6 Comparison between conventional 3D whole-heart acquisition with diaphragmatic navigator and the proposed bright-blood T$_2$Prep BOOST. Improved delineation of the RCA can be appreciated in Patient 01 with T$_2$Prep BOOST when compared to the conventional CMRA acquisition (arrows in **a**, **b**). Dilated aorta can be observed in Patient 06 due to the presence of hypertensive heart disease (**d**, **e**). Excellent coronary delineation was obtained with both sequences in Patient 10 (**g**, **h**). Furthermore, the complementary black-blood PSIR BOOST datasets for LGE assessment are shown in **c**, **f**, and **i**

blood dataset in the same acquisition time, whereas the overall acquisition of conventional CMRA and 2D PSIR sequences was about 20 min in our cohort of patients. This intrinsic efficiency of the BOOST framework holds potentials for reducing the scan time that is currently needed to perform a complete CMR examination. This might be particularly beneficial in the case of claustrophobic, anxious, or clinically unstable patients. Additionally, reducing the overall examination time would imply economic benefits and reduction of patients waiting lists. Future technical developments of the BOOST sequence will include the integration of acceleration techniques [36, 41, 42] to improve both the nominal acquisition time as well as the spatial resolution. Furthermore, improvements in the acquired spatial resolution might enable isotropic acquisitions that would, for instance, allow for more robust visualization of the mid and distal coronary arteries. Similarly, the achievement of higher

spatial resolution could benefit tissue characterization, allowing for a more accurate delineation of scar tissue and enabling a more accurate image fusion between the bright-blood T$_2$Prep BOOST and the black-blood PSIR BOOST datasets for the assessment of scar location and transmurality. Additionally, the framework will be integrated with algorithms for arrhythmia rejection that could further improve the image quality that was obtained in this study. Currently, BOOST is combined with image-based navigation enabling in-line translational motion correction along the SI and RL directions. However, the breathing pattern in patients is often more complex and involves translation, rotation, and non-rigid deformations [43–45]. Therefore, future technical developments will aim at combining the BOOST framework with strategies for non-rigid respiratory motion correction [46] that might be particularly beneficial in very sick patients who often have irregular

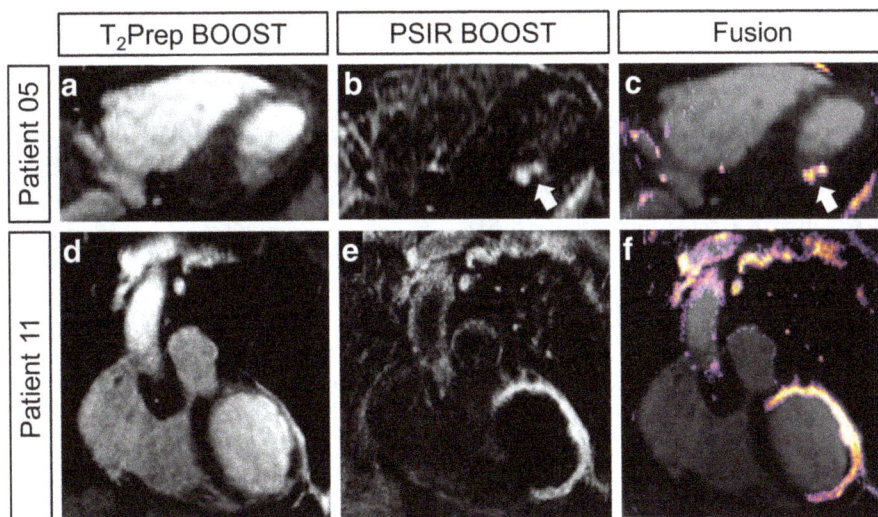

Fig. 7 Fusion of the bright-blood T$_2$Prep BOOST and the black blood PSIR BOOST datasets. Images correspond to two representative patients with positive LGE findings. Bright-blood images for visualization of the heart anatomy are shown in **a**, **d** (**T$_2$Prep-BOOST**). Complementary visualization of scar tissue (PSIR BOOST) is shown in **b**, **e**; these datasets could potentially be used for an easy scar segmentation, as unclear border between the surrounding tissues and the scar itself have disappeared. Fusion images, where the anatomical localization of the scar can be retrieved, are shown in **c**, **f**

breathing patterns [47]. In addition, the use of non-rigid respiratory motion correction may help to reduce ghosting artefacts that may originate from rigid translation of static tissues such as the chest wall and arms during the motion correction process. Similarly, a rigid registration between the T$_2$Prep-IR BOOST dataset and the T$_2$Prep BOOST dataset is currently performed prior PSIR computation to compensate for residual mis-registration errors; this may be also sub-optimal and the use of non-rigid registration could further improve the quality of the resulting PSIR BOOST dataset and additionally reduce the risk of phase errors that may originate in portions of the image where phases are not varying smoothly (e.g. in correspondence to the interface between different tissues).

In this study, the BOOST acquisition was performed at the end of a clinical CMR examination as it was considered unethical to potentially jeopardize the acquisition of conventional LGE data at the expense of a novel sequence at this stage. Injection timing was optimized to provide optimal contrast agent concentration during the acquisition of the clinical 2D PSIR sequences, thus providing suboptimal contrast conditions for the BOOST scan. This was noticed particularly in two specific cases (Patient 08 and Patient 10), where LGE uptake could not be depicted despite the absence of motion artefacts and the achievement of optimal blood signal suppression. Furthermore, as the BOOST acquisition was performed at the end of the clinical scan, there may have been more respiratory or heart-rate irregularities that might have had an additional detrimental effect on the image quality that was obtained with BOOST. However, scan time was

not prolonged by more than 15 min at most. Therefore, future studies are warranted to rigorously compare the proposed post-contrast 3D BOOST sequence and conventional 2D PSIR acquisitions by, for instance, randomizing the order of the two acquisitions and by performing separate Gd injections to ensure equivalent contrast conditions. Kellman et al. [19] demonstrated that black-blood LGE provides improved conspicuity of subendocardial infarcts; future studies will aim at investigating the accuracy of black-blood PSIR BOOST for the quantification of scar transmurality and, thus, regional viability assessment. Furthermore, accuracy in the detection and quantification of ischaemic scar will be validated. Similarly, further clinical validation of BOOST is needed in comparison to conventional CMRA in patients with angiographically confirmed coronary artery disease.

The improved contrast between blood pool and scar provided by the proposed black-blood PSIR BOOST images may facilitate scar segmentation. However, the nulling of the blood and viable myocardium signal reduces the depiction of the heart anatomy and might challenge the localization of the scar itself. This challenge can be addressed by fusing the co-registered black blood PSIR dataset with the bright blood whole heart dataset, which then allows both scar and myocardial anatomy visualization as shown in Fig. 7. This characteristic makes this framework particularly suitable for the planning of electrophysiology procedures. Similarly, the framework may be beneficial for the visualization of lesions after ablation and follow-up of patients. This further enlarges the spectrum of potential clinical applications of post-contrast

BOOST, that will be tested in dedicated studies in the upcoming future.

Conclusions

We demonstrated the feasibility of simultaneous black-blood LGE imaging and bright-blood visualization of cardiac anatomy, the great vessels, and the coronary artery lumen using a novel motion corrected multi-contrast 3D imaging sequence, referred to as BOOST. Data acquisition with BOOST was performed in free-breathing and ensures whole-heart coverage, 100% scan efficiency, and predictable scan time. The framework was validated in a group of cardiac patients and showed high quality depiction of the coronary arteries in comparison to standard CMRA and good agreement with 2D PSIR LGE scar visualization. This novel sequence has a broad spectrum of potential clinical applications.

Abbreviations

BOOST: Bright-blood and black-blood phase sensitive inversion recovery; bSSFP: Balanced steady state free precession; CMR: Cardiovascular magnetic resonance; CMRA: Coronary magnetic resonance angiography; CNR: Contrast to noise; EPG: Extended phase graph (simulation); FOV: Field of view; Gd: Gadolinium; GRAPPA: Generalized autocalibrating partially parallel acquisition; iNAV: Image-based navigator; IR: Inversion recovery; LAD: Left anterior descending coronary artery; LCX: Left circumflex coronary artery.; LGE: Late gadolinium enhancement; LM: Left main coronary artery; PSIR: Phase-sensitive inversion recovery; RCA: Right coronary artery; ROI: Region of interest; SNR: Signal to noise; T_2Prep: T_2-prepared; T_2Prep-IR: T_2-prepared inversion recovery\; TE: Echo time; TI: Inversion time; TR: Repetition time

Acknowledgements

The views expressed are those of the authors and not necessarily those of the National Health Service, the National Institute for Health Research, or the Department of Health.

Funding

This work was supported by the following grants: 1) EPSRC EP/N009258/1, EP/P001009/1, EP/P007619/1, MRC MR/L009676/1, and FONDECYT N° 1161051, 2) the Wellcome EPSRC Centre for Medical Engineering at King's College London (WT 203148/Z/16/Z) and 3) the Department of Health via the National Institute for Health Research (NIHR) comprehensive Biomedical Research Centre award to Guy's & St Thomas' NHS Foundation Trust in partnership with King's College London and King's College Hospital NHS Foundation Trust.

Authors' contributions

GG, RN, RMB, and CP designed the study. GG and RN implemented the acquisition and reconstruction framework on the scanner software. GG performed sequence simulations and phantom experiments. GG, IR, and TFI performed the data analysis. All the authors contributed to the acquisition of clinical research data. All the authors participated in drafting and revising the manuscript, and read and approved its final version.

Consent for publication

All the subjects provided written informed consent for the publication of accompanying images in this manuscript. The consent forms are held in the patients' clinical notes and are available to the Editor-in-Chief upon request.

Competing interests

R.N. is employed by Siemens Healthcare Limited. All the other Authors declare that they do not have competing interests.

Author details

[1]School of Biomedical Engineering and Imaging Sciences, King's College London, St Thomas' Hospital (Lambeth Wing), Westminster Bridge Rd, London SE1 7EH, UK. [2]MR Research Collaborations, Siemens Healthcare Limited, Sir William Siemens Square Frimley, Camberley GU16 8QD, UK. [3]Escuela de Ingeniería, Pontificia Universidad Católica de Chile, Vicuna Mackenna, 4860 Santiago, Chile.

References

1. Kim RJ, Fieno DS, Parrish TB, Harris K, Chen EL, Simonetti O, Bundy J, Finn JP, Klocke FJ, Judd RM. Relationship of MRI delayed contrast enhancement to irreversible injury, infarct age, and contractile function. Circulation. 1999; 100:1992–2002.
2. Fieno DS, Kim RJ, Chen EL, Lomasney JW, Klocke FJ, Judd RM. Contrast-enhanced magnetic resonance imaging of myocardium at risk: distinction between reversible and irreversible injury throughout infarct healing. J Am Coll Cardiol. 2000;36:1985–91.
3. Friedrich MG, Strohm O, Schulz-Menger J, Marciniak H, Luft FC, Dietz R. Contrast media-enhanced magnetic resonance imaging visualizes myocardial changes in the course of viral myocarditis. Circulation. 1998;97:1802–9.
4. Abdel-Aty H, Boye P, Zagrosek A, Wassmuth R, Kumar A, Messroghli D, Bock P, Dietz R, Friedrich MG, Schulz-Menger J. Diagnostic performance of cardiovascular magnetic resonance in patients with suspected acute myocarditis: comparison of different approaches. J Am Coll Cardiol. 2005; 45:1815–22.
5. Friedrich MG, Sechtem U, Schulz-Menger J, Holmvang G, Alakija P, Cooper LT, White JA, Abdel-Aty H, Gutberlet M, Prasad S, et al. Cardiovascular magnetic resonance in myocarditis: a JACC white paper. J Am Coll Cardiol. 2009;53:1475–87.
6. Lardo AC, McVeigh ER, Jumrussirikul P, Berger RD, Calkins H, Lima J, Halperin HR. Visualization and temporal/spatial characterization of cardiac radiofrequency ablation lesions using magnetic resonance imaging. Circulation. 2000;102:698–705.
7. Dickfeld T, Kato R, Zviman M, Lai S, Meininger G, Lardo AC, Roguin A, Blumke D, Berger R, Calkins H, Halperin H. Characterization of radiofrequency ablation lesions with gadolinium-enhanced cardiovascular magnetic resonance imaging. J Am Coll Cardiol. 2006;47:370–8.
8. Vergara GR, Marrouche NF. Tailored management of atrial fibrillation using a LGE-MRI based model: from the clinic to the electrophysiology laboratory. J Cardiovasc Electrophysiol. 2011;22:481–7.
9. Hunold P, Schlosser T, Vogt FM, Eggebrecht H, Schmermund A, Bruder O, Schuler WO, Barkhausen J. Myocardial late enhancement in contrast-enhanced cardiac MRI: distinction between infarction scar and non-infarction-related disease. AJR Am J Roentgenol. 2005;184:1420–6.
10. Bohl S, Wassmuth R, Abdel-Aty H, Rudolph A, Messroghli D, Dietz R, Schulz-Menger J. Delayed enhancement cardiac magnetic resonance imaging reveals typical patterns of myocardial injury in patients with various forms of non-ischemic heart disease. Int J Cardiovasc Imaging. 2008;24:597–607.
11. Ismail TF, Prasad SK, Pennell DJ. Prognostic importance of late gadolinium enhancement cardiovascular magnetic resonance in cardiomyopathy. Heart. 2012;98:438–42.
12. Gulati A, Jabbour A, Ismail TF, Guha K, Khwaja J, Raza S, Morarji K, Brown TD, Ismail NA, Dweck MR, et al. Association of fibrosis with mortality and sudden cardiac death in patients with nonischemic dilated cardiomyopathy. JAMA. 2013;309:896–908.
13. Simonetti OP, Kim RJ, Fieno DS, Hillenbrand HB, Wu E, Bundy JM, Finn JP, Judd RM. An improved MR imaging technique for the visualization of myocardial infarction. Radiology. 2001;218:215–23.
14. Kim RJ, Wu E, Rafael A, Chen EL, Parker MA, Simonetti O, Klocke FJ, Bonow RO, Judd RM. The use of contrast-enhanced magnetic resonance imaging to identify reversible myocardial dysfunction. N Engl J Med. 2000;343:1445–53.
15. Rutz T, Piccini D, Coppo S, Chaptinel J, Ginami G, Vincenti G, Stuber M, Schwitter J. Improved border sharpness of post-infarct scar by a novel self-navigated free-breathing high-resolution 3D whole-heart inversion recovery magnetic resonance approach. Int J Cardiovasc Imaging. 2016;32:1735–44.

16. Kellman P, Arai AE, McVeigh ER, Aletras AH. Phase-sensitive inversion recovery for detecting myocardial infarction using gadolinium-delayed hyperenhancement. Magn Reson Med. 2002;47:372–83.

17. Yamashita S, Sacher F, Mahida S, Berte B, Lim HS, Komatsu Y, Amraoui S, Denis A, Derval N, Laurent F, et al. Image integration to guide catheter ablation in scar-related ventricular tachycardia. J Cardiovasc Electrophysiol. 2016;27:699–708.

18. Kurzendorfer T, Forman C, Schmidt M, Tillmanns C, Maier A, Brost A. Fully automatic segmentation of left ventricular anatomy in 3-D LGE-MRI. Comput Med Imaging Graph. 2017;59:13–27.

19. Kellman P, Xue H, Olivieri LJ, Cross RR, Grant EK, Fontana M, Ugander M, Moon JC, Hansen MS. Dark blood late enhancement imaging. J Cardiovasc Magn Reson. 2016;18:77.

20. Liu CY, Wieben O, Brittain JH, Reeder SB. Improved delayed enhanced myocardial imaging with T2-prep inversion recovery magnetization preparation. J Magn Reson Imaging. 2008;28:1280–6.

21. Basha TA, Tang MC, Tsao C, Tschabrunn CM, Anter E, Manning WJ, Nezafat R. Improved dark blood late gadolinium enhancement (DB-LGE) imaging using an optimized jointinversion preparation and T2 magnetization preparation. Magn Reson Med. 2017. doi:10.1002/mrm.26692. [Epub ahead of print].

22. Kino A, Zuehlsdorff S, Sheehan JJ, Weale PJ, Carroll TJ, Jerecic R, Carr JC. Three-dimensional phase-sensitive inversion-recovery turbo FLASH sequence for the evaluation of left ventricular myocardial scar. AJR Am J Roentgenol. 2009;193:W381–8.

23. Kido T, Kido T, Nakamura M, Kawaguchi N, Nishiyama Y, Ogimoto A, Miyagawa M, Mochizuki T. Three-dimensional phase-sensitive inversion recovery sequencing in the evaluation of left ventricular myocardial scars in ischemic and non-ischemic cardiomyopathy: comparison to three-dimensional inversion recovery sequencing. Eur J Radiol. 2014;83:2159–66.

24. Ehman RL, Felmlee JP. Adaptive technique for high-definition MR imaging of moving structures. Radiology. 1989;173:255–63.

25. Keegan J, Drivas P, Firmin DN. Navigator artifact reduction in three-dimensional late gadolinium enhancement imaging of the atria. Magn Reson Med. 2014;72:779–85.

26. Ginami G, Neji R, Phinikaridou A, Whitaker J, Botnar RM, Prieto C. Simultaneous bright- and black-blood whole-heart MRI for noncontrast enhanced coronary lumen and thrombus visualization. Magn Reson Med. 2017. doi:10.1002/mrm.26815. [Epub ahead of print].

27. Henningsson M, Koken P, Stehning C, Razavi R, Prieto C, Botnar RM. Whole-heart coronary MR angiography with 2D self-navigated image reconstruction. Magn Reson Med. 2012;67:437–45.

28. Prieto C, Doneva M, Usman M, Henningsson M, Greil G, Schaeffter T, Botnar RM. Highly efficient respiratory motion compensated free-breathing coronary MRA using golden-step Cartesian acquisition. J Magn Reson Imaging. 2015;41:738–46.

29. Sussman MS, Wright GA. Factors affecting the correlation coefficient template matching algorithm with application to real-time 2-D coronary artery MR imaging. IEEE Trans Med Imaging. 2003;22:206–16.

30. Piccini D, Bonanno G, Ginami G, Littmann A, Zenge MO, Stuber M. Is there an optimal respiratory reference position for self-navigated whole-heart coronary MR angiography? J Magn Reson Imaging. 2016;43:426–33.

31. Weigel M. Extended phase graphs: dephasing, RF pulses, and echoes - pure and simple. J Magn Reson Imaging. 2015;41:266–95.

32. Kim WY, Danias PG, Stuber M, Flamm SD, Plein S, Nagel E, Langerak SE, Weber OM, Pedersen EM, Schmidt M, et al. Coronary magnetic resonance angiography for the detection of coronary stenoses. N Engl J Med. 2001; 345:1863–9.

33. Captur G, Gatehouse P, Keenan KE, Heslinga FG, Bruehl R, Prothmann M, Graves MJ, Eames RJ, Torlasco C, Benedetti G, et al. A medical device-grade T1 and ECV phantom for global T1 mapping quality assurance-the T1 mapping and ECV standardization in cardiovascular magnetic resonance (T1MES) program. J Cardiovasc Magn Reson. 2016;18:58.

34. Messroghli DR, Walters K, Plein S, Sparrow P, Friedrich MG, Ridgway JP, Sivananthan MU. Myocardial T1 mapping: application to patients with acute and chronic myocardial infarction. Magn Reson Med. 2007;58:34–40.

35. De Wilde JP, Lunt JA, Straughan K. Information in magnetic resonance images: evaluation of signal, noise and contrast. Med Biol Eng Comput. 1997;35:259–65.

36. Griswold MA, Jakob PM, Heidemann RM, Nittka M, Jellus V, Wang J, Kiefer B, Haase A. Generalized autocalibrating partially parallel acquisitions (GRAPPA). Magn Reson Med. 2002;47:1202–10.

37. Wang Y, Riederer SJ, Ehman RL. Respiratory motion of the heart: kinematics and the implications for the spatial resolution in coronary imaging. Magn Reson Med. 1995;33:713–9.

38. Amano Y, Onda M, Amano M, Kumazaki T. Magnetic resonance imaging of myelofibrosis. STIR and gadolinium-enhanced MR images. Clin Imaging. 1997;21:264–8.

39. Haase A, Frahm J, Hanicke W, Matthaei D. 1H NMR chemical shift selective (CHESS) imaging. Phys Med Biol. 1985;30:341–4.

40. Amano Y, Kiriyama T, Kobayashi Y, Tachi M, Matsumura Y, Kumita S. Simultaneous assessment of myocardial scar and coronary arteries using navigator-gated 3-dimensional fat-suppressed delayed-enhancement MRI at 3.0 T: a technical feasibility study. J Comput Assist Tomogr. 2012;36:72–6.

41. Sodickson DK, Manning WJ. Simultaneous acquisition of spatial harmonics (SMASH): fast imaging with radiofrequency coil arrays. Magn Reson Med. 1997;38:591–603.

42. Lustig M, Donoho D, Pauly JM. Sparse MRI: the application of compressed sensing for rapid MR imaging. Magn Reson Med. 2007;58:1182–95.

43. Manke D, Nehrke K, Bornert P, Rosch P, Dossel O. Respiratory motion in coronary magnetic resonance angiography: a comparison of different motion models. J Magn Reson Imaging. 2002;15:661–71.

44. Manke D, Nehrke K, Bornert P. Novel prospective respiratory motion correction approach for free-breathing coronary MR angiography using a patient-adapted affine motion model. Magn Reson Med. 2003;50:122–31.

45. Shechter G, Ozturk C, Resar JR, McVeigh ER. Respiratory motion of the heart from free breathing coronary angiograms. IEEE Trans Med Imaging. 2004;23: 1046–56.

46. Cruz G, Atkinson D, Henningsson M, Botnar RM, Prieto C. Highly efficient nonrigid motion-corrected 3D whole-heart coronary vessel wall imaging. Magn Reson Med. 2016; 10.1002/mrm.26274.

47. Ginami G, Bonanno G, Schwitter J, Stuber M, Piccini D. An iterative approach to respiratory self-navigated whole-heart coronary MRA significantly improves image quality in a preliminary patient study. Magn Reson Med. 2016;75:1594–604.

Ferumoxytol enhanced black-blood cardiovascular magnetic resonance imaging

Kim-Lien Nguyen[1,2,3], Eun-Ah Park[1,4], Takegawa Yoshida[1], Peng Hu[1,3] and J. Paul Finn[1,3*]

Abstract

Background: Bright-blood and black-blood cardiovascular magnetic resonance (CMR) techniques are frequently employed together during a clinical exam because of their complementary features. While valuable, existing black-blood CMR approaches are flow dependent and prone to failure. We aim to assess the effectiveness and reliability of ferumoxytol enhanced (FE) Half-Fourier Single-shot Turbo Spin-echo (HASTE) imaging without magnetization preparation pulses to yield uniform intra-luminal blood signal suppression by comparing FE-HASTE with pre-ferumoxytol HASTE imaging.

Methods: This study was IRB-approved and HIPAA compliant. Consecutive patients who were referred for FE-CMR between June 2013 and February 2017 were enrolled. Qualitative image scores reflecting the degree and reliability of blood signal suppression were based on a 3-point Likert scale, with 3 reflecting perfect suppression. For quantitative evaluation, homogeneity indices (defined as standard deviation of the left atrial signal intensity) and signal-to-noise ratios (SNR) for vascular lumens and cardiac chambers were measured.

Results: Of the 340 unique patients who underwent FE-CMR, HASTE was performed in 257. Ninety-three patients had both pre-ferumoxytol HASTE and FE-HASTE, and were included in this analysis. Qualitative image scores reflecting the degree and reliability of blood signal suppression were significantly higher for FE-HASTE images (2.9 [IQR 2.8–3.0] vs 1.8 [IQR 1.6–2.1], $p < 0.001$). Inter-reader agreement was moderate (k = 0.50, 95% CI 0.45–0.55). Blood signal suppression was more complete on FE-HASTE images than on pre-ferumoxytol HASTE, as indicated by lower mean homogeneity indices (24.5 [IQR 18.0–32.8] vs 108.0 [IQR 65.0–170.4], $p < 0.001$) and lower blood pool SNR for all regions (5.6 [IQR 3.2–10.0] vs 21.5 [IQR 12.5–39.4], $p < 0.001$).

Conclusion: FE-HASTE black-blood imaging offers an effective, reliable, and simple approach for flow independent blood signal suppression. The technique holds promise as a fast and routine complement to bright-blood cardiovascular imaging with ferumoxytol.

Keywords: USPIO, Ferumoxytol, Magnetic resonance imaging, Black-blood imaging, HASTE

Background

Black-blood cardiovascular magnetic resonance (CMR) imaging is important for depiction of vessel wall and intra-cardiac abnormalities. While the intensity and uniformity of luminal enhancement serve as the benchmark for bright blood CMR angiography, the completeness and uniformity of blood pool signal suppression set the complementary standard for black-blood imaging. A variety of strategies have been employed to suppress the blood signal [1], but most are to some degree flow dependent [2]. As a result, slow or inconsistent blood flow can result in persistence of signal within a patent vessel or cardiac chamber, mimicking a mass or thrombus.

Because of its speed, simplicity, and resistance to motion artifact, Half-Fourier Single-shot Turbo Spin-echo (HASTE) [3] imaging is widely used to complement bright blood techniques in CMR imaging [1]. The long echo train of HASTE (and related multi-echo spin echo techniques) supports efficient signal suppression for moderate to high velocity flow, but signal from slowly

* Correspondence: pfinn@mednet.ucla.edu
[1]Diagnostic Cardiovascular Imaging Laboratory, Department of Radiological Sciences, David Geffen School of Medicine at UCLA, Los Angeles, California, USA
[3]Physics and Biology in Medicine Interdepartmental Graduate Program, Department of Radiological Sciences, University of California at Los Angeles, Peter V. Ueberroth Building Suite 3371, 10945 Le Conte Ave, Los Angeles, CA 90095-7206, USA
Full list of author information is available at the end of the article

flowing blood can persist. For this reason, a dual inversion recovery magnetization preparation scheme is typically used to null the magnetization of blood which enters the imaging slice between the inversion and the readout [4]. Dual inversion recovery is effective as an adjunct for many black-blood applications and remains the most widely used scheme for black-blood conditioning of the great vessels and cardiac chambers. However, because of variable inflow speeds, electrocardiographic (ECG) gating with patient-specific adjustment of timing and imaging parameters may be necessary. Furthermore, for certain slice orientations and imaging parameters, timing conflicts within the cardiac cycle may undermine achievable image resolution or blood suppression, particularly in vessels with slow flow. Therefore, a flow-independent black-blood CMR technique would be desirable.

Recently, ferumoxytol has re-surfaced as an attractive CMR contrast agent [5, 6]. Although ferumoxytol is approved by the U.S. Food and Drug Administration (FDA) for intravenous treatment of iron deficiency anemia in adults with kidney disease, its pharmacokinetics and potent r_1 and r_2 effects ($r_1 = 15$ mM^{-1} s^{-1}, $r_2 = 89$ mM^{-1} s^{-1} at 1.5 T) [6, 7] can be exploited to support both bright blood angiography and flow independent, post-contrast black-blood imaging.

The purpose of our study is to evaluate the potential of ferumoxytol to generate reliable, flow independent, black-blood HASTE images, as a complement to bright-blood CMR angiography of the thorax, without the need for any magnetization preparation schemes, by comparing it with pre-ferumoxytol HASTE imaging.

Methods

Study population

This is a retrospective analysis of prospectively enrolled patients. All study procedures were approved by the local institutional review board and were compliant with the Health Insurance Portability and Accountability Act. Written informed consent was obtained from all patients or from their legal guardians. Consecutive patients age ≥ 3 years who were referred for ferumoxytol-enhanced (FE) magnetic resonance angiogram (MRA) from June 2013 to February 2017 and who had black-blood CMR were enrolled ($n = 257$). Figure 1 outlines the final patient population included in the analysis.

Image acquisition

Examinations were performed either on a 3 T (TIM Trio [$n = 161$], Prisma Fit [$n = 42$], Skyra [$n = 23$]; Siemens Healthineers, Erlangen, Germany) or a 1.5 T (Avanto [$n = 31$]; Siemens Healthineers) whole-body system. A combination of phased array body coils,

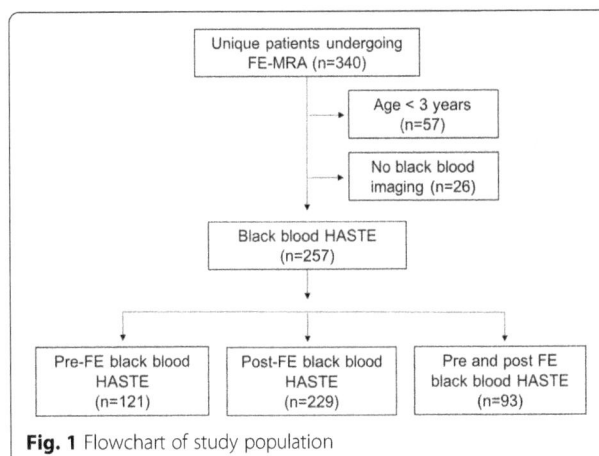

Fig. 1 Flowchart of study population

spine coils, head and neck coils or extremity coils were used depending on patient size.

Following initial localizer images, non-breath held HASTE images were acquired in the coronal plane [1, 8]. Typical acquisition parameters are outlined in Table 1. A dual inversion recovery, black blood magnetization preparation scheme was employed, but in most cases without ECG gating, such that the inflow time was not synchronized with or consistent within the cardiac cycle. The time between adjacent slice acquisitions (repetition time) was fixed at 3.0 s at 1.5 T and 4.0 s at 3 T. The reason for the longer than minimum repetition time was to allow for magnetization recovery within all tissues and to prevent cross talk and potential saturation between moving structures of adjacent slices. In one patient with a suspected left atrial mass on echocardiography, ECG gated pre-ferumoxytol HASTE imaging was performed in multiple planes, followed by post-ferumoxytol HASTE imaging. Typical slice thickness in adults was 7 mm at 1.5 T and 6 mm at 3 T. Stock ferumoxytol was diluted 6X –10X and administered as a slow infusion to a total dose of 4 mg /kg, as previously described [9]. Subsequently, breath-held, bright-blood, three-dimensional (3D) CMR

Table 1 Representative technical parameters for coronal HASTE

	3 Tesla	1.5 Tesla
Echo spacing (ms)	4.22	4.04
Echo time (ms)	68	51
Echo train length	123	98
Flip angle (°)	160	160
Bandwidth (Hz)	574	751
Acquisition matrix	512 × 374	512 × 358
Field of view (mm^2)	500 × 374	500 × 378
Slice thickness (mm)[a]	6	7
In-plane resolution (mm^2)	1.0 × 1.1	1.0 × 1.4

[a]For small children, the similar parameters were used with an effective slice thickness of 4 mm without interslice gaps

angiography was acquired during the steady state distribution of ferumoxytol. FE-HASTE images were acquired with identical parameters to the pre-ferumoxytol HASTE images, but without the dual inversion magnetization preparation scheme. All black-blood images were acquired during quiet breathing.

Image analysis

To qualitatively assess the effectiveness and reliability of blood signal suppression, two readers (T.Y. and E.A.P, each with 2 and 11 years of cardiovascular imaging experience, respectively) independently reviewed the pre-ferumoxytol and FE-HASTE images using a commercially available software platform (OsiriX, Pixmeo, Bernex, Switzerland). Images were de-identified and presented to reviewers in random order. The datasets were scored using a 3-point Likert grading scale: 3 = complete suppression of the blood signal within the vascular lumen on all slices; 2 = persistent, bright-blood signal within some part of the lumen on one or more slices; and 1 = persistent, bright-blood signal within a considerable part of the lumen on many or all slices. Ten cardiovascular regions within the chest cavity were scored: superior vena cava, both atria, both ventricles, the pulmonary trunk, the right and left pulmonary arteries, and the mid-ascending and mid-descending thoracic aorta. A final image quality score was calculated for each region by averaging the results of primary readers. In cases where the scores differed by 2 points between reader 1 and 2, a third reader (K.L.N., 5 years cardiovascular imaging experience) served as the consensus reader.

In patients with both pre-ferumoxytol and FE-HASTE images ($n = 93$), quantitative proxies of blood signal suppression were determined by calculating the signal-to-noise ratios (SNR) and generating a homogeneity index for each image dataset. Circular regions of interest (ROIs) measuring at least 1.0 cm^2 were drawn in the blood pool of the vascular lumen on coronal images. Coronal HASTE image datasets were chosen because 1) all 93 patients had at least coronal HASTE datasets and 2) the coronal datasets represent the orientation in which all of the cardiovascular ROIs were included. Ten representative vascular and intra-cardiac regions were scored: superior vena cava, both atria, both ventricles, pulmonary trunk, right and left pulmonary arteries, ascending aorta, and descending thoracic aorta. Image noise was determined by averaging the standard deviation of four ROIs drawn in the background air located within the image field of view. SNRs for each region were calculated by dividing signal intensities by image noise. The homogeneity index reflecting blood signal suppression was defined as the standard deviation of signal in the left atrium. Lower homogeneity indices reflect greater homogeneous suppression of blood signal in the

vascular lumen. The contrast-to-noise ratio (CNR) was calculated as the difference between the mean left ventricular signal intensity of the blood pool and myocardium divided by the standard deviation of noise in air.

Statistical analysis

Data were tested for normality using the D'Agostino-Pearson test and log transformed where needed. Descriptive statistics are expressed as means and standard deviations (SD) or medians and interquartiles (IQR) or as absolutes and percentages. The SNR for both HASTE datasets were compared using analysis of variance (ANOVA) for repeated measurements. Image noise and CNRs were compared using the Wilcoxon-signed rank sum test for paired samples. To evaluate for inter-reader agreement, a kappa (k) value was calculated for qualitative image scores: poor (k < 0.20), fair (k = 0.21–0.40), moderate (k = 0.41–0.60), good (k = 0.61–0.80), and excellent (k = 0.81–1.00). Analyses were performed using MedCalc (Version 16.8.4, Belgium). Two-tailed p values less than 0.05 were considered statistically significant and Bonferroni corrected where appropriate.

Results

Of the 340 patients who underwent FE-CMR between June 2013 to February 2017, a total of 257 patients (age 49 [IQR 16–67] years, 46% females) were ≥3 years old and had black-blood HASTE imaging. Ninety-three patients had both pre-ferumoxytol and FE-HASTE imaging. Characterization of the study population and clinical indications are outlined in Fig. 1 and Table 2, respectively. All studies were completed successfully and without major adverse events.

Qualitative analysis

Compared to pre-ferumoxytol HASTE, the image quality scores reflecting effectiveness and reliability of blood signal suppression for FE-HASTE images were significantly higher ($p < 0.001$, Fig. 2). Using a 3-point Likert scale with grade 3 representing complete and uniform blood signal suppression, FE- HASTE images had an overall image quality score of 2.9 (IQR 2.8–3.0). The overall image quality score for pre-ferumoxytol HASTE was 1.8 (IQR 1.6–2.1). Inter-reader agreement was moderate (k = 0.50, 95% CI 0.45–0.55).

Figures 3 and 4 provide comparative multislice examples of pre-ferumoxytol HASTE and FE-HASTE images. Both patients in Figs. 3 and 4 have critical aortic stenosis and had FE-CMR in the setting of renal impairment. Pre-ferumoxytol HASTE images (Fig. 3 and Fig. 4, upper panel, a-c) show incomplete and variable luminal signal suppression across all three coronal slices. In contrast, FE-HASTE images (Fig. 3 and Fig. 4, lower panel, a-c) demonstrate uniform and complete luminal blood signal

Table 2 Patient characteristics and clinical indications[a]

	All with HASTE (n = 257)	Pre-FE HASTE (n = 121)	Post-FE HASTE (n = 229)	Pre- and post-FE HASTE (n = 93)
Age, y	49 (16–67)	39 (13–65)	48 (16–67)	44 (16–67)
Gender (female)	118 (46%)	52 (43%)	95 (41%)	40 (43%)
Pre-CMR creatinine (mg/dL)	1.9 (1.2–2.9)	1.9 (1.0–3.0)	1.9 (0.99–2.8)	1.7 (0.95–2.85)
Clinical indications				
Aneurysm /dissection	18 (8%)	6 (5%)	18 (8%)	6 (6%)
AVMs	2 (1%)	0	2 (1%)	0
CHD	40 (16%)	15 (12%)	36 (16%)	11 (12%)
Embolus /thrombus	15 (6%)	7 (6%)	14 (6%)	6 (6%)
Interventional planning	28 (11%)	16 (13%)	26 (11%)	14 (15%)
Mass	19 (7%)	13 (11%)	19 (8%)	13 (14%)
Other	10 (4%)	4 (3%)	9 (4%)	3 (3%)
Placenta	4 (2%)	4 (3%)	4 (2%)	4 (4%)
Post-renal transplant	21 (8%)	12 (10%)	20 (9%)	11 (12%)
Pre-renal transplant	12 (5%)	6 (5%)	8 (3%)	2 (2%)
Vascular mapping	22 (9%)	12 (10%)	14 (6%)	4 (4%)
Vascular thrombosis	66 (26%)	26 (21%)	59 (26%)	19 (20%)

AVMs arteriovenous malformations, CHD congenital heart disease, CKD chronic kidney disease, eGFR estimated glomerular filtration rate, FE ferumoxytol enhanced, y years
[a]Values are reported as median and interquartile range or absolutes and frequencies

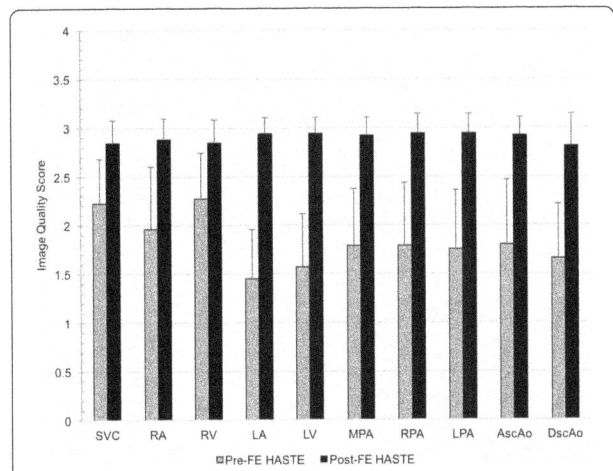

Fig. 2 Qualitative comparison between pre-ferumoxytol HASTE and FE-HASTE images. A 3-point Likert grading scale was employed: 3 = complete suppression of the blood signal within the vascular lumen on all slices; 2 = persistent, bright blood signal within some part of the lumen on one or more slices; and 1 = persistent, bright blood signal within a considerable part of the lumen on many or all slices. Compared to pre-ferumoxytol HASTE images, the mean image quality scores for all 10 cardiovascular regions on FE-HASTE images were significantly higher (p < 0.001). AscAo ascending aorta; DscAo descending aorta; LA left atrium; LPA left pulmonary artery; LV left ventricle; MPA main pulmonary artery; RA right atrium; RPA right pulmonary artery; RV right ventricle; SVC superior vena cava

suppression across multiple slices. Complex atherosclerotic plaques can be confidently visualized on T2-weighted FE-HASTE image (Fig. 3a, lower panel, white arrow). Despite the severely dilated left atrium and differences in the flow pattern between the great vessels and the left atrium, there is uniform blood signal suppression on FE-HASTE images in all structures (Fig. 3, lower panel, a-c). Note the sharp left atrial myocardial edge definition on FE-HASTE images (Fig. 3b-c, lower panel). Although there is slight blurring of the myocardial edge in Fig. 4 (lower panel), the luminal blood signal suppression is uniform.

Two patients with abdominal aneurysms post endovascular repair are presented in Figs. 5 and 6. In both examples, the complementarity of black blood FE-HASTE and bright-blood 3D CMR angiography was helpful for demonstrating stent patency, characterizing the aneurysm sac, and determining whether an endoleak was present. In Fig. 5, FE-HASTE allowed for high contrast discrimination between perfused lumen and thrombus. The lack of enhancement within the aneurysm sac suggests the absence of an endoleak. Conversely, the combination of FE-HASTE and bright-blood CMR angiogram in Fig. 6 showed near circumferential contrast leakage into the aneurysm sac, suggesting a Type II endoleak. The complementarity of FE-HASTE and bright-blood CMR angiogram also allowed for confident identification of diffuse, eccentric, and ulcerated atherosclerotic plaques along the aorta. Notable is

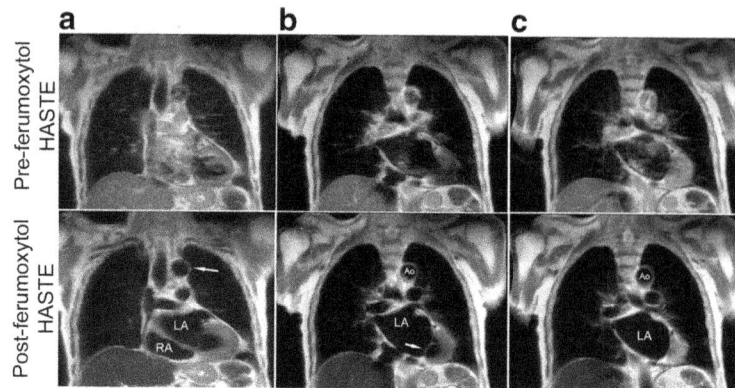

Fig. 3 Pre- and post-ferumoxytol coronal CMR images (3 T) belonging to a 94-year old male with critical aortic stenosis who had vascular mapping prior to transcatheter aortic valve replacement. Pre-ferumoxytol HASTE images (**a-c**, upper panel) illustrate poor blood signal suppression. FE-HASTE images (**a-c**, lower panel) at approximately the same region demonstrate uniform blood signal suppression in all vascular regions and intra-cardiac chambers within the imaged field of view. A multi-slice comparison of pre-ferumoxytol HASTE and FE-HASTE images is available as Additional file 1: Video S1. Thin scallops of the mitral valve (**b**, lower panel) are well depicted against the uniformly dark left atrium. Atherosclerotic plaques along the vessel wall of the transverse aortic arch (**a**, lower panel, white arrow) are present. *Ao* aorta; *LA* left atrium; *RA* right atrium

the uniform and complete blood signal suppression depicted on the FE-HASTE images.

The effectiveness of FE-HASTE is further illustrated in Fig. 7 and Fig. 8. In Fig. 7, FE-CMR was performed to evaluate known coronary aneurysms in a 4-year old child with Kawasaki disease. On pre-ferumoxytol HASTE images, the thrombosed portion (Fig. 7, red T) of the left coronary artery aneurysm and the perfused lumen have similar signal. However, blood signal suppression on FE-HASTE clearly differentiated the perfused lumen from the superior thrombosed portion (Fig. 7, green arrows). These findings correlate closely with the bright-blood CMR angiogram. In the setting of cardiomegaly and very slow flow, FE-HASTE images provided more reliable and complete blood signal suppression in the left atrium

(Fig. 8). ECG-gating during pre-ferumoxytol HASTE imaging (Fig. 8, panel b) failed to provide effective blood signal suppression whereas FE-HASTE succeeded fully, even without ECG-gating.

Quantitative analysis

Compared to pre-ferumoxytol HASTE images, intra-luminal blood signal suppression was more effective on FE-HASTE (Table 3). The median homogeneity index for FE-HASTE images was at least five times lower than pre-ferumoxytol HASTE images ($p < 0.001$), indicating more effective signal suppression post-ferumoxytol. Similarly, the mean SNR for all ten cardiovascular regions (superior vena cava, both atria, both ventricles, pulmonary trunk, right and left pulmonary arteries,

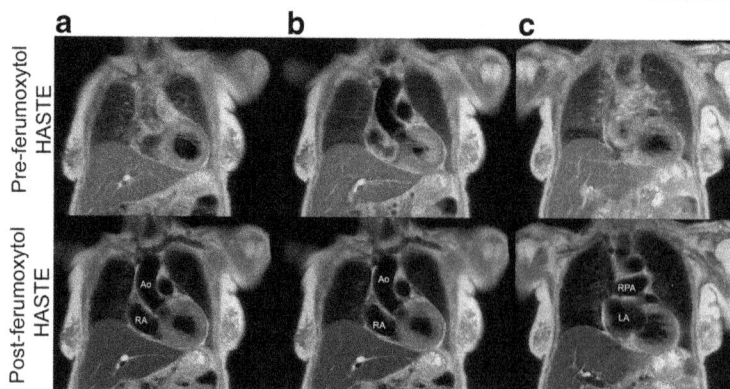

Fig. 4 Pre and post-ferumoxytol coronal CMR images (3 T) belonging to a 93-year-old female with critical aortic stenosis who had FE-CMR for vascular mapping in the setting of renal impairment. Pre-ferumoxytol HASTE images (image quality score 1–2) illustrate inconsistent blood signal suppression across multiple slices (upper panel, **a-c**). The blood signal in FE HASTE images (image quality 3) is consistently and uniformly suppressed in both vascular lumen and intra-cardiac chambers and across multiple slices (lower panel, **a-c**) compared to pre-ferumoxytol HASTE images. *Ao* aorta; *LA* left atrium; *RA* right atrium; *RPA* right pulmonary artery

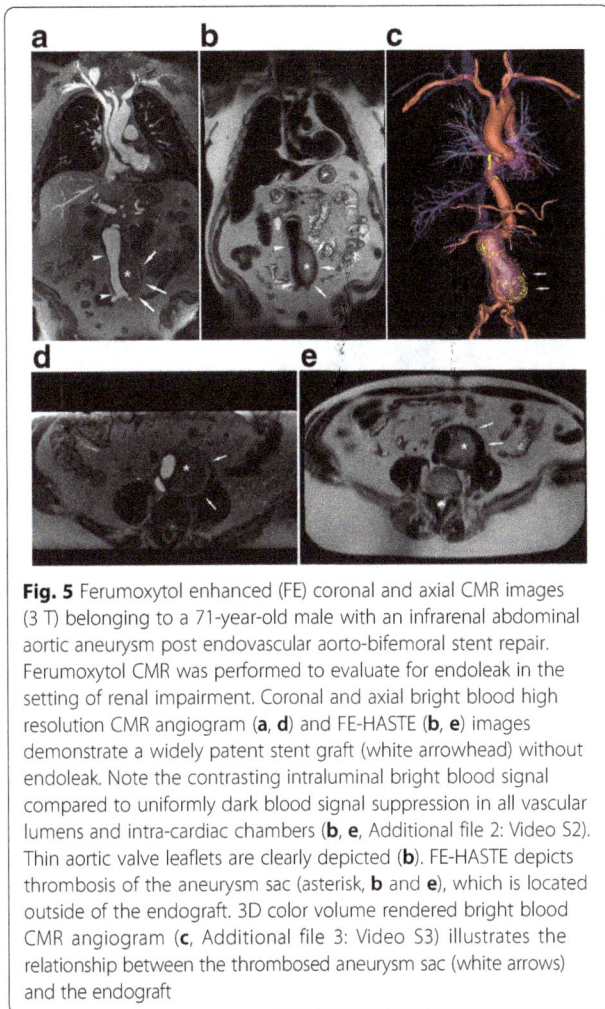

Fig. 5 Ferumoxytol enhanced (FE) coronal and axial CMR images (3 T) belonging to a 71-year-old male with an infrarenal abdominal aortic aneurysm post endovascular aorto-bifemoral stent repair. Ferumoxytol CMR was performed to evaluate for endoleak in the setting of renal impairment. Coronal and axial bright blood high resolution CMR angiogram (**a**, **d**) and FE-HASTE (**b**, **e**) images demonstrate a widely patent stent graft (white arrowhead) without endoleak. Note the contrasting intraluminal bright blood signal compared to uniformly dark blood signal suppression in all vascular lumens and intra-cardiac chambers (**b**, **e**, Additional file 2: Video S2). Thin aortic valve leaflets are clearly depicted (**b**). FE-HASTE depicts thrombosis of the aneurysm sac (asterisk, **b** and **e**), which is located outside of the endograft. 3D color volume rendered bright blood CMR angiogram (**c**, Additional file 3: Video S3) illustrates the relationship between the thrombosed aneurysm sac (white arrows) and the endograft

ascending aorta, and descending thoracic aorta) was significantly lower for FE-HASTE images (5.6 [IQR 3.2–10.0] vs 21.5 [IQR 12.5–39.4], $p < 0.001$). Comparison of SNR for each region is outlined in Table 3. The CNR for FE-HASTE images (28.3 [IQR 16.6–46.8]) was higher than pre-ferumoxytol (20.5 [IQR 10.9–42.9]), but this was not statistically significant ($p = 0.14$).

Discussion

Our study demonstrates that FE-HASTE is a simple and effective technique that overcomes many limitations associated with conventional black-blood imaging. FE-HASTE produced reliable, flow independent, uniform suppression of blood signal in the vascular lumen and cardiac chambers. Compared to pre-ferumoxytol HASTE, FE-HASTE yielded more consistent and greater homogeneity in blood signal suppression. In conventional black-blood imaging, the effectiveness of dual inversion is attributable to the longer duration available for inflow of the out-of-slice inverted spins into the imaged volume. With the use of ECG gating and appropriate adjustment of the inflow time

within the cardiac cycle, the effectiveness of blood signal suppression can be increased. However, the requirement for cardiac gating imposes limits on the duration of the image acquisition window and on spatial resolution, particularly for slow flow where the inflow time may occupy a substantial portion of the cardiac cycle. Further, ECG gating at 3 T can be problematic and prone to inconsistency.

In our study, the dual inversion module of the pre-ferumoxytol HASTE images was in most cases positioned randomly within the cardiac cycle and this may help explain the frequent persistence of intravascular signal. It is well recognized that with pulsatile blood flow, the image acquisition window may encompass anywhere from maximum velocity to zero velocity flow on various slices. Therefore, ours was not a comparison between an optimal pre-ferumoxytol dual inversion HASTE and FE-HASTE, but rather a study of how well FE-HASTE, with parameters chosen to provide high resolution images and prevent inter-slice cross-talk, supports complete blood signal suppression without any magnetization preparation schemes. That said, even with ECG gating, dual inversion black blood imaging may fail if timing is not optimal or if flow is very slow, as we found in the patient illustrated in Fig. 8.

Blood signal suppression with ferumoxytol is independent of blood flow because, beyond a threshold TE, the blood signal will decay because of its T2. In our study, the TEs employed at both 1.5 T and 3 T were clearly at or beyond the minimum to ensure full blood signal suppression, although we did not explore what the threshold minimum TE was. Our study confirmed that, with appropriate T2 weighting, FE-HASTE can be leveraged to complement bright-blood CMR for characterization of cardiovascular pathology.

Multiple strategies have been explored for blood signal suppression in MRI, including spatial presaturation, long train radiofrequency pulses such as RARE (rapid acquisition with relaxation enhancement) [10], inversion recovery magnetization preparation techniques [4, 11], or T2* shortening of deoxygenated blood (susceptibility weighted imaging). Other black-blood techniques and their variants such as presaturation of inflowing blood by slab-selective radiofrequency pulses [12], motion-sensitizing magnetization preparation gradient echo sequences [13], multislice motion-sensitized driven-equilibrium (MSDE) turbo spin-echo sequences [14], free breath 3D whole heart MSDE [15], and radial steady-state free precession [16] have been also been introduced. Despite these efforts, black-blood imaging remains challenging in clinical practice due to troublesome artifacts and flow dependency. Frequently, sufficient image quality can be achieved through selection of imaging parameters on an individualized patient basis and is influenced by the skill and experience of clinicians and technologists. With FE-HASTE, customized imaging parameters and

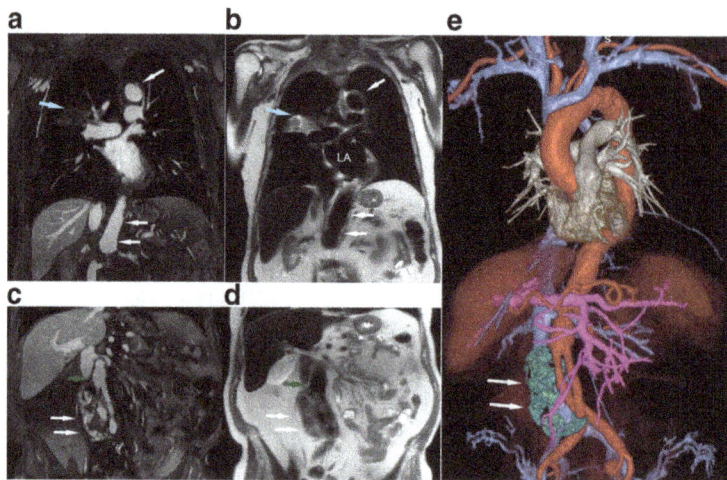

Fig. 6 Post-ferumoxytol 3D CMR angiogram multiplanar reformat (**a**, **c**) and T2 FE-HASTE (**b**, **d**) coronal CMR images (3 T) belonging to an 85-year old male with infrarenal abdominal aortic aneurysm post endovascular aorto and bilateral iliac stent graft repair. The CMR exam was performed to evaluate for endoleak. There is diffuse atherosclerosis of the transverse and abdominal aorta with eccentric and ulcerated plaques (**a-b**, white arrow; Additional file 4: Video S4). An incidental heterogeneous lesion with serpiginous border (**a-b**, blue arrow) is present in the right middle lobe and is well demarcated on FE-HASTE. Coronal FE-HASTE (**b**, **d**) demonstrates uniformly suppressed blood signal throughout the lumen. The aneurysm sac (**c-e**, white arrows) has circumferential contrast leakage (**c-d**), suggestive of a Type II endoleak. Relationships between the endoleak (**e**, white arrow, segmented green) and stent grafts are depicted on the 3D color volume rendered bright blood CMR angiogram image (**e**). Compared to the bright blood CMR angiogram image (**c**, green arrow), the intra-luminal blood signal is completely suppressed in the patent iliac stent graft (**d**, green arrow). Comparison of aortic vessel wall characteristics and endoleak tissue characteristics on FE-HASTE and bright blood 3D CMR angiogram is available as Additional file 5: Video S5. LA, left atrium; MPR, multiplanar reformat

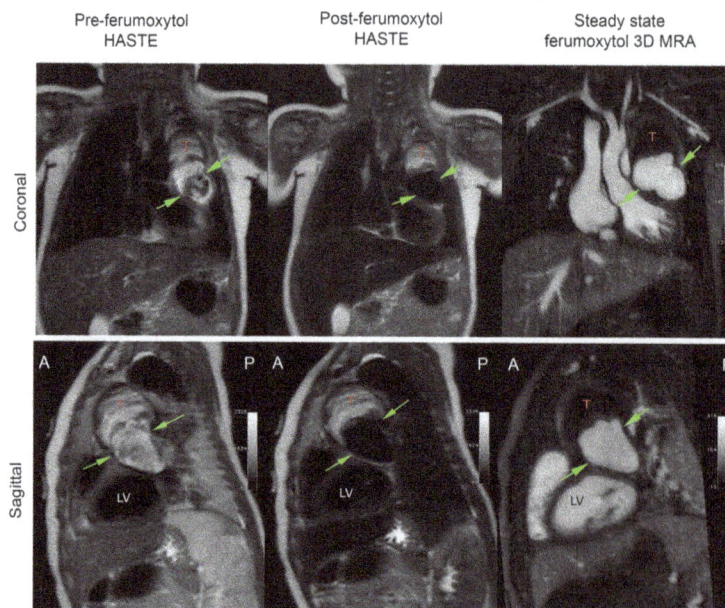

Fig. 7 Pre- and post-ferumoxytol CMR images (3 T) belonging to a 4-year-old girl with Kawasaki disease. CMR was performed to evaluate left and right coronary aneurysms. Compared to pre-ferumoxytol HASTE images, excellent blood signal suppression of intracardiac chambers and vascular segments is demonstrated on FE-HASTE images. The thrombosed portion of the left coronary aneurysm (T) and the lumen (green arrows) are well-demarcated on FE-HASTE and 3D high resolution CMR angiogram images. The distinction between the partially thrombosed coronary aneurysm and the perfused lumen is not well depicted due to complex flow patterns on pre-ferumoxytol HASTE

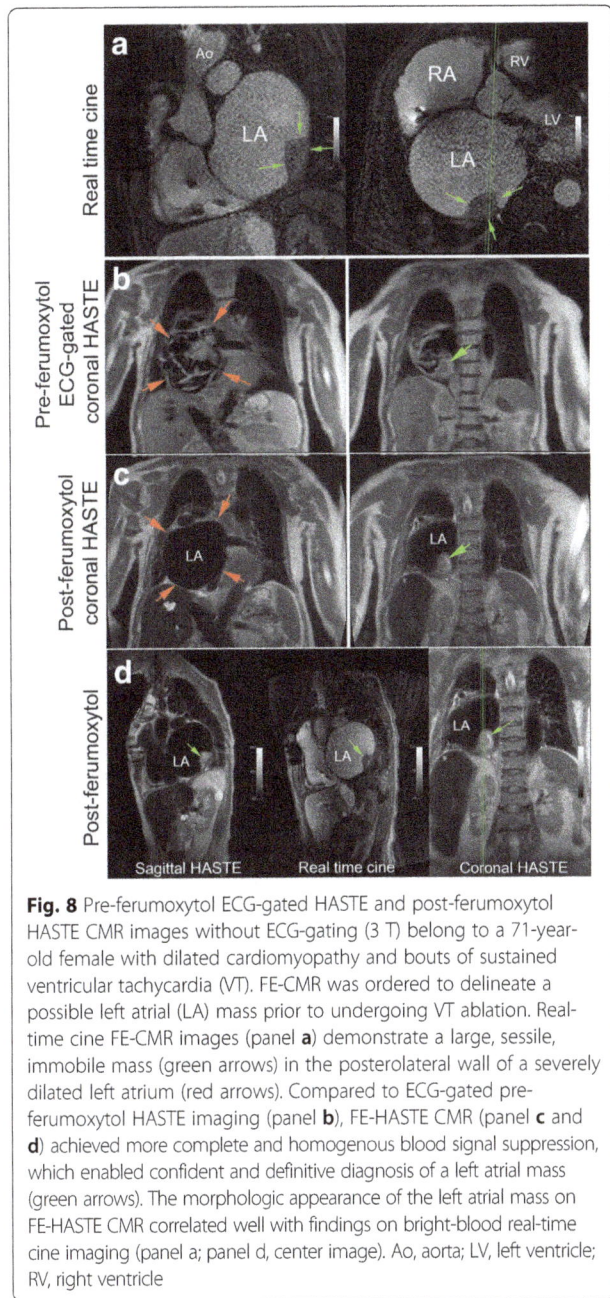

Fig. 8 Pre-ferumoxytol ECG-gated HASTE and post-ferumoxytol HASTE CMR images without ECG-gating (3 T) belong to a 71-year-old female with dilated cardiomyopathy and bouts of sustained ventricular tachycardia (VT). FE-CMR was ordered to delineate a possible left atrial (LA) mass prior to undergoing VT ablation. Real-time cine FE-CMR images (panel **a**) demonstrate a large, sessile, immobile mass (green arrows) in the posterolateral wall of a severely dilated left atrium (red arrows). Compared to ECG-gated pre-ferumoxytol HASTE imaging (panel **b**), FE-HASTE CMR (panel **c** and **d**) achieved more complete and homogenous blood signal suppression, which enabled confident and definitive diagnosis of a left atrial mass (green arrows). The morphologic appearance of the left atrial mass on FE-HASTE CMR correlated well with findings on bright-blood real-time cine imaging (panel a; panel d, center image). Ao, aorta; LV, left ventricle; RV, right ventricle

Table 3 Comparison of SNR measurements as a proxy for uniform intra-luminal blood signal suppression ($n = 93$)

	Pre-FE HASTE DIR	Post-FE HASTE	P value
Image noise	10.0 (6.7–16.5)	9.7 (6.2–15.1)	0.344*
Homogeneity index	108.0 (65.0–170.4)	24.5 (18.0–32.8)	<0.001*
Signal-to-noise ratio (SNR)			
Overall	21.5 (12.5–39.4)	5.6 (3.2–10.0)	<0.001**
SVC	11.2 (5.6–23.0)	6.2 (3.5–13.0)	<0.001**
RA	11.3 (5.1–23.6)	3.3 (2.2–6.2)	<0.001**
RV	6.4 (2.7–12.3)	2.7 (1.6–6.0)	<0.001**
LA	27.5 (10.8–47.0)	4.3 (2.4–7.1)	<0.001**
LV	22.4 (5.1–44.3)	3.7 (2.0–5.6)	<0.001**
MPA	18.5 (8.1–38.0)	6.2 (2.9–10.9)	<0.001**
RPA	22.3 (6.9–37.2)	5.4 (2.9–12.3)	<0.001**
LPA	22.0 (8.0–47.1)	6.1 (3.4–11.7)	<0.001**
Asc Ao	12.4 (5.0–29.6)	5.1 (2.9–9.2)	<0.001**
Dsc Ao	33.2 (15.3–67.6)	6.9 (3.4–15.1)	<0.001**

Values are reported as median and interquartile range

Asc Ao ascending aorta, *DIR* double-inversion recovery, *Dsc Ao* descending aorta, *FE* ferumoxytol enhanced, *LA*, left atrium, *LPA* left pulmonary artery, *LV* left ventricle, *MPA* main pulmonary artery, *RA* right atrium, *RPA* right pulmonary artery, *RV* right ventricle, *SNR* signal-to-noise ratio, *SVC* superior vena cava

*Wilcoxon rank sum test; **ANOVA for repeated measures

magnetization preparation schemes are not required for effective blood signal suppression, and less restrictive parameters can be prescribed to optimize other aspects of image quality. Based on our findings, FE-HASTE is a simple strategy for discrimination between flow artifact and true vessel wall pathology such as thrombus, tumor, or plaque.

Although ferumoxytol is FDA approved for treatment of iron deficiency anemia in adults with kidney disease, it has several promising attributes for diagnostic CMR imaging [5, 6, 17, 18]. First, unlike gadolinium-based contrast agents (GBCAs), ferumoxytol is not cleared by the kidneys, but is metabolized by the reticuloentholelial

system and the iron core is incorporated into the body for biologic use. Second, although the longitudinal r_1 relaxivity of ferumoxytol is similar to gadofosveset, its intravascular half-life is substantially longer (> 15 h). With a molecular weight of 750 kD and particle size of 30 nm, ferumoxytol has excellent fidelity as an intravascular contrast agent with both strong T1 and T2* shortening effects [7]. The dual potential of ferumoxytol was previously highlighted by Li et al. [19] in a pilot study of lower extremity deep venous thrombosis. With the exception of an abstract by Vu AT et al. describing ferumoxytol black-blood cine imaging [20], the more general use of ferumoxytol as a black-blood imaging agent has not previously been described.

A recent FDA warning highlighted the occurrence of rare, but serious hypersensitivity reactions associated with the therapeutic use of ferumoxytol [21], some of which were associated with fatal outcomes. Based on therapeutic use data from post-marketing trials [22–26], the calculated aggregate risk of anaphylactic reaction is 0.03%. Suggestions to minimize hypersensitivity reactions include dilution and slow infusion. Monitoring of vital signs up to 30 min post-infusion is also recommended and should be standard practice. Compared to other USPIOs, the outer carbohydrate shell of ferumoxytol was designed to have lower free-iron release [27], decreased immunologic allergic reaction, and an improved safety profile [28]. To date, no severe adverse events have been directly associated with the diagnostic use of ferumoxytol CMR in both small and large cohort single-center safety studies [9, 29–31].

Our study has several limitations. First, although images were evaluated in a blind and random way, the apparent difference in the uniformity of the blood signal suppression on FE-HASTE images made it challenging to truly blind the readers. Second, not all images received perfect image quality scores even though blood signal suppression was excellent on FE-HASTE images. This observation may relate to the intrinsic limitations of HASTE imaging, and also the lack of cardiac gating which may result in occasional blurring along vessel or endocardial borders. However, black-blood imaging is rarely used alone, but in conjunction with bright blood imaging techniques, which is where the complementary duality of FE imaging may be of considerable value. Our study was also not designed to assess the diagnostic accuracy of FE-HASTE, but rather to gauge its effectiveness for flow independent blood signal suppression. More extensive work will be required to address the broader question of diagnostic accuracy. Lastly, because of ferumoxytol's long intravascular half-life, imagers need to be aware that ferumoxytol may influence CMR tissue contrast for days or weeks, and should interpret follow up studies appropriately. While the issue of iron overload has been raised, this is rarely a practical clinical concern, because iron overload is a long-term process and is uncommon other than in hemochromatosis. Moreover, the majority of the world's population is iron deficient [32, 33] and the amount of iron available for physiologic use is tightly regulated [34, 35]. Nevertheless, careful screening and appropriate candidate selection are encouraged.

Conclusions

FE-HASTE imaging provides a simple, fast, and reliable strategy for uniform, flow independent blood signal suppression at 3 T and 1.5 T. Compared to pre-contrast HASTE, FE-HASTE obviates the need for magnetization preparation schemes and ECG gating, which add complexity and may limit achievable resolution. In those already undergoing clinical FE-CMR for bright-blood applications, black-blood FE-HASTE is a simple and practical technique that can be used in conjunction with bright-blood imaging for further characterization of cardiovascular pathology.

Additional files

Additional file 1: Video S1. Coronal multi-slice comparison of pre-ferumoxytol HASTE and ferumoxytol-enhanced HASTE images.

Additional file 2: Video S2. Coronal multi-slice ferumoxytol-enhanced black blood HASTE in a patient with a repaired infrarenal abdominal aortic aneurysm.

Additional file 3: Video S3. 3D color volume-rendered bright blood ferumoxytol-enhanced CMRA of a thrombosed aneurysm sac and endograft.

Additional file 4: Video S4. Coronal multi-slice ferumoxytol-enhanced black blood HASTE in a patient with infrarenal abdominal aortic aneurysm and bilateral iliac stent graft repair.

Additional file 5: Video S5. Comparison of aortic vessel wall characteristics and endoleak tissue characteristics on ferumoxytol-enhanced HASTE and bright blood 3D CMRA.

Abbreviations
Ao: Aorta; CMR: Cardiovascular magnetic resonance; CNR: Contrast-to-noise ratio; DICOM: Digital Imaging and Communication in Medicine; ECG: Electrocardiogram; FDA: United States Food and Drug Administration; FE: Ferumoxytol-enhanced; GBCA: Gadolinium-based contrast agent; HASTE: Half-Fourier Acquisition Single-shot Turbo Spin-echo; LA: Left atrium; LPA: Left pulmonary artery; LV: Left ventricle/left ventricular; MPA: Main pulmonary artery; RA: Right atrium; RPA: Right pulmonary artery; RV: Right ventricular; ROI: Region-of interest; SI: Signal intensity; SNR: Signal-to-noise ratio; USPIO: Ultrasmall superparamagnetic iron oxide

Acknowledgements
The authors thank Dr. Jiaxin Shao (Assistant Project Scientist, Department of Radiological Sciences, David Geffen School of Medicine at UCLA) for providing technical consultation.

Funding
None.

Authors' contributions
KLN participated in its design, scored the studies, performed the statistical analysis, interpreted the data, and drafted the manuscript. EAP participated in its design, scored the studies, interpreted the data, and revised the manuscript. TY scored the studies, and revised the manuscript. PH participated in the design, interpreted the data, and revised the manuscript. JPF conceived the study, participated in its design, acquired the images, and revised the manuscript. All authors read and approved the final manuscript.

Consent for publication
Written informed consent was obtained from the patient (or guardian) for publication of their individual details and accompanying images in this manuscript. The consent form is held by the authors /the authors' institution and is available for review by the Editor-in-Chief.

Competing interests
Dr. J. Paul Finn serves on the Scientific Advisory Board for AMAG, Bracco, and Bayer. The other authors declare they have no competing interests.

Author details
[1]Diagnostic Cardiovascular Imaging Laboratory, Department of Radiological Sciences, David Geffen School of Medicine at UCLA, Los Angeles, California, USA. [2]Division of Cardiology, David Geffen School of Medicine at UCLA and VA Greater Los Angeles Healthcare System, Los Angeles, California, USA. [3]Physics and Biology in Medicine Interdepartmental Graduate Program, Department of Radiological Sciences, University of California at Los Angeles, Peter V. Ueberroth Building Suite 3371, 10945 Le Conte Ave, Los Angeles, CA 90095-7206, USA. [4]Department of Radiology and The Institute of Radiation Medicine, Seoul National University Hospital, Seoul 110-744, South Korea.

References

1. Finn JP, Nael K, Deshpande V, Ratib O, Laub G. Cardiac MR imaging: state of the technology. Radiology. 2006;241:338–54.
2. Bradley WG Jr. Carmen lecture. Flow phenomena in MR imaging. AJR Am J Roentgenol. 1988;150:983–94.
3. Patel MR, Klufas RA, Alberico RA, Edelman RR. Half-fourier acquisition single-shot turbo spin-echo (HASTE) MR: comparison with fast spin-echo MR in diseases of the brain. AJNR Am J Neuroradiol. 1997;18:1635–40.
4. Edelman RR, Chien D, Kim D. Fast selective black blood MR imaging. Radiology. 1991;181:655–60.
5. Finn JP, Nguyen KL, Han F, Zhou Z, Salusky I, Ayad I, Hu P. Cardiovascular MRI with ferumoxytol. Clin Radiol. 2016;71:796–806.
6. Bashir MR, Bhatti L, Marin D, Nelson RC. Emerging applications for ferumoxytol as a contrast agent in MRI. J Magn Reson Imaging. 2015;41:884–98.
7. Bashir MR, Mody R, Neville A, Javan R, Seaman D, Kim CY, Gupta RT, Jaffe TA. Retrospective assessment of the utility of an iron-based agent for contrast-enhanced magnetic resonance venography in patients with endstage renal diseases. J Magn Reson Imaging. 2014;40:113–8.
8. Winterer JT, Lehnhardt S, Schneider B, Neumann K, Allmann KH, Laubenberger J, Langer M. MRI of heart morphology. Comparison of nongradient echo sequences with single- and multislice acquisition. Investig Radiol. 1999;34:516–22.
9. Nguyen KL, Yoshida T, Han F, Ayad I, Reemtsen BL, Salusky IB, Satou GM, Hu P, Finn JP. MRI with ferumoxytol: a single center experience of safety across the age spectrum. J Magn Reson Imaging. 2017;45(3):804–12. [Epub 2016 Aug 2]
10. Hennig J, Nauerth A, Friedburg H. RARE imaging: a fast imaging method for clinical MR. Mag Reson Med. 1986;3:823–33.
11. Simonetti OP, Finn JP, White RD, Laub G, Henry DA. "black blood" T2-weighted inversion-recovery MR imaging of the heart. Radiology. 1996;199:49–57.
12. Edelman RR, Mattle HP, Wallner B, Bajakian R, Kleefield J, Kent C, Skillman JJ, Mendel JB, Atkinson DJ. Extracranial carotid arteries: evaluation with "black blood" MR angiography. Radiology. 1990;177:45–50.
13. Nguyen TD, de Rochefort L, Spincemaille P, Cham MD, Weinsaft JW, Prince MR, Wang Y. Effective motion-sensitizing magnetization preparation for black blood magnetic resonance imaging of the heart. J Magn Reson Imaging. 2008;28:1092–100.
14. Wang J, Yarnykh VL, Hatsukami T, Chu B, Balu N, Yuan C. Improved suppression of plaque-mimicking artifacts in black-blood carotid atherosclerosis imaging using a multislice motion-sensitized driven-equilibrium (MSDE) turbo spin-echo (TSE) sequence. Mag Reson Med. 2007;58:973–81.
15. Srinivasan S, Hu P, Kissinger KV, Goddu B, Goepfert L, Schmidt EJ, Kozerke S, Nezafat R. Free-breathing 3D whole-heart black-blood imaging with motion sensitized driven equilibrium. J Magn Reson Imaging. 2012;36:379–86.
16. Edelman RR, Botelho M, Pursnani A, Giri S, Koktzoglou I. Improved dark blood imaging of the heart using radial balanced steady-state free precession. J Cardiovasc Magn Reson. 2016;18:69.
17. Neuwelt EA, Hamilton BE, Varallyay CG, Rooney WR, Edelman RD, Jacobs PM, Watnick SG. Ultrasmall superparamagnetic iron oxides (USPIOs): a future alternative magnetic resonance (MR) contrast agent for patients at risk for nephrogenic systemic fibrosis (NSF)? Kidney Int. 2009;75:465–74.
18. Finn JP, Nguyen KL and Hu P. Ferumoxytol vs. Gadolinium agents for contrast-enhanced MRI: Thoughts on evolving indications, risks, and benefits. J Magn Reson Imaging. 2017. doi:10.1002/jmri.25580.
19. Li W, Salanitri J, Tutton S, Dunkle EE, Schneider JR, Caprini JA, Pierchala LN, Jacobs PM, Edelman RR. Lower extremity deep venous thrombosis: evaluation with ferumoxytol-enhanced MR imaging and dual-contrast mechanism–preliminary experience. Radiology. 2007;242:873–81.
20. Vu AT, Li W, Tutton S, Pierchala L, Prasad P, Edelman RR. Robust and efficient whole heart black blood cine imaging. Proc Intl Soc Mag Reson Med. 2005;13:1638.
21. U.S. Food and Drug Administration. FDA Drug Safety Communication: FDA strengthens warnings and changes prescribing instructions to decrease the risk of serious allergic reactions with anemia drug Feraheme (ferumoxytol). http://www.fda.gov/Drugs/DrugSafety/ucm440138.htm. Accessed 30 Mar 2015.
22. Hetzel D, Strauss W, Bernard K, Li Z, Urboniene A, Allen LF. A phase III, randomized, open-label trial of ferumoxytol compared with iron sucrose for the treatment of iron deficiency anemia in patients with a history of unsatisfactory oral iron therapy. Am J Hematol. 2014;89:646–50.
23. Vadhan-Raj S, Strauss W, Ford D, Bernard K, Boccia R, Li J, Allen LF. Efficacy and safety of IV ferumoxytol for adults with iron deficiency anemia previously unresponsive to or unable to tolerate oral iron. Am J Hematol. 2014;89:7–12.
24. Macdougall IC, Strauss WE, McLaughlin J, Li Z, Dellanna F, Hertel J. A randomized comparison of ferumoxytol and iron sucrose for treating iron deficiency anemia in patients with CKD. Clin J Am Soc Nephrol. 2014;9:705–12.
25. Schiller B, Bhat P, Sharma A. Safety and effectiveness of ferumoxytol in hemodialysis patients at 3 dialysis chains in the United States over a 12-month period. Clin Ther. 2014;36:70–83.
26. Auerbach M, Strauss W, Auerbach S, Rineer S, Bahrain H. Safety and efficacy of total dose infusion of 1,020 mg of ferumoxytol administered over 15 min. Am J Hematol. 2013;88:944–7.
27. Balakrishnan VS, Rao M, Kausz AT, Brenner L, Brenner L, Pereira BJG, Frigo TB, Lewis JM. Physicochemical properties of ferumoxytol, a new intravenous iron preparation. Eur J Clin Investig. 2009;39:489–96.
28. Provenzano R, Schiller B, Rao M, Coyne D, Brenner L, Pereira BJ. Ferumoxytol as an intravenous iron replacement therapy in hemodialysis patients. Clin J Am Soc Nephrol. 2009;4:386–93.
29. Ning P, Zucker EJ, Wong P, Vasanawala SS. Hemodynamic safety and efficacy of ferumoxytol as an intravenous contrast agents in pediatric patients and young adults. Magn Reson Imaging. 2016;34:152–8.
30. Muehe AM, Feng D, von Eyben R, Luna-Fineman S, Link MP, Muthig T, Huddleston AE, Neuwelt EA, Daldrup-Link HE. Safety report of Ferumoxytol for magnetic resonance imaging in children and young adults. Investig Radiol. 2016;51:221–7.
31. Varallyay CG, Toth GB, Fu R, Netto JP, Firkins J, Ambady P and Neuwelt EA. What Does the Boxed Warning Tell Us? Safe Practice of Using Ferumoxytol as an MRI Contrast Agent. AJNR Am J Neuroradiol. 2017. doi:10.3174/ajnr.A5188.
32. Clark SF. Iron deficiency anemia. Nutr Clin Pract. 2008;23:128–41.
33. Lopez A, Cacoub P, Macdougall IC, Peyrin-Biroulet L. Iron deficiency anaemia. Lancet. 2016;387:907–16.
34. Nemeth E, Ganz T. The role of hepcidin in iron metabolism. Acta Haematol. 2009;122:78–86.
35. Bradbury MW. Transport of iron in the blood-brain-cerebrospinal fluid system. J Neurochem. 1997;69:443–54.

12

Quantitative assessment of symptomatic intracranial atherosclerosis and lenticulostriate arteries in recent stroke patients using whole-brain high-resolution cardiovascular magnetic resonance imaging

Mengnan Wang[1], Fang Wu[2], Yujiao Yang[3], Huijuan Miao[1], Zhaoyang Fan[4], Xunming Ji[5], Debiao Li[4], Xiuhai Guo[1*] and Qi Yang[2,4*]

Abstract

Background: It has been shown that intracranial atherosclerotic stenosis (ICAS) has heterogeneous features in terms of plaque instability and vascular remodeling. Therefore, quantitative information on the changes of intracranial atherosclerosis and lenticulostriate arteries (LSAs) may potentially improve understanding of the pathophysiological mechanisms underlying stroke and may guide the treatment and work-up strategies. Our present study aimed to use a novel whole-brain high-resolution cardiovascular magnetic resonance imaging (WB-HRCMR) to assess both ICAS plaques and LSAs in recent stroke patients.

Methods: Twenty-nine symptomatic and 23 asymptomatic ICAS patients were enrolled in this study from Jan 2015 through Sep 2017 and all patients underwent WB-HRCMR. Intracranial atherosclerotic plaque burden, plaque enhancement volume, plaque enhancement index, as well as the number and length of LSAs were evaluated in two groups. Enhancement index was calculated as follows: ([Signal intensity (SI)$_{plaque}$/SI$_{normal\ wall}$ on post-contrast imaging] − [SI$_{plaque}$/SI$_{normal\ wall}$ on matched pre-contrast imaging])/(SI$_{plaque}$ / SI$_{normal\ wall}$ on matched pre-contrast imaging). Logistic regression analysis was used to investigate the independent high risk plaque and LSAs features associated with stroke.

Results: Symptomatic ICAS patients exhibited larger enhancement plaque volume (20.70 ± 3.07 mm^3 vs. 6.71 ± 1.87 mm^3 $P = 0.001$) and higher enhancement index (0.44 ± 0.08 vs. 0.09 ± 0.06 $P = 0.001$) compared with the asymptomatic ICAS. The average length of LSAs in symptomatic ICAS (20.95 ± 0.87 mm) was shorter than in asymptomatic ICAS (24.04 ± 0.95 mm) ($P = 0.02$). Regression analysis showed that the enhancement index (100.43, 95% CI − 4.02-2510.96; $P = 0.005$) and the average length of LSAs (0.80, 95% CI − 0.65-0.99; $P = 0.036$) were independent factors for predicting of stroke.

Conclusion: WB-HRCMR enabled the comprehensive quantitative evaluation of intracranial atherosclerotic lesions and perforating arteries. Symptomatic ICAS had distinct plaque characteristics and shorter LSA length compared with asymptomatic ICAS.

Keywords: Intracranial atherosclerotic stenosis, High-resolution cardiovascular magnetic resonance imaging, Stroke, Lenticulostriate arteries

* Correspondence: guoxhxuan@126.com; qi.yang@cshs.org; yangyangqiqi@gmail.com
[1]Department of Neurology, Xuanwu Hospital, Capital Medical University, Beijing 100053, China
[2]Department of Radiology, Xuanwu Hospital, Capital Medical University, Beijing 100053, China
Full list of author information is available at the end of the article

Background

Intracranial atherosclerotic stenosis (ICAS) is one of the most common causes of ischemic stroke, which is associated with high morbidity and mortality rates in Asian countries [1–4]. The initial and follow-up assessment of stroke patients rely mostly upon the evaluation of luminal stenosis via several methods, including transcranial Doppler (TCD), computed tomography angiography (CTA) and magnetic resonance angiography (MRA) [5–8]. Recently, high-resolution cardiovascular magnetic resonance imaging (HR-CMR) has been used to directly depict intracranial vessel wall plaques [9, 10]. Two-dimensional imaging techniques were commonly used for HR-CMR to assess intracranial atherosclerotic plaque morphology and plaque composition [11–13]. However, limited spatial temporal resolution hampered its application in quantitative measurement of vessel wall dimensions and visualization of lenticulostriate arteries (LSAs). Several studies have demonstrated that flow-sensitive black blood magnetic resonance angiography (FSBB-MRA) based on 3D gradient-echo sequence can be specifically used to visualize LSAs [14–16]. Our recent studies have demonstrated the feasibility of whole-brain high-resolution magnetic resonance imaging (WB-HRCMR),which enables combined evaluation of plaque and LSAs in one image setting [17, 18]. Thus, in this study, we aimed to use WB-HRCMR to quantitatively investigate different features of plaque and LSAs in symptomatic versus asymptomatic ICAS groups.

Methods
Study population

From January 2015 to September 2017, consecutive symptomatic and asymptomatic ICAS patients who were admitted to or visit the Department of Neurology of our hospital were consecutively recruited. The inclusion criteria: (1) age 18–80 years old; (2) symptomatic ICAS referred to first time acute ischemic stroke in the middle cerebral artery (MCA) territory identified by diffusion weighted imaging (DWI) performed within 72 h of symptom onset, and asymptomatic ICAS referred to patients who were diagnosed with other diseases without history of stroke but had MCA stenosis confirmed on image screening; (3) All enrolled subjects had moderate (stenosis: 50–69%) or severe (stenosis: 70–99%) MCA stenosis, confirmed by MRA, CTA, or digital subtraction angiography. The exclusion criteria included: (1) DWI with lacunar infarction: cerebral infarction in LSAs territory involving less than two layers or the diameter of the infarction < 15 mm; (2) coexistent ipsilateral internal carotid stenosis; (3) preexisting conditions such as vasculitis, moyamoya disease, dissection, reversible cerebral vasoconstriction syndrome (RCVS); (4) evidence of cardioembolism (e.g., arterial fibrillation, mechanical prosthetic valve disease, sick sinus syndrome, dilated cardiomyopathy). All patients underwent WB-HRCMR within 2 weeks of symptom onset. Informed consent was obtained from all participants, and all protocols were approved by the Institutional Review Board.

WB-HRCMR

All patients underwent WB-HRCMR with a 3-Tesla system (Magnetom Verio; Siemens Healthineers, Erlangen, Germany) and a standard 32-channel head coil. WB-HRCMR was performed at both pre-contrast and post-contrast states by using a 3D T1-weighted whole-brain vessel wall CMR technique known as inversion-recovery (IR) prepared SPACE (Sampling Perfection with Application-optimized Contrast using different flip angle Evolutions) [17, 18], with the following parameters: TR/TE = 900/15 ms; field of view = 170×170 mm^2; 240 slices with slice thickness of 0.53 mm; voxel size = $0.53 \times 0.53 \times 0.53$ mm^3; scan time = 8 min. The CMR contrast agent, gadopentetate dimeglumine (Magnevist; Schering, Berlin, Germany), was injected through an antecubital vein (0.1 mmol per kilogram of body weight), and WB-HRCMR was repeated 5 min after injection was performed.

WB-HRCMR image analysis

Evaluation of WB-HRCMR was conducted in consensus by two experienced neuroradiologists blinded to the patient's clinical details. Commercial software (Vessel Analysis, Oak Medical Imaging Technologies, Inc.) with 3D multi-planar reformation and region-of-interest (ROI) signal measurement functionalities was used for quantitative analysis. A plaque was defined as thickening of the vessel wall using its adjacent proximal, distal, or contralateral vessel segment as a reference. A culprit plaque was defined as (1) the only lesion within the vascular vicinity of the stroke or (2) the most stenotic lesion when multiple plaques were present within the same vascular territory of the stroke. The vessel area (VA) and lumen area were measured by manually tracing vessel and lumen boundaries. The difference between VA and lumen area was the wall area (WA). Stenosis degree was defined as (1-lesion lumen area/reference lumen area) × 100%. The remodeling index (RI) was calculated as the ratio of the lesion VA to the reference VA. The wall area index was defined as the ratio of the lesion WA to the reference WA. And the plaque burden was calculated as WA/VA × 100%. The mean signal intensity (SI) values of culprit plaques and reference vessel wall were measured on pre- and post-contrast WB-HRCMR images.

Pre- and post-contrast WB-HRCMR were first co-registered and two-dimensional short-axis images were then generated for the measurement of MCA plaque enhancement. Care was taken to ensure that the short-axis views of the plaque were perpendicular to the M1 segment of MCA. Fusion image of pre- and post-contrast WB-HRCMR have been utilized for the segmentation of the enhanced area of plaque and the enhancement volume was then calculated (Fig. 1). Enhancement index was calculated as follows: ([$SI_{plaque}/SI_{normal\ wall}$ on postcontrast imaging] – [$SI_{plaque}/SI_{normal\ wall}$ on matched precontrast imaging])/(SI_{plaque} / $SI_{normal\ wall}$ on matched precontrast imaging).

LSAs images were generated using five to six slices of minimum intensity projection (MinIP) in coronal direction with 10–15 mm thickness on pre-contrast WB-HRCMR. LSA branches longer than 5 mm were traced and analyzed by using these images [14]. When LSA branches less than 5 mm from the MCA origin, each branch was counted and measured separately, because more than 70% of branches were found to originate from common trunks [19].

Statistical analysis

All quantitative data were expressed as means ± standard deviations. Categorical variables were analyzed using Chi-square test and continuous variables were compared using t-test between the two groups. A logistic regression analysis with the method of enter stepwise was used to look for independent predictors of stroke. A P-value of less than 0.05 indicated statistical significance. All statistical analyzes were performed by using commercial software (SPSS 22.0, International Business Machnines, Armonk, New York, USA).

Results
Patient characteristics

One hundred and one patients were consecutively recruited in the study and forty-nine patients were excluded from analysis due to poor image quality ($N = 5$), < 50% MCA stenosis ($N = 4$), evidence of cardio embolism ($N = 7$), patients with other etiologies ($N = 13$), and patients with lacunar infarction ($N = 20$). The remaining 52 patients were enrolled of which 29 were symptomatic. The demographic data was illustrated in Table 1. No statistically significant differences in patient demographics and the main clinical characteristics were found.

ICAS plaque location

A total of seventy-nine ICAS plaques were observed. In symptomatic ICAS group, 29 (61.7%) plaques were found in MCA and 18 (38.3%) were in intracranial ICA. In asymptomatic ICAS group, 23 (71.8%) plaques were detected in MCA, 9 (28.2%) were in intracranial ICA. No statistically significant differences in MCA plaque distribution were found ($P = 0.469$) between the two groups. All culprit plaques in MCA were included for the final analysis.

ICAS plaque characteristics

A total of fifty-two MCA plaques were included for the final analysis. The degrees of stenoses, RI, WA, and plaque burden did not differ significantly between two groups. Symptomatic MCA demonstrated greater plaque enhancement, including larger enhancement volume (20.70 ± 3.07 mm³ vs. 6.71 ± 1.87 mm³, $P = 0.001$) and higher enhancement index (0.44 ± 0.08 vs. 0.09 ± 0.06, $P = 0.001$)

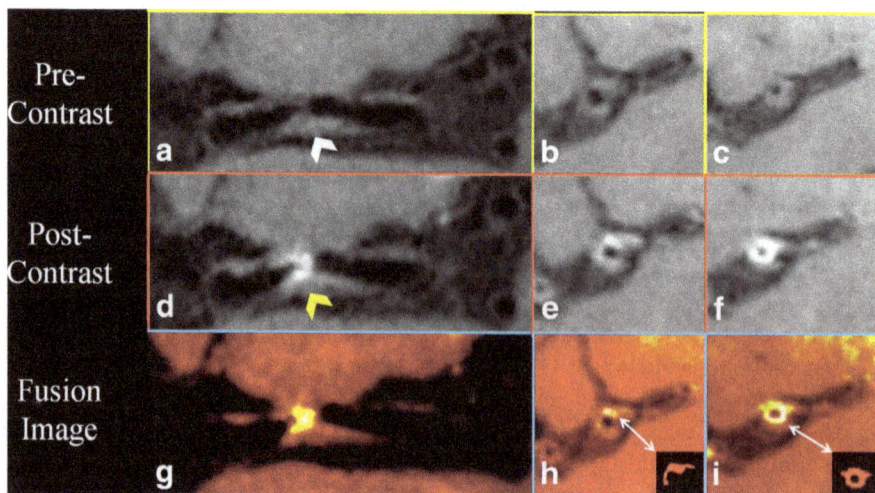

Fig. 1 Pre-contrast coronal and cross-sectional whole brain high resolution cardiovascular magnetic resonance (WB-HRCMR) images showed diffused plaque (**a-c**, white arrow) located on middle cerebral artery (MCA). Partial enhancement of the plaque was observed (**d-f**, yellow arrow). The enhancement plaque area was segmented through fusion images (**h, i**). The plaque enhanced volume was 11.02mm³

Table 1 Demographic in symptomatic and asymptomatic ICAS patients

	Symptomatic ICAS ($N = 29$)	Asymptomatic ICAS ($N = 23$)	P value
Age (mean ± SD, years)	46.00 ± 2.32	50.30 ± 2.36	0.397
Male No. (%)	20(69)	13 (56.5)	0.632
Body mass index (mean ± SD, kg/cm^2)	24.86 ± 1.08	24.75 ± 0.74	0.939
Hypertension No. (%)	12(41.4)	11(47.8)	0.780
Diabetes No. (%)	4(13.8)	4(17.4)	1
Hyperlipidemia No (%)	10(34.5)	9(39.1)	0.778
Smoker No. (%)	15(51.7)	11(47.8)	0.477
LDL-c (mean ± SD, mmol/L)	2.23 ± 0.14	2.32 ± 0.15	0.274
HDL-c (mean ± SD, mmol/L)	1.04 ± 0.05	1.08 ± 0.08	0.203
Triglycerides (mean ± SD, mmol/L)	1.45 ± 0.12	1.43 ± 0.17	0.380
Total cholesterol (mean ± SD, mmol/L)	3.80 ± 0.17	3.67 ± 0.22	0.451

LDL-c Low Density Lipoprotein-cholesterol, *HDL-c* High Density Lipoprotein-cholesterol

(Fig. 2). Two representative cases of symptomatic and asymptomatic MCA are presented in Figs. 3 and 4.

The LSAs features

In order to compare the several features of LSAs, twenty age-and sex-matched healthy subjects were included as normal controls. The mean number of LSAs was 3.65 ± 0.18 in symptomatic group, 3.87 ± 0.21 in asymptomatic group and 4.55 ± 0.19 on normal controls, respectively. There was significant difference between symptomatic group and normal controls ($P = 0.002$), and asymptomatic group also had statistical differences in LSAs branches compared with normal controls ($P = 0.020$). Symptomatic group had significant shorter total length of LSAs than normal controls ($P < 0.001$) but no difference was found between asymptomatic and normal

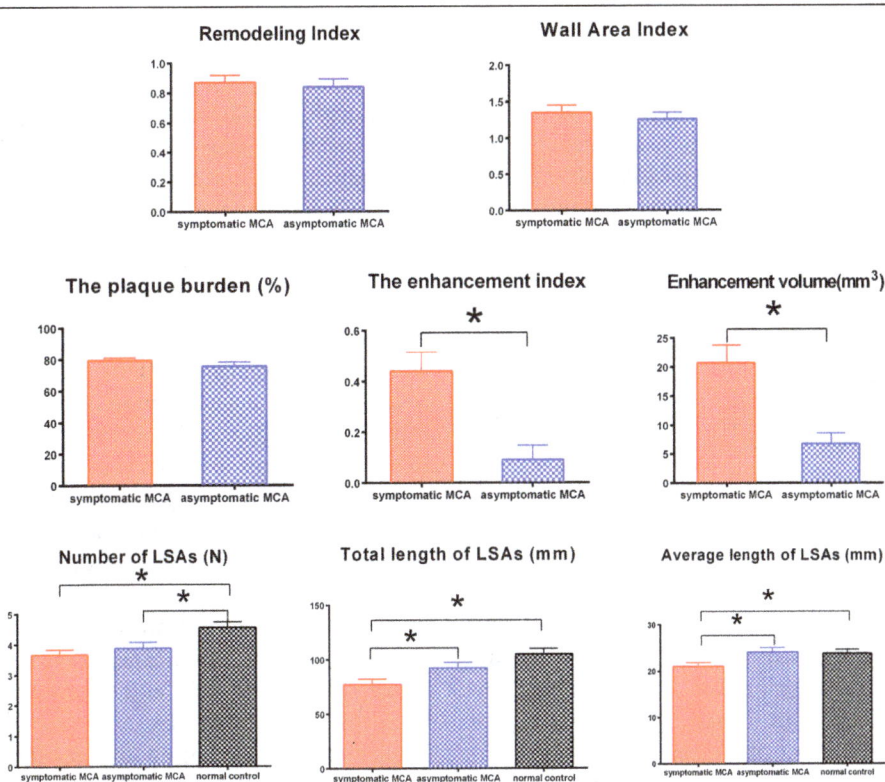

Fig. 2 Comparison of remodeling index, wall area index, plaque burden, enhancement index, enhanced volume, number of lenticulostriate arteries (LSAs) and length of LSAs in symptomatic and asymptomatic MCA groups

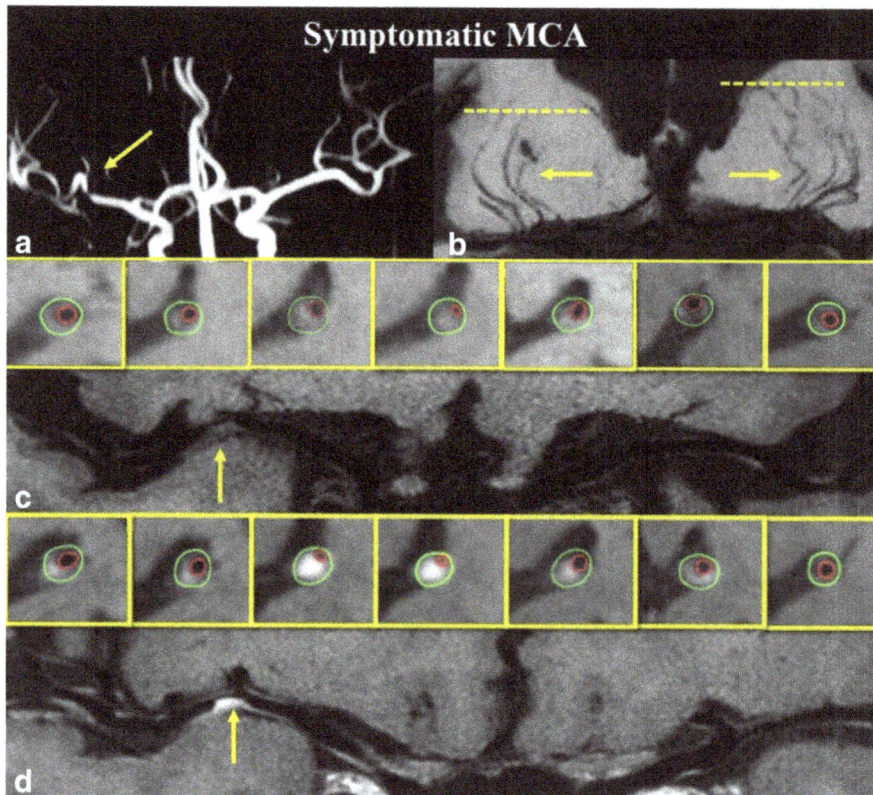

Fig. 3 A 61 years old symptomatic ICAS patient with severe stenosis on right MCA (**a**), coronal MinIP revealed the decrease of right LSA branches compared to the left side (**b**); pre-contrast curved WB-HRCMR and cross-sectional images showed a plaque (**c**, arrow) on the MCA wall; Post-contrast WB-HRCMR showed extensive enhanced plaque volume which can be measured on corresponding cross-sectional images

groups ($P = 0.111$). The symptomatic group had shorter average length than both the asymptomatic groups ($P = 0.02$) and the normal controls ($P = 0.034$). Table 2 summarizes detailed characteristics of the two groups.

Multivariate analysis

In a logistic regression analysis, the higher enhancement index and shorter average length of LSAs were independently associated with stroke. Odds ratios for enhancement index and average length of LSAs were 100.43 and 0.80 (95% confidence interval 4.02–2510.96 and 0.65–0.99; $P = 0.005$ and 0.036) respectively.

Discussion

In this study, we found that symptomatic MCA plaques exhibited a higher enhancement index and larger enhancement volume than the asymptomatic group. Furthermore, a significant reduction in the average number and length of LSAs in symptomatic ICAS groups was also found. To the best of our knowledge, this is the first study using WB-HRCMR to quantitatively explore the intracranial high risk plaque characteristics and LSA features in one imaging setting in ICAS patients.

Although variable refocusing flip angle sequences have been the most extensively studied 3D techniques for intracranial vessel wall imaging to date, it is still associated with inadequate suppression of cerebrospinal fluid (CSF) signals and limited field of view. Some lesions may be missed, especially in the more distally vessels. This may cause an underestimation of the true intracranial plaque burden. WB-HRCMR technique allows for whole brain coverage, relatively high and isotropic spatial resolution, and more importantly, remarkable suppression of CSF and enhanced T1 contrast weighting. It enables the measurement of total intracranial plaque burden, plaque morphology and perforating arteries together.

Previous studies found that enhancement of an intracranial atherosclerotic plaque is associated with a recent ischemic event, and is independent of plaque thickness [20–24]. However, in most studies, the extent of plaque enhancement was not quantitatively measured [21, 24–26] and qualitative methods have been used to categorize the degree of plaque enhancement by comparing the enhancement of plaque and the pituitary on MR [25]. Our findings are in line with the these studies, however, with a step forward quantitative method. We registered and fused the

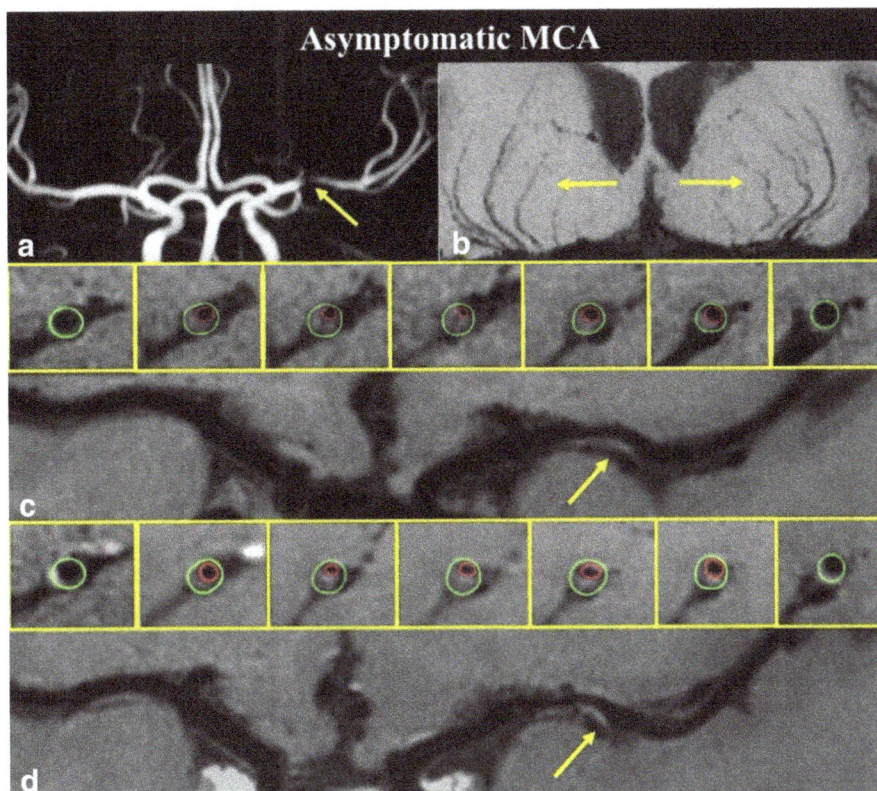

Fig. 4 A 65 years old asymptomatic ICAS patient with severe stenosis on left MCA (**a**), coronal minimum intensity projection (MinIP) revealed symmetrical LSAs of the left and right hemispheres (**b**); pre-contrast curved WB-HRCMR and cross-sectional images showed a plaque (**c**, arrow) on the ventral and inferior side of MCA wall; post-contrast WB-HRCMR showed no enhancement

pre- and post-contrast WB-HRCMR images and contour the enhanced plaque volume, accordingly. Thus, WB-HRCMR enables more accurate measurements of intracranial atherosclerosis plaques characteristics, such as enhancement index and the enhancement volume. We observed that symptomatic MCAs had higher enhancement index and larger enhanced volume of intracranial atherosclerosis plaques.

Recent studies have demonstrated that FSBB-MRA can be used to visualize LSAs [14–16, 27]. Our recent studies proved the feasibility of using whole-brain intracranial vessel wall imaging to depict LSA branches

Table 2 Plaque features and logistic regression analyses in symptomatic and asymptomatic ICAS

	Symptomatic ICAS (N = 29)	Asymptomatic ICAS (N = 23)	P value	Univariate Analysis OR(95%CI)	P value	Multivariable Analysis OR(95%CI)	P value
Degree of stenoses (mean ± SD, %)	63.60 ± 2.80	63.94 ± 3.02	0.936	1.01 (0.99–1.04)	0.424	–	–
Remodeling index (mean ± SD,)	0.87 ± 0.05	0.84 ± 0.06	0.868	1.57(0.18–13.64)	0.681	–	–
Wall area index (mean ± SD)	1.35 ± 0.10	1.26 ± 0.09	0.517	1.46(0.47–4.50)	0.509	–	–
Plaque burden (mean ± SD, %)	79.39 ± 1.64	75.71 ± 2.68	0.227	1.03(0.98–1.09)	0.238	–	–
Enhancement volume (mean ± SD, mm³)	20.70 ± 3.07	6.71 ± 1.87	0.001	1.02(1.02–1.18)	0.005	–	–
Enhancement index (mean ± SD)	0.44 ± 0.08	0.09 ± 0.06	0.001	23.65(2.63–213.02)	0.005	100.43 (4.02–2510.96)	0.005
Number of LSA (mean ± SD, N)	3.65 ± 0.18	3.87 ± 0.21	0.433	0.80(0.44–1.41)	0.425	–	–
Total length of LSA (mean ± SD,mm)	77.12 ± 5.16	92.16 ± 5.15	0.047	0.98(0.96–1.00)	0.054	–	–
Average length of LSA(mean ± SD,mm)	20.95 ± 0.87	24.04 ± 0.95	0.020	0.86(0.76–0.98)	0.027	0.80(0.65–0.99)	0.036

OR Odds ratio, *CI* Confidence interval

[17, 18]. The mean number of LSA branches on normal controls in our study was 4.55, which is consistent with Okuchi's and Kang's previous studies [15, 28]. Compared with normal controls, symptomatic MCAs had a significant decrease in the number and the length of LSAs.

There were several limitations in our study. First, this is an observational study and longitudinal studies are warranted to investigate and expound on the usage of WB-HRCMR in the prediction of stroke outcome and the risk of recurrent stroke. Secondly, the mechanism of plaque enhancement remains unclear and there is no pathological validation of the intracranial plaque vulnerability. Finally, due to the relatively limited spatial resolution used, it is difficult to evaluate the distal small perforating arteries. Partial volume effect of the volume measurement can be overcome by further optimizing imaging parameters or applying with higher field strength.

Conclusions

WB-HRCMR enabled the comprehensive quantitative evaluation of vessel wall lesions and the LSAs in stroke patients. Symptomatic MCAs have larger enhanced plaque volume, higher enhancement plaque index, and shorter length of LSAs compared with asymptomatic MCAs.

Abbreviations

CSF: Cerebrospinal fluid; CTA: Computed tomography angiography; DWI: Diffusion weighted imaging; FSBB-MRA: Flow-sensitive black blood magnetic resonance angiography; HDL: High density lipoprotein; HR-CMR: High-resolution cardiovascular magnetic resonance imaging; ICAS: Intracranial atherosclerotic stenosis; IR: Inversion-recovery; LDL: Low density lipoprotein ; LSA: Lenticulostriate artery ; MCA: Middle cerebral artery; MinIP: Minimum intensity projection; MRA: Magnetic resonance angiography; RCVS: Reversible cerebral vasoconstriction syndrome; RI: Remodel index; ROI: Region-of-interest; SI: Signal intensity; SPACE: Sampling Perfection with Application-optimized Contrast using different flip angle Evolutions; TCD: Transcranial Doppler; VA: Vessel area; WA: Wall area; WB-HRCMR: Whole-brain high-resolution cardiovascular magnetic resonance

Acknowledgements

The authors thank Dr. Haiqing Song, Dr. Qingfeng Ma from Xuanwu Hospital, Capital Medical University for patients recruitment.

Funding

The study was partially support by National Institutes of Health grant number (5 R01 HL096119–07), National Key R&D Program of China (2016YFC1301702,2017YFC1307903), Capital Health Research and Development of Special (2016-1-1031),National Science Foundation of China (NSFC 91749127).

Authors' contributions

Drs QY and XG had full access to all the data in the study and took responsibility for the integrity of the data and the accuracy of the data analysis. Study concept and design: DL, XJ, and QY. Acquisition, analysis, or interpretation of data: MW, HM, YY, ZF, FW. Drafting of the manuscript: MW, QY, XG. Critical revision of the manuscript for important intellectual content: QY. Statistical analysis: HM. Administrative, technical, or material support: DL, XJ. Study supervision: QY, XG. All authors read and approved the final manuscript.

Consent for publication

All individual person's data has consent for publication obtained from that person.

Competing interests

The authors declare that they have no competing interests.

Author details

[1]Department of Neurology, Xuanwu Hospital, Capital Medical University, Beijing 100053, China. [2]Department of Radiology, Xuanwu Hospital, Capital Medical University, Beijing 100053, China. [3]Department of Neurology, Sanbo Brain Hospital, Capital Medical University, Beijing 100093, China. [4]Biomedical Imaging Research Institute, Cedars Sinai Medical Center, Los Angeles, CA 90048, USA. [5]Department of Neurosurgery, Xuanwu Hospital, Capital Medical University, Beijing 100053, China.

References

1. Li H, Wong KS. Racial distribution of intracranial and extracranial atherosclerosis. J Clin Neurosci. 2003;10(1):30–4.
2. Qureshi AI, Caplan LR. Intracranial atherosclerosis. Lancet. 2014;383(9921): 984–98.
3. Feldmann E, Daneault N, Kwan E, Ho KJ, Pessin MS, Langenberg P, Caplan LR. Chinese-white differences in the distribution of occlusive cerebrovascular disease. Neurology. 1990;40(10):1541–5.
4. Wityk RJ, Lehman D, Klag M, Coresh J, Ahn H, Litt B. Race and sex differences in the distribution of cerebral atherosclerosis. Stroke. 1996;27: 1974–80.
5. Kasner SE, Chimowitz MI, Lynn MJ, Howlett-Smith H, Stern BJ, Hertzberg VS, Frankel MR, Levine SR, Chaturvedi S, Benesch CG, et al. Predictors of ischemic stroke in the territory of a symptomatic intracranial arterial stenosis. Circulation. 2006;113(4):555–63.
6. Carvalho M, Oliveira A, Azevedo E, Bastos-Leite AJ. Intracranial arterial stenosis. J Stroke Cerebrovasc Dis. 2014;23(4):599–609.
7. Dubow JS, Salamon E, Greenberg E, Patsalides A. Mechanism of acute ischemic stroke in patients with severe middle cerebral artery atherosclerotic disease. J Stroke Cerebrovasc Dis. 2014;23:1191–4.
8. Sada S, Reddy Y, Rao S, Alladi S, Kaul S. Prevalence of middle cerebral artery stenosis in asymptomatic subjects of more than 40 years age group: a transcranial Doppler study. Neurol India. 2014;62(5):510–5.
9. Mossa-Basha M, Hwang WD, De Havenon A, Hippe D, Balu N, Becker KJ, Tirschwell DT, Hatsukami T, Anzai Y, Yuan C. Multicontrast high-resolution vessel wall magnetic resonance imaging and its value in differentiating intracranial vasculopathic processes. Stroke. 2015;46(6):1567–73.
10. Xu W-H, Li M-L, Gao S, Ni J, Zhou L-X, Yao M, Peng B, Feng F, Jin Z-Y, Cui L-Y. In vivo high-resolution MR imaging of symptomatic and asymptomatic middle cerebral artery atherosclerotic stenosis. Atherosclerosis. 2010;212:507–11.
11. Chen XY, Wong KS, Lam WW, Zhao HL, Ng HK. Middle cerebral artery atherosclerosis: histological comparison between plaques associated with and not associated with infarct in a postmortem study. Cerebrovasc Dis. 2008;25(1–2):74–80.
12. Turan TN, Rumboldt Z, Granholm AC, Columbo L, Welsh CT, Lopes-Virella MF, Spampinato MV, Brown TR. Intracranial atherosclerosis: correlation between in-vivo 3T high resolution MRI and pathology. Atherosclerosis. 2014;237(2):460–3.
13. Teng Z, Peng W, Zhan Q, Zhang X, Liu Q, Chen S, Tian X, Chen L, Brown AJ, Graves MJ, et al. An assessment on the incremental value of high-resolution magnetic resonance imaging to identify culprit plaques in atherosclerotic disease of the middle cerebral artery. Eur Radiol. 2016;26(7):2206–14.
14. Gotoh K, Okada T, Miki Y, Ikedo M, Ninomiya A, Kamae T, Togashi K. Visualization of the lenticulostriate artery with flow-sensitive black-blood acquisition in comparison with time-of-flight MR angiography. J Magn Reson Imaging. 2009;29(1):65–9.
15. Okuchi S, Okada T, Ihara M, Gotoh K, Kido A, Fujimoto K, Yamamoto A, Kanagaki M, Tanaka S, Takahashi R, et al. Visualization of lenticulostriate arteries by flow-sensitive black-blood MR angiography on a 1.5 T MRI system: a comparative study between subjects with and without stroke. AJNR Am J Neuroradiol. 2013;34(4):780–4.

16. Okuchi S, Okada T, Fujimoto K, Fushimi Y, Kido A, Yamamoto A, Kanagaki M, Dodo T, Mehemed TM, Miyazaki M, et al. Visualization of lenticulostriate arteries at 3T: optimization of slice-selective off-resonance sinc pulse-prepared TOF-MRA and its comparison with flow-sensitive black-blood MRA. Acad Radiol. 2014;21(6):812–6.
17. Fan Z, Yang Q, Deng Z, Li Y, Bi X, Song S, Li D. Whole-brain intracranial vessel wall imaging at 3 tesla using cerebrospinal fluid-attenuated T1-weighted 3D turbo spin echo. Magn Reson Med. 2017;77(3):1142–50.
18. Yang Q, Deng Z, Bi X, Song SS, Schlick KH, Gonzalez NR, Li D, Fan Z. Whole-brain vessel wall MRI: a parameter tune-up solution to improve the scan efficiency of three-dimensional variable flip-angle turbo spin-echo. J Magn Reson Imaging. 2017;46(3):751–7.
19. Marinkovic S, Gibo H, Milisavljevic M, Cetkovic M. Anatomic and clinical correlations of the Lenticulostriate arteries. Clin Anat. 2001;14:190–5.
20. Choi YJ, Jung SC, Lee DH. Vessel Wall imaging of the intracranial and cervical carotid arteries. J Stroke. 2015;17(3):238–55.
21. Skarpathiotakis M, Mandell DM, Swartz RH, Tomlinson G, Mikulis DJ. Intracranial atherosclerotic plaque enhancement in patients with ischemic stroke. AJNR Am J Neuroradiol. 2013;34(2):299–304.
22. Natori T, Sasaki M, Miyoshi M, Ito K, Ohba H, Miyazawa H, Narumi S, Kabasawa H, Harada T, Terayama Y. Intracranial plaque characterization in patients with acute ischemic stroke using pre- and post-contrast three-dimensional magnetic resonance Vessel Wall imaging. J Stroke Cerebrovasc Dis. 2016;25(6):1425–30.
23. Ryu CW, Kwak HS, Jahng GH, Lee HN. High-resolution MRI of intracranial atherosclerotic disease. Neurointervention. 2014;9(1):9–20.
24. Vakil P, Vranic J, Hurley MC, Bernstein RA, Korutz AW, Habib A, Shaibani A, Dehkordi FH, Carroll TJ, Ansari SA. T1 gadolinium enhancement of intracranial atherosclerotic plaques associated with symptomatic ischemic presentations. AJNR Am J Neuroradiol. 2013;34(12):2252–8.
25. Qiao Y, Zeiler SR, Mirbagheri S, Leigh R, Urrutia V, Wityk R, Wasserman BA. Intracranial plaque enhancement in patients with cerebrovascular events on high- spatial-resolution MR images. Radiology. 2014;271;271(2):534–42.
26. Kim J-M, Jung K-H, Sohn C-H, Moon J, Shin J-H, Park J, Lee S-H, Han MH, Roh J-K. Intracranial plaque enhancement from high resolution vessel wall magnetic resonance imaging predicts stroke recurrence. Int J Stroke. 2016; 11(2):171–9.
27. Akashi T, Taoka T, Ochi T, Miyasaka T, Wada T, Sakamoto M, Takewa M, Kichikawa K. Branching pattern of lenticulostriate arteries observed by MR angiography at 3.0 T. Jpn J Radiol. 2012;30(4):331–5.
28. Kang CK, Park CA, Park CW, Lee YB, Cho ZH, Kim YB. Lenticulostriate arteries in chronic stroke patients visualised by 7 T magnetic resonance angiography. Int J Stroke. 2010;5(5):374–80.

13

Cardiovascular magnetic resonance imaging of aorto-iliac and ilio-femoral vascular calcifications using proton density-weighted in-phase stack of stars

Ali Serhal[1,2], Ioannis Koktzoglou[2,3], Pascale Aouad[1], James C. Carr[1], Shivraman Giri[4], Omar Morcos[5] and Robert R. Edelman[1,2]* [iD]

Abstract

Background: Comparing cardiovascular magnetic resonance (CMR) angiography with computed tomography angiography (CTA), a major deficiency has been its inability to reliably image peripheral vascular calcifications that may impact the choice of interventional strategy and influence patient prognosis. Recently, MRI using a proton density-weighted, in-phase stack of stars (PDIP-SOS) technique has proved capable of detecting these calcifications. The goal of the present study was two-fold: (1) to determine whether magnetic field strength impacts the apparent size and conspicuity of ilio-femoral arterial calcifications; and (2) to determine whether the technique can be accurately applied to image aorto-iliac arterial calcifications.

Main body: Two patient cohorts were studied. For the first cohort, ilio-femoral arterial calcifications were imaged at 1.5 Tesla in 20 patients and at 3 Tesla in 12 patients. For the second cohort, aorto-iliac arterial calcifications were imaged in 10 patients at 3 Tesla and one patient at 1.5 Tesla. Qualitative image analysis as well as quantitative analysis using a semi-automated technique were performed using CTA as the reference standard. Qualitatively, most PDIP-SOS CMR images showed good-to-excellent confidence to detect vascular calcifications, with good-to-excellent inter-reader agreement ($\kappa = 0.67$ for ilio-femoral region, $P < 0.001$; $\kappa = 0.80$ for aorto-iliac region, $P < 0.01$). There was an overall excellent correlation ($r = 0.98$, $P < 0.001$) and agreement (intraclass correlation coefficient $= 0.97$, $P < 0.001$) between PDIP-SOS CMR and CTA measures of calcification volume in both regions, with no overt difference in performance at 1.5 Tesla vs. 3 Tesla for ilio-femoral calcifications. CMR lesion volumes were slightly lower than those measured for CTA.

Conclusion: Using PDIP-SOS CMR, aorto-iliac and ilio-femoral calcifications could be simultaneously evaluated at 3 Tesla in less than six minutes with excellent correlation and agreement to CTA. Our results suggest that PDIP-SOS CMR provides a reliable alternative to CT for pre-interventional evaluation of peripheral vascular calcium burden.

Keywords: Vascular calcification, Stack of stars, Magnetic resonance imaging, Quiescent-interval slice-selective, CT angiography, Peripheral arterial disease

* Correspondence: redelman999@gmail.com
[1]Radiology, Northwestern Memorial Hospital, Chicago, IL, USA
[2]Radiology, Northshore University HealthSystem, Walgreen Building, G534, 2650 Ridge Avenue, Evanston, IL 60201, USA
Full list of author information is available at the end of the article

Background

Both computed tomography angiography (CTA) and cardiovascular magnetic resonance (CMR) angiography are accurate tests for the cross-sectional assessment of peripheral arterial disease (PAD) [1, 2]. Compared with CMR angiography, CTA offers higher speed, lower cost, and fewer drawbacks overall. Nonetheless, peripheral CMR angiography remains in widespread use, in part because it avoids exposure to ionizing radiation and, given that patients with PAD often suffer from poor renal function [3], offers the option of imaging without an exogenous contrast agent [4].

In diabetic patients, CMR angiography is advantageous compared with CTA because of the high prevalence of peripheral vascular calcifications [5]. With CTA, these calcifications confound the evaluation of small caliber vessels due to blooming artifact that obscures the vessel lumen [6]. Since vascular calcifications are unapparent and do not cause image artifacts with CMR angiography, it is often preferred to CTA in this patient group. However, important information deriving from the presence of vascular calcifications, including the impact on interventional strategy and patient prognosis, is then lost [7–10]. For instance, dense arterial wall calcifications should be avoided when choosing a percutaneous access site, and their presence is a major determinant of failure for percutaneous endovascular aneurysm repair [10].

The inability to image vascular calcifications remains an important and unaddressed deficiency of CMR angiography. For instance, in the largest clinical trial to evaluate the association of plaque characteristics with functional performance in patients with PAD, investigators were unable to reliably identify vascular calcifications [11]. The only way to recover this information would be to perform an additional CT scan, which is inconvenient and costly.

Vascular calcifications have negligible signal intensity with standard CMR pulse sequences due to low free water concentration and short T2* [12]. While this property makes them difficult to visualize with CMR angiography, a recent study demonstrated the feasibility of using "neutral contrast" 3D gradient-echo techniques to depict peripheral vascular calcifications on minimum intensity projection CMR images [13]. However, a major unknown with using CMR to image vascular calcifications is the potential impact of field strength on apparent lesion volumes. Just as calcifications can show blooming artifact with CT, diamagnetic susceptibility and T2* effects have the potential to cause field strength-dependent blooming artifact with CMR. Vascular calcifications are strongly diamagnetic - as much as ten times that of the vessel wall – which results in field strength-dependent phase shifts [14]. Moreover, the signal-to-noise ratio (SNR), R2*, chemical shift and off-resonance effects all increase with field strength.

Another unknown is whether CMR can reliably image vascular calcifications in the abdomen and pelvis. In these regions, respiratory motion as well as presence of peristalsing, air-containing bowel loops have the potential to cause blurring and off-resonance effects, thereby obscuring vessel calcifications.

To address these concerns, the goals of the present study were two-fold: (1) to determine whether magnetic field strength impacts the apparent size and conspicuity of ilio-femoral arterial calcifications; and (2) to determine whether the technique can be applied to accurately image aorto-iliac arterial calcifications.

Methods

This prospective study was approved by the Institutional Review Boards of two academic centers and informed consent was obtained. Two cohorts of patients were studied. For the first cohort, 32 patients (52–84 years, 10 female) were consecutively recruited from those in whom CTA performed within the preceding three months demonstrated vascular calcifications in at least one ilio-femoral vessel segment. At one institution, 20 patients were imaged using a 1.5 Tesla MAGNETOM Aera scanner (Siemens Healthineers, Erlangen, German), while at the other institution 12 patients were imaged using a 3.0 Tesla MAGNETOM Skyra Fit scanner (Siemens Healthineers). For the second cohort, 11 patients (57–83 years, 2 female) were recruited from those in whom CTA demonstrated vascular calcifications in the region of the aorto-iliac bifurcation; ten patients in this cohort were imaged at 3 Tesla, while one patient was imaged at 1.5 Tesla.

Nonenhanced quiescent-interval slice-selective (QISS) CMR angiography [15] of the peripheral arteries was used as the scout for positioning the proton density-weighted, in-phase stack-of-stars (PDIP-SOS) spoiled gradient-echo pulse sequence. This sequence provides nearly isotropic images in which muscle, fat, and intravascular signal show intermediate signal intensity, whereas vascular calcifications appear uniformly dark [16]. Unlike a Cartesian 3D acquisition, in which chemical shift artifacts at fat/water interfaces appear as discrete dark lines that can obscure or be confounded with vascular calcifications in minimum intensity projections, these interfaces are less distinct with the in-phase stack-of-stars radial k-space trajectory so that they are invisible in the projection images.

For the first cohort of patients, the PDIP-SOS sequence used a legacy encoding scheme whereby all radial views were collected in rapid sequence as a single shot. For the second cohort of patients, the k-space sampling strategy was updated so that all slice partitions, rather than radial views, were collected in rapid sequence.

PDIP-SOS images were acquired in an oblique coronal plane. Body and peripheral phased array coils were used for signal reception. There were some differences in the imaging parameters between the two magnetic field strengths, due primarily to the in-phase echo time at 1.5 Tesla being twice the value at 3 Tesla and the use of a lower sampling bandwidth to improve the SNR, in turn lengthening the repetition time. Consequently, some compromises in spatial resolution were needed at 1.5 Tesla to avoid increasing scan time and to maintain adequate SNR despite the lower field strength. Slice thickness was 1.3-mm at 1.5 Tesla and 1.0-mm at 3 Tesla, with 128 reconstructed slices per 3D slab and in-plane resolution at both field strengths of 1.0-mm × 1.0-mm prior to interpolation. For the second patient cohort using the updated k-space sampling strategy, PDIP-SOS CMR encompassing both the aorto-iliac and ilio-femoral regions was acquired with 1200 radial views in a scan time of 5 min 49 s. The PDIP-SOS images were processed into thin (4 to 15-mm) minimum intensity projections for qualitative display of the vascular calcifications.

The CTA studies were acquired on three different scanners: SOMATOM Force, SOMATOM Definition AS and SOMATOM Definition (Siemens Healthineers, Forchheim, Germany) with standard technique using either iterative reconstruction or filtered back projection according to clinical routine. Typical slice thickness was on the order of 0.6-mm to 1-mm. kVp was selected according to the pre-determined body mass index-based institutional protocol.

Quantitative image analysis

Quantification of the calcification volumes was done using in-house software executed within ImageJ (version 1.51p, National Institutes of Health, Bethesda, Maryland, USA). For analysis of the ilio-femoral region, on each lower limb extremity, two segments of the femoral artery were analyzed: the proximal segment which covered 5 cm of the common femoral artery immediately above the femoral bifurcation, and the distal segment which covered 5 cm of the superficial femoral artery immediately below the bifurcation. For analysis of the aorto-iliac region, five segments of the aorta and iliac vessels were analyzed: the most distal 5 cm segment of the aorta, the left and right common iliac arteries, and the left and right external iliac arteries. The segmentation algorithm volumetrically segmented the calcifications using thresholds based on Hounsfield units for CTA images and on signal intensity for CMR images. Using this algorithm, we have previously found that a threshold of 560

Hounsfield units was optimal for distinguishing calcifications on CTA from contrast-enhanced lumen. For CMR images of the ilio-femoral region, voxels having a signal intensity more than three standard deviations below the mean were classified as calcifications. A CMR threshold of two (instead of three) standard deviations was used in the aorto-iliac region due to slightly increased background signal variability in this region from bowel and respiratory motion. Bicubic interpolation was used to scale all CMR and CTA data to 0.5 mm isotropic resolution before measurement of calcification volume.

Qualitative image analysis

Two cardiovascular radiology fellows (AS, PA), blinded to clinical information, qualitatively reviewed source images and multi-planar reformats for both CTA and CMR. CTA images were taken as a reference and the PDIP-SOS CMR images were analyzed for degree of confidence to detect calcification, matching size, shape and location of calcification with the CTA images. Images were scored using a 5-point Likert scale as: 1- very poor, 2- poor, 3- fair, 4- good, 5- excellent.

Data and statistical analysis

Correlation between volume of vascular calcification shown by PDIP-SOS and CTA was assessed by linear regression and Pearson's correlation analysis (with correlation coefficient, r). Agreement of vascular calcification volume was assessed by intraclass correlation coefficient (ICC). Sub-analyses of data in the ilio-femoral region were performed by stratifying according to magnetic field strength (1.5 Tesla and 3 Tesla), and severity of calcification (none or mild, moderate, severe) based on calcification volume measures on CTA. Group 1 included patients with no or mild vascular calcification (volume 0–99 mm^3), group 2 included patients with moderate vascular calcification (volume 100–299 mm^3), and group 3 included patients with severe vascular calcification (volume ≥ 300 mm^3). Weighted Cohen's kappa (κ) coefficient was used to assess inter-rater agreement of qualitative scores. Pearson correlation (r), ICC, and κ coefficients were interpreted as follows: < 0.40 – poor, 0.40–0.59 – fair, 0.60–0.74 – good, ≥ 0.75 – excellent [17]. Bland-Altman analysis was used to compute mean bias (MR volume minus CTA volume) and 95% limits of agreement. Statistical analyses were performed in R software (version 3.4.2, R Foundation for Statistical Computing, Vienna, Austria).

Results
Cohort 1 (Ilio-femoral vessels)

Of 128 ilio-femoral vessel segments available for analysis, 6 were excluded (4 due to magnetic susceptibility artifact from hip prosthesis or stent and 2 due to artifact relating to recent bypass graft), leaving a total of 122 vessel segments that were analyzed.

Qualitatively, PDIP-SOS CMR images showed good-to-excellent confidence to detect ilio-femoral vascular calcifications with a mean score of 4.1 (range 3–5) for the first reader and 4.3 (range 3–5) for the second reader. Inter-rater agreement was good (κ=0.67, 95% confidence interval (CI): 0.54–0.80, $P < 0.001$). The size, shape and location of the calcifications by PDIP-SOS CMR matched CTA findings in all patients regardless of lesion volume (Fig. 1).

Figure 2 shows scatter plots of calcification volume in the ilio-femoral region stratified by magnetic field strength and severity of calcification. There was an overall excellent correlation ($r = 0.98$, 95% CI: 0.97–0.99, $P < 0.001$) and agreement (ICC = 0.97, 95% CI: 0.96–0.98, $P < 0.001$) between PDIP-SOS CMR and CTA measures of calcification volume (Fig. 2a). The average volume was 124 mm^3 (range 0–953 mm^3) by CTA and 109 mm^3 (range 0–914 mm^3) by CMR. When comparing the results of CMR exams done on 1.5 Tesla and 3 Tesla, the correlation coefficients were $r = 0.98$ (95% CI: 0.97–

0.99, $P < 0.001$) and 0.99 (95% CI: 0.98–0.99, $P < 0.001$), while ICC values were 0.96 (95% CI: 0.94–0.97, $P < 0.001$) and 0.99 (95% CI: 0.98–0.99, $P < 0.001$), respectively (Figs. 2b and c). Bland-Altman mean biases and 95% limits of agreement (CMR minus CTA calcification volume) at both magnetic field strengths, 1.5 Tesla, and 3 Tesla were – 15.7 [– 95.2, 63.8] mm^3, – 20.3 [– 107.9, 67.3] mm^3, and – 7.0 [– 65.4, 51.4] mm^3, respectively.

The Pearson correlation coefficients of calcification volume for patients with no-to-mild, moderate and severe vascular calcifications were $r = 0.83$ (95% CI: 0.74–0.89), 0.90 (95% CI: 0.80–0.95), and 0.88 (95% CI: 0.69–0.96) ($P < 0.001$ for all), respectively (Figs. 2d-f). Corresponding ICC values for agreement in these three strata remained in the excellent range and were 0.82 (95% CI: 0.73–0.88), 0.77 (95% CI: 0.58–0.89), and 0.84 (95% CI: 0.63–0.94) ($P < 0.001$ for all), respectively. Bland-Altman mean biases [95% limits of agreement] for patients with no-to-mild, moderate, and severe vascular calcifications were – 1.7 [– 30.0, 26.6] mm^3, – 30.3 [– 80.5, 19.9] mm^3, and – 53.4 [– 223.1, 116.3] mm^3, respectively.

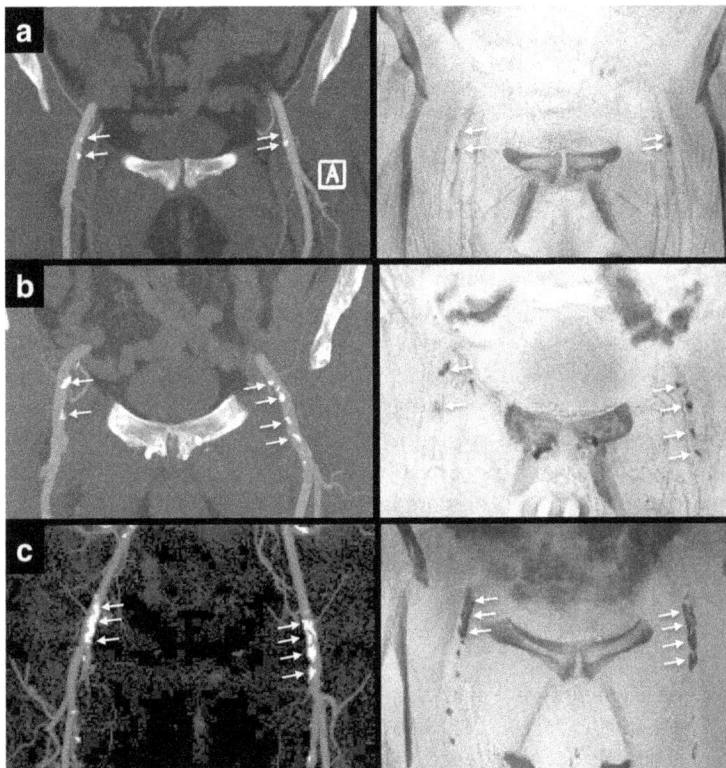

Fig. 1 Examples of PDIP-SOS CMR (right) in comparison to CTA (left) for: (**a**) 66-year-old female imaged at 1.5 Tesla showing mild vascular calcifications (Group 1), (**b**) 80-year-old male imaged at 1.5 Tesla showing moderate vascular calcifications (Group 2), and (**c**) 68-year-old female imaged at 3 Tesla showing severe vascular calcifications (Group 3). Vascular calcifications (arrows) appear dark with PDIP-CMR (presented as thin minimum intensity projections), and bright with CTA (presented as thin maximum intensity projections). There is excellent correlation between CMR and CTA irrespective of lesion severity

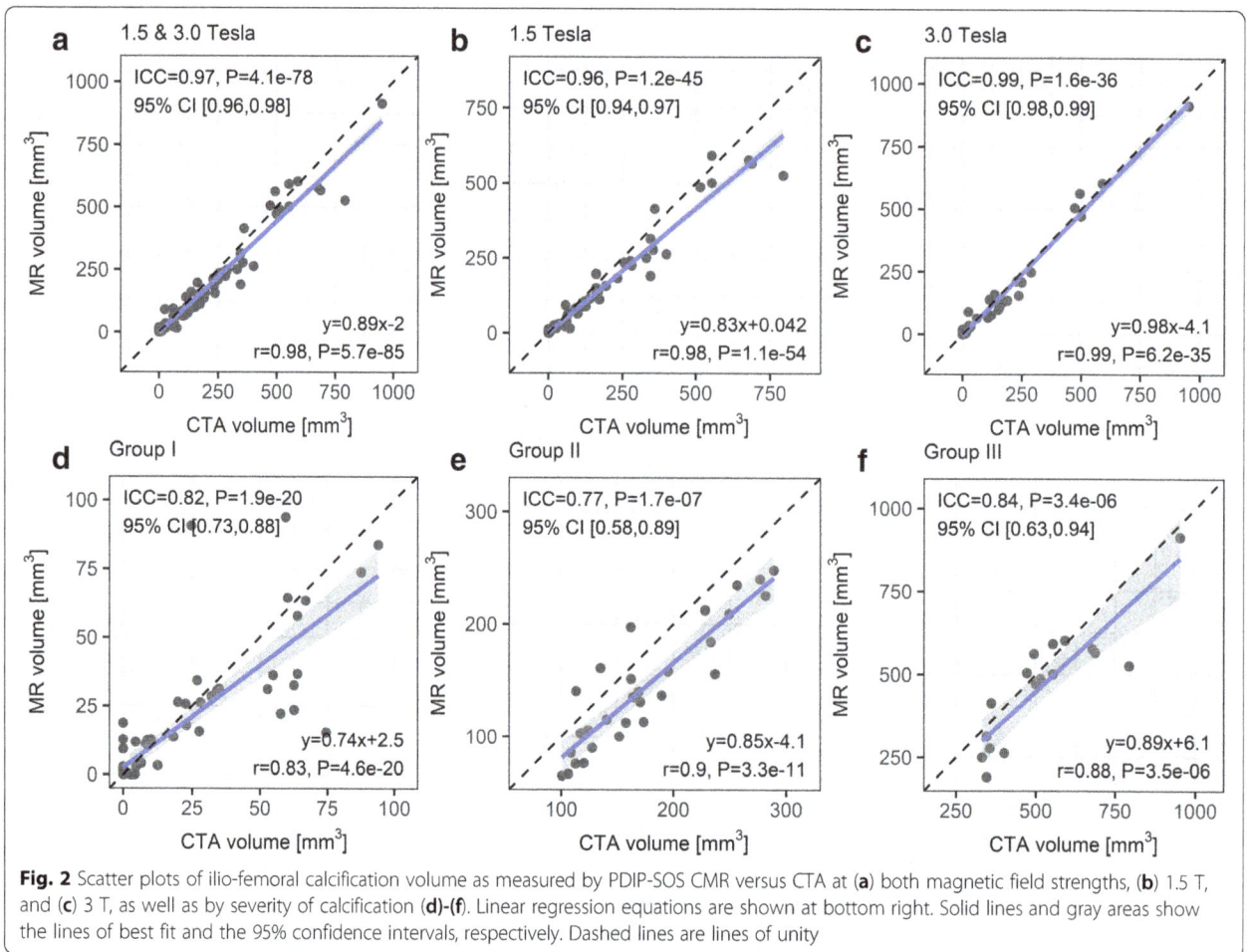

Fig. 2 Scatter plots of ilio-femoral calcification volume as measured by PDIP-SOS CMR versus CTA at (**a**) both magnetic field strengths, (**b**) 1.5 T, and (**c**) 3 T, as well as by severity of calcification (**d**)-(**f**). Linear regression equations are shown at bottom right. Solid lines and gray areas show the lines of best fit and the 95% confidence intervals, respectively. Dashed lines are lines of unity

Cohort 2 (aorto-iliac vessels)

Initial studies demonstrated that the order in which the slice partitions and radial views were collected, while largely irrelevant for the ilio-femoral vessels, had a profound effect on image quality for the aorto-iliac vessels. Acquisitions using a legacy k-space encoding strategy in which the radial views were collected in rapid sequence as a single shot typically showed extensive artifacts relating to air-containing bowel loops which often obscured the distal aorta and pelvic arteries. In contrast, these artifacts were largely absent when the slice partitions were collected in rapid sequence as a single shot allowing for unambiguous identification of vascular calcifications (Fig. 3).

A total of 55 aorto-iliac vessel segments were analyzed, and none were excluded. Qualitatively, most PDIP-SOS CMR images showed good-to-excellent confidence to detect aorto-iliac vascular calcifications with a mean score of 4.1 (range 3–5) for the first reader and 4.0 (range 3–5) for the second reader. Inter-rater agreement was excellent (κ=0.80, 95% confidence interval (CI): 0.57–1.00, $P < 0.01$).

Figure 4 shows a scatter plot of calcification volume in the aorto-iliac region. There was an overall excellent correlation ($r = 0.98$, 95% CI: 0.97–0.99, $P < 0.001$) and agreement (ICC = 0.97, 95% CI: 0.96–0.98, $P < 0.001$) between PDIP-SOS CMR and CTA measures of calcification volume. The average volume was 450 mm^3 (range 0–2750 mm^3) by CTA and 391 mm^3 (range 0–2854 mm^3) by CMR. The Bland-Altman (CMR minus CTA calcification volume) mean bias was − 58.5 mm^3, while the 95% limits of agreement were [− 261.8, 144.7] mm^3.

Discussion

Prior work has shown that CMR using a PDIP-SOS pulse sequence is accurate for ilio-femoral vascular calcifications [16]. The present work differs in three significant ways from this prior work. First, the present study was sufficiently powered to examine the impact of magnetic field strength (1.5 Tesla vs. 3 Tesla) on sequence performance and apparent lesion size for ilio-femoral calcifications. Second, we used a new motion-resistant k-space trajectory to additionally enable evaluation of

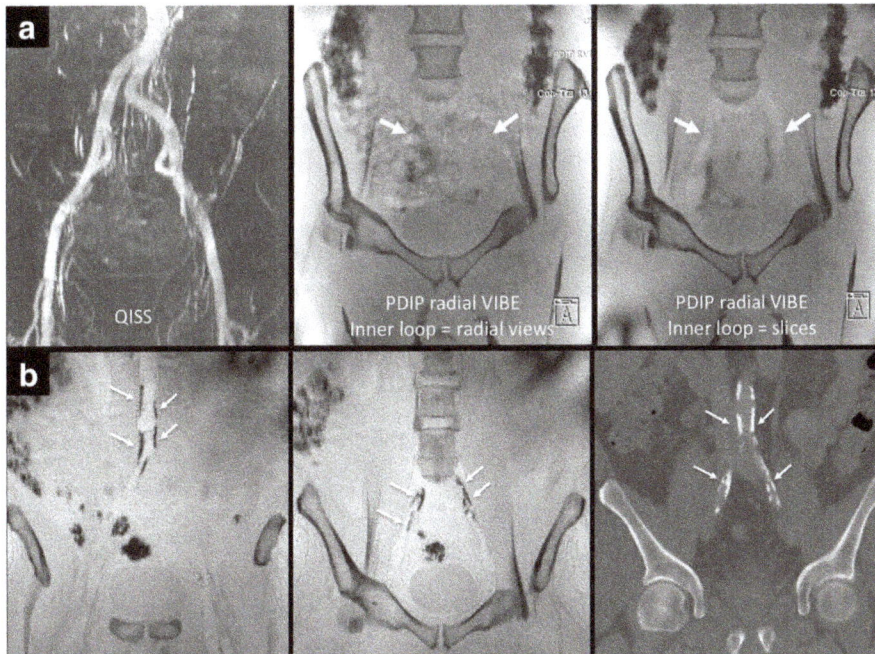

Fig. 3 Evaluation of the aorto-iliac vessels using PDIP-SOS CMR. (a) Healthy volunteer. Left: QISS nonenhanced CMR angiogram used for positioning the stack of stars imaging slab. Middle: PDIP-SOS CMR using the legacy k-space encoding approach of acquiring all radial views in rapid sequence. There are severe ghost artifacts arising from centrally-located bowel loops that obscure the iliac vessels (arrows). Right: Identical PDIP-SOS acquisition except that all slice partitions (instead of radial views) were acquired in rapid sequence. The bowel-related artifacts are eliminated, so that the iliac vessels are well shown (arrows). Note that both the aorto-iliac and ilio-femoral regions are encompassed in the field of view, allowing simultaneous assessment of both regions. (b) Patient with aorto-iliac calcifications. Left, middle: 4-mm thick minimum intensity projections from PDIP-SOS CMR clearly depict vascular calcifications involving the distal aorta and proximal iliac vessels. Right: Thin-slab maximum intensity coronal projection from the CT shows excellent correspondence with the PDIP-SOS CMR

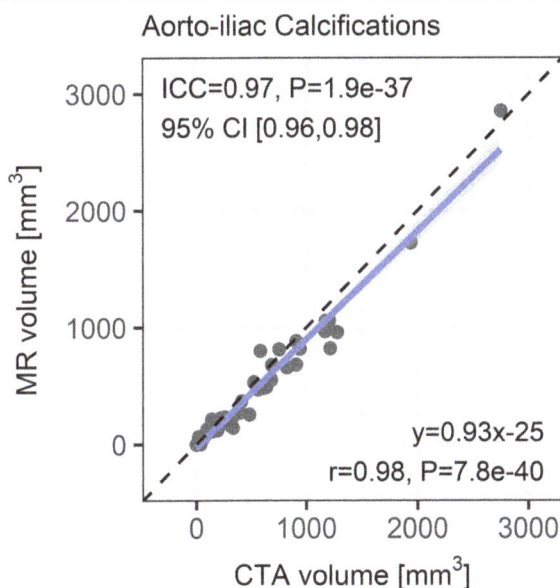

Fig. 4 Scatter plot of aorto-iliac calcification volume as measured by PDIP-SOS CMR versus CTA. Linear regression equation is shown at bottom right. The solid line and gray area show the line of best fit and the 95% confidence interval, respectively. Dashed line shows the line of unity

aorto-iliac calcifications, which was not possible with earlier versions of the technique due to excessive respiratory and bowel motion artifacts. Third, a new cohort of patients with PAD was used for the present study with no overlap to the prior study.

Our results indicate that CMR using a PDIP-SOS pulse sequence depicts ilio-femoral and aorto-iliac calcifications with excellent correlation ($r \geq 0.98$) and agreement (ICC ≥ 0.97) to CTA over a wide range of lesion volumes. The correlation and agreement to CTA for ilio-femoral calcifications were similar at 1.5 Tesla and 3 Tesla, suggesting that lesion volumes as measured by PDIP-SOS CMR are not substantially dependent on magnetic field strength. Regardless of field strength, in no case did CMR miss large calcifications that might adversely impact the outcome of a percutaneous procedure, nor falsely suggest significant calcifications where none existed in the CTA.

Given that CMR is generally considered to be insensitive to vascular calcifications, it is notable that the PDIP-SOS imaging technique could detect calcifications over a wide range of lesion volumes, including small vascular calcifications that spanned only a few pixels. However, the use of a very small voxel (e.g. ~ 1 mm^3 in the current study) and adequate SNR are essential for confidently detecting small lesions.

The stack of stars k-space trajectory has the benefit of being less sensitive to artifacts from respiratory motion than a Cartesian 3D acquisition, due to extensive over-sampling of the center of k-space [18]. Nonetheless, we found that our legacy k-space encoding approach for PDIP-SOS, in which all radial views were acquired in rapid sequence as a single shot, often showed severe image artifacts in the pelvic and abdominal regions due to respiratory and peristaltic motion of bowel loops. These bowel-related artifacts often obscured nearby vascular calcifications. In order to overcome these artifacts, we modified the k-space sampling strategy to acquire all slice partitions in rapid sequence rather than radial views. A similar sampling strategy has previously been reported to reduce respiratory motion artifact in the upper abdomen [19], and we found it to be highly effective at suppressing artifacts from bowel motion in the lower abdomen and pelvis as well. With this updated PDIP-SOS CMR technique, it is now possible to simultaneously and accurately assess vascular calcifications in both the aorto-iliac and ilio-femoral regions with a single, < 6-min oblique coronal acquisition.

Across all patients at both magnetic field strengths, CMR slightly underestimated calcification volumes (linear regression slopes of ~ 0.89 and ~ 0.93 for ilio-femoral and aorto-iliac regions) compared with CTA. This discrepancy might be explained by the fact that blooming artifact artifactually enlarges dense calcifications on CT images [20]. Alternatively, it is conceivable that the surface regions of a calcification contain mobile water spins that produce detectable signal intensity, which would decrease their apparent volume with PDIP-SOS CMR.

A limitation of our study was that contrast-enhanced CTA was used as a reference standard, whereas non-contrast CT would be preferred. However, at the two institutions used for this study, non-contrast CT series were acquired at 3 to 5-mm slice thickness, too thick for volumetric evaluation, compared with 0.6 to 1-mm slice thickness for CTA. Also, PDIP-SOS CMR scan times were substantially longer than is the case with CT. Scan time can be greatly reduced (e.g. to 30 s or less) by acquiring thicker slices and using fewer radial views at the expense of more partial volume averaging, decreased SNR and increased radial streak artifacts. While this accelerated approach would reduce sensitivity for very small calcifications, it is unlikely that detection of bulky, clinically significant calcifications would be adversely affected. Finally, our study demonstrated that imaging of both aorto-iliac and ilio-femoral calcifications is accurate at 3 Tesla. While imaging of ilio-femoral calcifications is also accurate at 1.5 Tesla, the study was underpowered ($n = 1$) at this field strength to draw any conclusions about aorto-iliac calcifications.

Conclusion

Using PDIP-SOS CMR, aorto-iliac and ilio-femoral calcifications could be simultaneously evaluated at 3 Tesla in less than six minutes with excellent correlation and agreement to CTA. Lesion size was not substantially affected by magnetic field strength. Our results suggest that PDIP-SOS CMR provides a reliable alternative to CT for pre-interventional evaluation of peripheral vascular calcium burden.

Abbreviations
CMR: cardiovascular magnetic resonance; CT: computed tomography; CTA: computed tomographic angiography; PAD: peripheral arterial disease; PDIP-SOS: proton density-weighted, in-phase stack-of-stars; QISS: Quiescent-Interval Slice-Selective; SNR: signal-to-noise ratio

Acknowledgements
We would like to thank Dr. Wei Li and Maria Carr for assisting with data collection and analysis.

Funding
Research support, NIH grants R01 HL130093 and R21 HL126015. Research support, Siemens Healthineers. Research support, Department of Radiology, NorthShore University HealthSystem.

Authors' contributions
RE: participated in all aspects of the study and is the guarantor of study integrity. AS: assisted with image analysis and manuscript review. PA: assisted with image analysis and manuscript review. JC: assisted with patient recruitment and manuscript review. OM: assisted with patient recruitment and manuscript review. SG: assisted with pulse sequence implementation and manuscript review. IK: assisted with pulse sequence implementation, statistical analysis and manuscript review. All authors read and approved the manuscript.

Consent for publication
Consent for publication of their individual details and accompanying images in this manuscript was prospectively provided in all 43 subjects. No protected health information for any subject is given in this manuscript. The tables and figures are all original and have never been submitted or published elsewhere.

Competing interests
RE: Research support and invention licensing agreement, Siemens Healthcare. SG: Employee, Siemens Healthineers. There were no potential financial conflicts for the other authors. There were no non-financial. conflicts of interest for any of the authors.

Author details
[1]Radiology, Northwestern Memorial Hospital, Chicago, IL, USA. [2]Radiology, Northshore University HealthSystem, Walgreen Building, G534, 2650 Ridge Avenue, Evanston, IL 60201, USA. [3]Radiology, University of Chicago Pritzker School of Medicine, Chicago, IL, USA. [4]Siemens Healthineers, Chicago, IL, USA. [5]Surgery, Northshore University HealthSystem, Evanston, IL, USA.

References

1. Met R, Bipat S, Legemate DA, Reekers JA, Koelemay MJ. Diagnostic performance of computed tomography angiography in peripheral arterial disease: a systematic review and meta-analysis. JAMA. 2009;301:415–24.

2. Menke J, Larsen J. Meta-analysis: accuracy of contrast-enhanced magnetic resonance angiography for assessing steno-occlusions in peripheral arterial disease. Ann Intern Med. 2010;153:325–34.

3. Tranche-Iparraguirre S, Marín-Iranzo R, Fernández-de Sanmamed R, Riesgo-García A, Hevia-Rodríguez E, García-Casas JB. Peripheral arterial disease and kidney failure: a frequent association. Nefrologia. 2012;32:313–20. https://doi.org/10.3265/Nefrologia.pre2011.Nov.11172. Epub 2012 Jan 27

4. Miyazaki M, Lee VS. Nonenhanced MR angiography. Radiology. 2008;248:20–43. https://doi.org/10.1148/radiol.2481071497.

5. Singh DK, Winocour P, Summerhayes B, Kaniyur S, Viljoen A, Sivakumar G, Farrington K. Prevalence and progression of peripheral vascular calcification in type 2 diabetes subjects with preserved kidney function. Diabetes Res Clin Pract. 2012;97:158–65. https://doi.org/10.1016/j.diabres.2012.01.038. Epub 2012 Mar 3

6. Ouwendijk R, Kock MC, van Dijk LC, van Sambeek MR, Stijnen T, Hunink MG. Vessel wall calcifications at multi-detector row CT angiography in patients with peripheral arterial disease: effect on clinical utility and clinical predictors. Radiology. 2006;241:603–8.

7. Niskanen L, Siitonen O, Suhonen M, Uusitupa MI. Medial artery calcification predicts cardiovascular mortality in patients with NIDDM. Diabetes Care. 1994;17:1252–6.

8. Guzman RJ, Brinkley DM, Schumacher PM, Donahue RM, Beavers H, Qin X. Tibial artery calcification as a marker of amputation risk in patients with peripheral arterial disease. J Am Coll Cardiol. 2008;51:1967–74.

9. Pentecost MJ, Criqui MH, Dorros G, et al. Guidelines for peripheral percutaneous transluminal angioplasty of the abdominal aorta and lower extremity vessels. A statement for health professionals from a special writing group of the councils on cardiovascular radiology, arteriosclerosis, cardio-thoracic and vascular surgery, clinical cardiology, and epidemiology and prevention, the American Heart Association. Circulation. 1994;89:511–31.

10. Manunga JM, Gloviczki P, Oderich GS, Kalra M, Duncan AA, Fleming MD, Bower TC. Femoral artery calcification as a determinant of success for percutaneous access for endovascular abdominal aortic aneurysm repair. J Vasc Surg. 2013 Jul 2.

11. McDermott MM, Liu K, Carroll TJ, et al. Superficial femoral artery plaque and functional performance in peripheral arterial disease: walking and leg circulation study (WALCS III). JACC Cardiovasc Imaging. 2011;4:730–9. https://doi.org/10.1016/j.jcmg.2011.04.009.

12. Tenner MS, Spiller M, Koenig SH, Valsamis MP, Childress S, Brown RD 3rd, Kasoff SS. Calcification can shorten T2, but not T1, at magnetic resonance imaging fields. Investig Radiol. 1995;30(6):345–53.

13. Edelman RR, Flanagan O, Giri S, Koktzoglou I. Neutral contrast MRI for the detection of peripheral arterial wall calcifications. J Cardiovasc Magn Reson. 2014;16(Suppl 1):O76. https://doi.org/10.1186/1532-429X-16-S1-O76.

14. Yang Q, Liu J, Barnes SRS, et al. Imaging the vessel wall in major peripheral arteries using susceptibility weighted imaging. J Magn Reson Imaging. 2009;30(2):357–65.

15. Edelman RR, Sheehan JJ, Dunkle E, Schindler N, Carr J, Koktzoglou I. Quiescent-interval single-shot unenhanced magnetic resonance angiography of peripheral vascular disease: technical considerations and clinical feasibility. Magn Reson Med. 2010;63:951–8.

16. Ferreira Botelho MP, Koktzoglou I, Collins JD, Giri S, Carr JC, Gupta N, Edelman RR. MR imaging of iliofemoral peripheral vascular calcifications using proton density-weighted, in-phase three-dimensional stack-of-stars gradient echo. Magn Reson Med 2017 Jun;77(6):2146–2152. https://doi.org/10.1002/mrm.26295. Epub 2016 Jun 14.

17. Cicchetti DV. Guidelines, criteria, and rules of thumb for evaluating normed and standardized assessment instruments in psychology. Psychological Assessment. 1994;6:284–90. https://doi.org/10.1037/1040-3590.6.4.284.

18. Glover GH, Pauly JM. Projection reconstruction techniques for reduction of motion effects in MRI. Magn Reson Med. 1992;28:275–89.

19. Block KT, Chandarana H, Milla S, et al. Towards routine clinical use of radial stack-of-stars 3D gradient-echo sequences for reducing motion sensitivity. Journal of the Korean Soc Magnet Resona in Med. 2014;18(2):87–106.

20. Fleischmann D, Hallett RL, Rubin GD. CT angiography of peripheral arterial disease. J Vasc Interv Radiol. 2006 Jan;17(1):3–26.

14

Feasibility of 3D black-blood variable refocusing angle fast spin echo cardiovascular magnetic resonance for visualization of the whole heart and great vessels in congenital heart disease

Markus Henningsson[1]*(iD), Riad Abou Zahr[2], Adrian Dyer[2], Gerald F. Greil[2], Barbara Burkhardt[2], Animesh Tandon[2] and Tarique Hussain[2]

Abstract

Background: Volumetric black-blood cardiovascular magnetic resonance (CMR) has been hampered by long scan times and flow sensitivity. The purpose of this study was to assess the feasibility of black-blood, electrocardiogram (ECG)-triggered and respiratory-navigated 3D fast spin echo (3D FSE) for the visualization of the whole heart and great vessels.

Methods: The implemented 3D FSE technique used slice-selective excitation and non-selective refocusing pulses with variable flip angles to achieve constant echo signal for tissue with T1 (880 ms) and T2 (40 ms) similar to the vessel wall. Ten healthy subjects and 21 patients with congenital heart disease (CHD) underwent 3D FSE and conventional 3D balanced steady-state free precession (bSSFP). The sequences were compared in terms of ability to perform segmental assessment, local signal-to-noise ratio (SNR_l) and local contrast-to-noise ratio (CNR_l).

Results: In both healthy subjects and patients with CHD, 3D FSE showed superior pulmonary vein but inferior coronary artery origin visualisation compared to 3D bSFFP. However, in patients with CHD the combination of 3D bSSFP and 3D FSE whole-heart imaging improves the success rate of cardiac morphological diagnosis to 100% compared to either technique in isolation (3D FSE, 23.8% success rate, 3D bSSFP, 5% success rate). In the healthy subjects SNR_l for 3D bSSFP was greater than for 3D FSE (30.1 ± 7.3 vs 20.9 ± 5.3; $P = 0.002$) whereas the CNR_l was comparable (17.3 ± 5.6 vs 17.4 ± 4.9; $P = 0.91$) between the two scans.

Conclusions: The feasibility of 3D FSE for whole-heart black-blood CMR imaging has been demonstrated. Due to their high success rate for segmental assessment, the combination of 3D bSSFP and 3D FSE may be an attractive alternative to gadolinium contrast enhanced morphological CMR in patients with CHD.

Keywords: Black-blood CMR, Volumetric CMR, Fast spin-echo, Whole-heart imaging

* Correspondence: markus.henningsson@kcl.ac.uk
[1]School of Biomedical Engineering and Imaging Sciences, King's College London, London, UK
Full list of author information is available at the end of the article

Background

Three-dimensional (3D) cardiovascular magnetic resonance (CMR) can be used for visualization of the whole heart and great vessel morphology in patients with congenital heart disease (CHD) [1]. This is commonly achieved using cardiac and respiratory gated whole-heart 3D balanced steady-state free precession (3D bSSFP) which provides bright-blood contrast [2, 3]. However, 3D bSSFP is susceptible to signal loss due to flow-related dephasing, particularly during turbulent or rapid blood-flow [4]. Contrast-enhanced cardiovascular magnetic resonance angiography (CE CMRA) may be used to obtain volumetric, time-resolved morphological information in a much shorter scan time than 3D bSSFP. However, CE CMRA typically has lower spatial resolution than 3D bSSFP and is not synchronized with the cardiac cycle leading to motion-induced blurring. Furthermore, CE CMRA typically requires the administration of gadolinium-based contrast agents which has known (nephrogenic systemic fibrosis) and undetermined risks (related to potential retention). An alternative approach to visualize morphology in CHD is black-blood CMR, which allows for visualization of myocardium and vessel wall with positive contrast without using exogenous contrast agents by suppressing blood signal [5]. However, the conventional approach – double inversion recovery (DIR) – is limited to two-dimensional (2D) acquisitions with non-isotropic resolution [6]. Furthermore, insufficient blood-suppression with suboptimal contrast often results from slowly flowing blood or flow perpendicular to the 2D DIR slice direction.

In recent years, 3D black-blood techniques have been proposed to allow high-resolution imaging of the aortic vessel wall [7–9]. This includes fast spin echo (FSE) using variable flip angle refocusing pulses which relies on the motion sensitivity of the spin echo pulse sequence to suppress signal from flowing blood [10]. Following the 90° excitation radiofrequency (RF) pulse, a few (5–10) dummy/startup RF refocusing pulses are performed during which moving/flowing spins rapidly de-phase. The amplitude of the refocusing pulses is typically modulated during the echo-train to obtain a constant vessel wall signal [11]. To achieve short echo-spacing, non-selective refocusing pulses can be used for 3D FSE [12]. However, this may lead to artifacts arising from signal outside the field-of-view (FOV) which is excited by the non-selective refocusing pulses, and subsequently generate a free induction decay (FID) signal [13]. To avoid these artifacts, oversampling in the slice direction can be employed at the expense of increasing the scan time. Alternatively, signal averaging can be used [14], again leading to a longer total scan duration. Three-dimensional FSE of the cardiovascular system may be particularly susceptible to outer volume

artifacts as it is surrounded by a significant volume of tissue from the chest and arms including subcutaneous fat. However, prolonging scan time is also undesirable due to the increased likelihood of physiological motion artifacts. Due to these technical challenges, whole-heart black-blood imaging has so far mainly employed less efficient but more motion tolerant and flow independent gradient echo acquisitions [15, 16]. A few studies have described cardiac and respiratory motion compensated black-blood 3D FSE [8, 17]. To the authors' knowledge no systematic evaluation or optimization has been performed of important 3D FSE parameters for cardiovascular black-blood imaging.

In this study we describe a new 3D FSE protocol for black-blood CMR of the whole heart and great vessels. Although the flow sensitivity of 3D FSE is well-documented in the literature [11, 18, 19], in this study we investigate the flow suppression performance of a specific cardiovascular 3D FSE protocol in simulations and in vivo. Furthermore, we investigate if the proposed 3D FSE protocol can be performed in the absence of averaging or slice-oversampling without FID artifacts from the outer volume. The main purpose of this study was to assess the feasibility of black-blood 3D FSE for the visualization of the whole heart and great vessels in patients with CHD. We compare the new 3D FSE technique to the conventional techniques for volumetric morphological CMR – bright-blood 3D bSSFP.

Methods

CMR studies were performed on a 1.5 T Philips scanner (Philips Healthcare, Best, The Netherlands) using a 32-channel torso coil. All participants provided written informed consent, and the study was approved by the local ethics committee (IRB STU 032016–009).

3D FSE pulse sequence

The 3D FSE sequence used a slice-selective 90° excitation pulse and non-selective refocusing pulses [13]. The refocusing flip angles of the FSE were modulated to yield constant transverse magnetisation across the echo train for a specific T1 (880 ms) and T2 (40 ms) combination, assumed to be similar to those of the aortic vessel wall based on a previous study of the carotid vessel wall [20]. The first echo spacing (ESP1), from excitation pulse to the first echo, was longer than the following echo spacing (ESP2) to account for the longer duration of the slice-selective excitation pulse. ESP2 was defined as the shortest possible duration to reduce scan time and maximise vessel wall signal which has a short T2. The refocusing flip angle for one shot and the resulting transverse magnetisation for the vessel wall, static blood and flowing blood are shown in Fig. 1. A centric view-ordering scheme was used to ensure the highest temporal correlation between the respiratory navigator

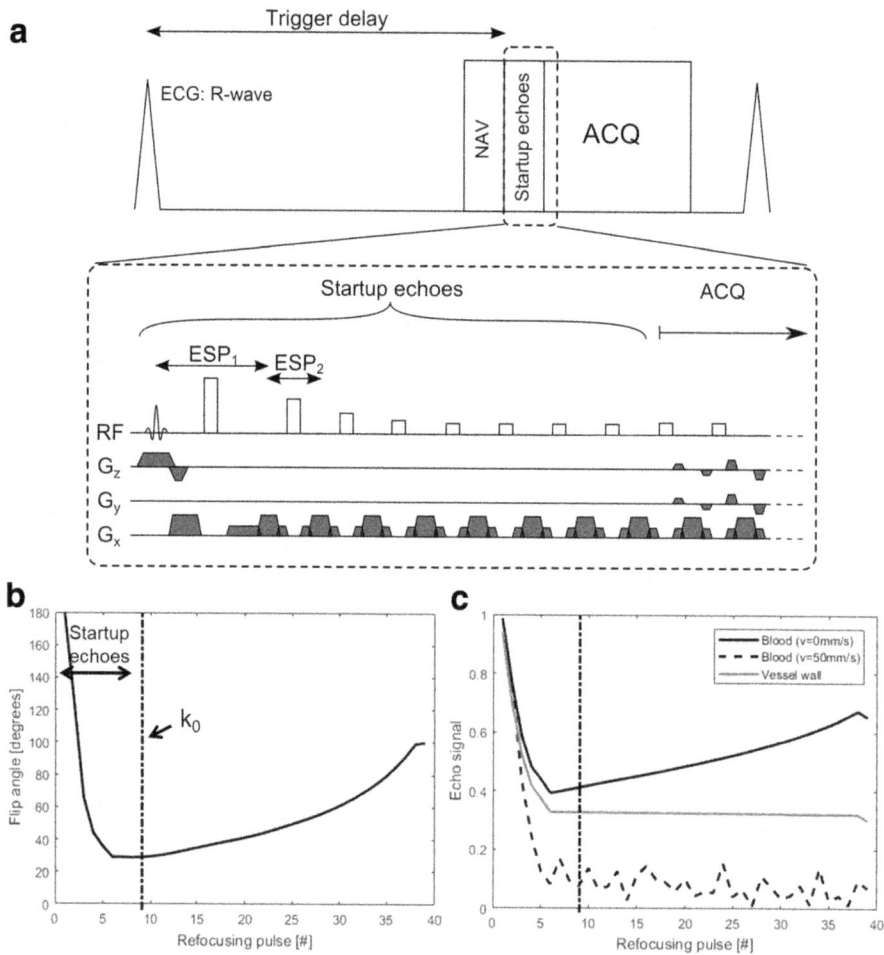

Fig. 1 Pulse sequence diagram of 3D fast spin echo (FSE) sequence, using electrocardiogram (ECG)-triggering and respiratory navigator (NAV) for motion compensation (**a**). The slab-selective 90 excitation pulse is followed by a series of non-selective refocusing pulses, modulated to generate a constant transverse magnetisation for vessel wall tissue (T1 = 880 ms, T2 = 40 ms) (**b**). Eight startup echoes are used to discard varying signal early in the echo train, while allowing signal from flowing blood to de-phase (blood v = 0 mm/s versus v = 50 mm/s) (**c**). During the startup echoes gradients are only performed in the readout direction leading to flow-induced dephasing primarily along this direction. A centric k-space view ordering scheme is used, whereby the centre of k-space (k_0) is acquired after the startup echoes at the 9th echo (dashed line in (**b**) and (**c**). A longer echo spacing (ESP$_1$) was used between the excitation pulse and first echo compared to subsequent echoes (ESP$_2$) to account for the longer duration of the slab-selective excitation pulse

motion measurements and the acquisition of the centre of k-space. Eight startup echoes were used, during which no data was collected, to avoid the rapidly changing transverse magnetisation at the start of the echo train, and allow the signal from flowing blood to de-phase as shown in Fig. 1. Although the 90° excitation pulse is slab-selective, the refocusing pulses are non-selective. In practice, this means gradients are only performed in the readout-direction during the startup echoes as shown in Fig. 1a, leading to flow-induced de-phasing only along this direction. As a result, the orientation of the FOV relative to the direction of the blood flow is important to achieve black-blood contrast [21]. A coronal orientation with readout along

foot-head direction was used to maximise blood signal suppression in the aorta, as determined in a small pilot study shown in Additional file 1: Figure S1.

Simulations

To investigate the influence of flow velocity on the ability to suppress blood signal, simulations were performed using the extended phase graph algorithm. The algorithm was implemented in MatLab 2017a (MathWorks, Natick, Massachusetts, USA) with an additional phase term to simulate flow of constant velocity during the 3D FSE pulse sequence. The details of this algorithm have been described by Weigel, including the incorporation of flow [21]. Velocities from 0 mm/s to 100 mm/s were simulated to determine the flow sensitivity of the 3D FSE sequence. Acquisition parameters were identical as for those described for 3D FSE in Table 1. Relaxation times of blood at 1.5 T were used for these simulations (T1 = 1600 ms; T2 = 250 ms).

CMR studies: Outer volume artifacts

To investigate the susceptibility to outer volume artifacts of the 3D FSE sequence without signal averaging, CMR experiments were performed in a T1 phantom [22] and 3 healthy subjects (29 ± 4 years). In these experiments the slab-selective pulse excited a volume of tissue half of the size of the encoded field-of-view. The experiments aimed to spatially encode potential FID artifacts arising from tissue outside the excited FOV which only experience the non-selective refocusing pulses. Encoding a volume twice the size of the slab-selection profile is the equivalent to using a slice oversampling factor of 2. Although the slices outside the excited volume are typically discarded, in these experiments the outer slices were visually inspected for potential FID artifacts. The imaging parameters for the scans were: encoded FOV = $330 \times 330 \times 200$ mm^3, RF excitation profile width = 100 mm, effective echo time = 30 ms, echo-spacing = 2.7 ms, voxel size = $1.5 \times 1.5 \times 1.5$, echo train length = 35 (plus 8 startup echoes), number of averages = 1, coronal orientation, SENSE acceleration = 2 left-right (LR). The in vivo scan were electrocardiogram (ECG)-triggered to the

mid-diastolic rest period and used a diaphragmatic navigator with 7 mm gating window and 0.6 tracking factor for respiratory motion compensation.

Healthy subject experiments: 3D FSE versus 3D bSSFP

A study was performed in 10 healthy subjects (28 ± 4 years) to compare 3D FSE and bright-blood 3D bSSFP in terms of ability to visualise cardiovascular anatomical structures. The two scans were performed in a randomized order for each subject and the imaging parameters are summarized in Table 1. The scans were ECG-triggered to coincide with the diastolic rest period, as visually determined from a time-resolved 2D cine scan. The FOV of 3D FSE and 3D bSSFP were identical, covering the whole heart and great vessels. All scans were acquired with a pencil beam navigator for respiratory motion compensation, including a 7 mm gating window and 0.6 tracking factor.

Patient studies: 3D FSE versus 3D bSSFP

Patients with CHD referred for CMR examination at Children's Medical Center, Dallas, Texas, USA, between September 2017 and January 2018 were considered for inclusion in this prospective study. Patients were scanned with the proposed 3D FSE scan and the findings were compared to 3D bSSFP. As these were clinically indicated CMR examinations, 3D bSSFP was often performed after any administration of gadolinium as per clinical routine in order for improved image quality. CE CMRA was not performed in all cases and so not available for comparison. Reasons for a clinical protocol of selective CE CMRA include restriction of gadolinium to cases where it is absolutely required and because, in cases where coronary anatomy is required as paramount, this information is not available on CE CMRA. The 3D FSE imaging parameters were: encoded FOV = (250–350), number of slices 120 to 180, effective echo time = 30 ms, echo-spacing = 2.7 ms, voxel size = $1.3 \times 1.3 \times 1.3$ mm, echo train length = 18 to 35 (plus 8 startup echoes), number of averages = 1, coronal orientation, SENSE acceleration = 2 (LR). Fat suppression was performed using spectral presaturation with inversion recovery (SPIR). The 3D bSSFP imaging parameters were: encoded FOV = (250–350), number of slices 120 to 180, echo time = 2 ms, voxel size = 1.3 mm^3 to 1.8 mm^3, echo train length = 22 to 40 (plus 10 startup echoes), number of averages = 1, coronal orientation, SENSE acceleration = 2 (LR). SPIR was used for fat suppression. Both 3D FSE and 3D bSSFP scans were ECG-triggered to the mid-diastolic rest period or end-systolic rest period (depending on which was longer and more consistent) and used a diaphragmatic navigator with 3–7 mm gating window (dependent on patient size) and 0.6 tracking factor for

Table 1 Imaging Parameters for healthy subject CMR studies

	3D FSE	3D bSSFP
TR	RR-interval	4.2 ms
TE$_{eff}$ (ms)	30.0	2.1
Echo-spacing (ms)	3.0	–
FOV (mm^3)	$300 \times 300 \times 110$	$300 \times 300 \times 110$
Voxel size (mm^3)	$1.3 \times 1.3 \times 1.3$	$1.3 \times 1.3 \times 1.3$
Slice oversampling	1.2	1.2
Number of startup echoes	8	10
Pixel bandwidth (Hz)	1657	1238
Number of averages	1	1
Orientation	Coronal	Coronal
SENSE acceleration	2 (PE)	2 (PE)
Respiratory gating	7 mm G + 0.6 T	7 mm G + 0.6 T
Acquisition window (ms)	140	140
Fat suppression	SPIR	SPIR
Nominal scan time	4 min 7 s	4 min 16 s

bSSFP balanced steady state free precession, *FH* foot-head, *FOV* field of view, *FSE* fast spin echo, *PE* phase encoding, *SENSE* sensitivity encoding, *G* gating, *T* tracking, *TE* echo time, *TR* repetition time, *SPIR* spectral presaturation with inversion recovery

respiratory motion compensation. The scan times for both 3D FSE and 3D bSSFP were recorded.

Image analysis

For the healthy subjects and CHD patient scans using whole-heart 3D FSE and 3D bSSFP, the relative success rates of achieving a full sequential segmental diagnosis (i.e. identifying all thoracic cardiovascular morphological elements – superior vena cava (e); inferior vena cava; coronary sinus; right atrium; left atrium; right ventricle; left ventricle; aorta; main pulmonary artery; pulmonary artery branches; pulmonary veins; aorta and head & neck branches; coronary artery origins) was compared between 3D FSE and 3D bSSFP. A structure was recorded as visualized if its connections were identified and there was no more than mild image blurring affecting that structure. More specifically, using a previously validated scoring system, the image quality score was greater than or equal to 3 out of 4 [23].

Acquisition of a noise image required for global signal to noise ratio (SNR) and contrast to noise ratio (CNR) calculations with parallel imaging was not considered practical due to time constraints [24]. Furthermore SNR and CNR between bright blood (3D bSSFP) and black blood sequences (3D FSE) have different signals of interest. Nevertheless, comparisons are provided in order to provide insight and, by ensuring imaging parameters such as the patient position, field-of-view, phase encoding direction and acceleration factor were unchanged between sequences, and by selecting identical regions-of-interest (ROIs) in both sets of resulting images, a local SNR (SNR_l) and local CNR (CNR_l) were calculated as detailed:

3D bSSFP SNR_l = IB / SD (L).
3D FSE SNR_l = IM / SD (L).
3D bSSFP CNR_l = (IB − IM) / SD (L).
3D FSE CNR_l = (IM − IB) / SD (L).

where IB and IM refers to the mean signal-intensity in an ROI in the blood-pool (proximal ascending aorta) and myocardium (mid ventricular septum) respectively, and SD (L) refers to the standard deviation of an ROI of air in the lungs (chosen to contain a minimum of 100pixels while avoiding any visible vascular structures).

Statistical analysis

All continuous variables are presented as mean ± standard deviation, while non-continuous variables are presented as median [25th percentile, 75th percentile]. Differences in continuous variables were statistically compared using paired t-test with a significance thresh-hold of 0.05. Non-continuous variables were compared using Wilcoxon sign-rank test, also with a 0.05 significance thresh-hold. To account for multiple comparisons, Holm-Bonferroni correction was used.

Results
Simulations

Simulated transverse magnetisation across the echo train for the 3D FSE for blood with different velocities are shown in Fig. 2a. Flowing blood rapidly de-phase during the initial startup echoes leading to black-blood contrast. The echo signal at the acquisition of the centre of k-space are shown in Fig. 2b, where good blood signal suppression for velocities higher than 30 mm/s can be seen.

Outer-volume suppression experiments

The phantom experiment using twice the size of encoded FOV in slice direction compared to the excited FOV and resulting 3D FSE is shown in Additional file 1: Figure S2. Excellent suppression of signal for all vials (which ranged in T1 from 250 ms to 1500 ms) was achieved outside the volume of the 90° excitation pulse. Good outer volume suppression was also achieved in the in-vivo experiments in three healthy subjects where a similar experiment was performed with increased encoded FOV relative to the excited FOV. The 3D FSE images from two healthy subjects are shown in Fig. 3. Signal profiles in the slice excitation direction show practically no measureable signal in tissue outside the excited FOV, highlighting the excellent outer volume suppression of this technique.

Healthy subject studies: 3D FSE versus 3D bSSFP

Three-dimensional bSSFP failed to achieve diagnostic accuracy in all cases (0% success rate). Failure was due to more than mild blurring of one or more pulmonary veins (PV's) in 10 out of 10 cases (6 right lower, 9 right upper, 9 left upper and 4 left lower PV's were inadequately visualized). This was invariably due to dephasing artefacts in the PVs. Two healthy subjects had poor image quality of head and neck vessels (left common carotid, n = 1; left subclavian artery, n = 1).

3D FSE achieved full segmental diagnoses in 1 case (10% success rate). All failed cases were due to inadequate quality of coronary origins while PV visualization was successful in all apart from 1 case (90% success). Additionally, the left subclavian artery appeared with more than mild blurring in 2 cases, the right subclavian artery failed in 2 cases, and the branch pulmonary arteries were inadequate in 1 case. However, the combination of 3D bSSFP and 3D FSE was able to provide the full segmental morphological diagnosis for 9 out of 10 cases (90% success). Images from one healthy subject are shown in Fig. 4, demonstrating excellent visualization of the right coronary artery (RCA) and left anterior descending coronary artery (LAD) using 3D bSSFP, while only the proximal course of the RCA and LAD are visualized with 3D FSE. However, the pulmonary veins could

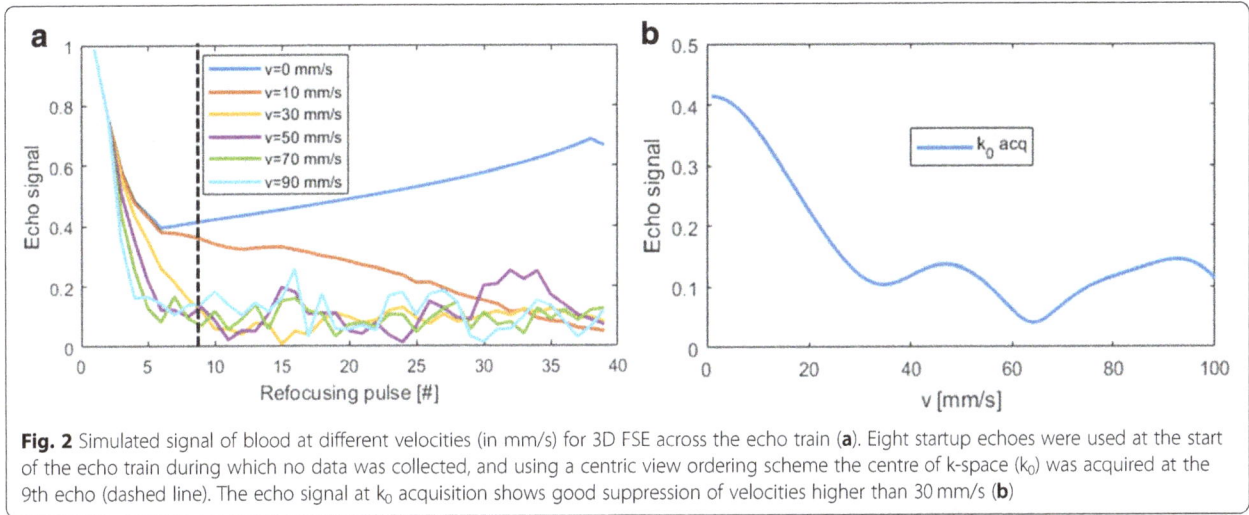

Fig. 2 Simulated signal of blood at different velocities (in mm/s) for 3D FSE across the echo train (**a**). Eight startup echoes were used at the start of the echo train during which no data was collected, and using a centric view ordering scheme the centre of k-space (k_0) was acquired at the 9th echo (dashed line). The echo signal at k_0 acquisition shows good suppression of velocities higher than 30 mm/s (**b**)

be visualized with 3D FSE but not 3D bSSFP. The scan time for 3D FSE was similar to 3D bSSFP (9:21 ± 2:8 vs 8:36 ± 1:54; $P = 0.19$). 3D bSSFP SNR_l was greater than 3D FSE SNR_l of the sequence (30.1 ± 7.3 vs 20.9 ± 5.3; $P = 0.002$) whereas the CNR_l was comparable (17.3 ± 5.6 vs 17.4 ± 4.9; $P = 0.91$).

Patient studies: 3D FSE versus 3D bSSFP
Twenty one CHD patients underwent CMR (12 female; age 9.6 ± 7.4 years (range 9 months to 26 years)). The mean heart rate was 84 ± 15 bpm for 3D FSE and 87 ± 16 bpm for 3D bSSFP. There was no significant difference between heart rates between sequences ($P = 0.49$).

The scan time for 3D FSE was similar to 3D bSSFP (3D FSE = 5:17 ± 1:33 vs 3D bSSFP = 4:48 ± 1:55; $P = 0.46$). The main indication for imaging was coronary anatomy in 5 cases, PV anatomy in 4 cases, aortic root anatomy in 1 case and complex single ventricle anatomy in 3 cases. The remaining cases received imaging for follow-up of repaired truncus arteriosus, tetralogy or transposition.

In patients with CHD, 3D bSSFP failed to achieve full segmental diagnoses in all but 1 case (5% success rate). Failure was due to more than mild blurring of one or more PV's in 15 out of 21 cases (12 right lower, 9 right upper, 6 left upper and 3 left lower PV's were inadequately visualized). This was invariably due to dephasing artifacts

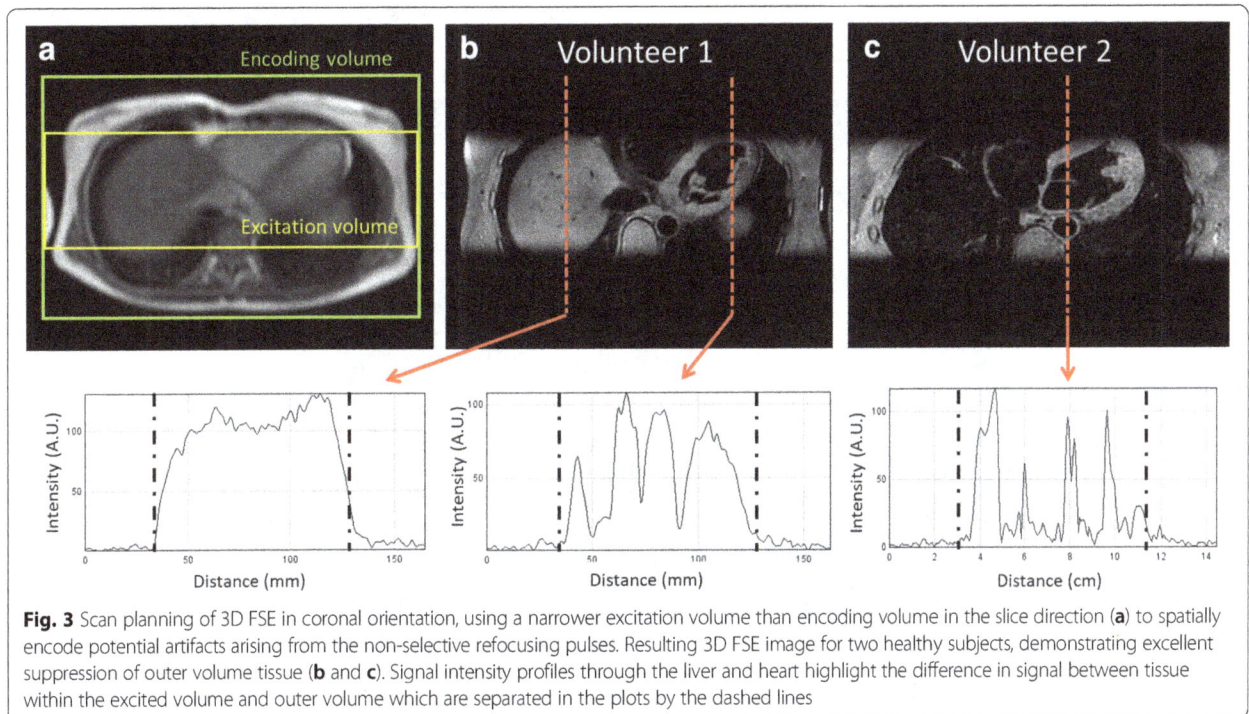

Fig. 3 Scan planning of 3D FSE in coronal orientation, using a narrower excitation volume than encoding volume in the slice direction (**a**) to spatially encode potential artifacts arising from the non-selective refocusing pulses. Resulting 3D FSE image for two healthy subjects, demonstrating excellent suppression of outer volume tissue (**b** and **c**). Signal intensity profiles through the liver and heart highlight the difference in signal between tissue within the excited volume and outer volume which are separated in the plots by the dashed lines

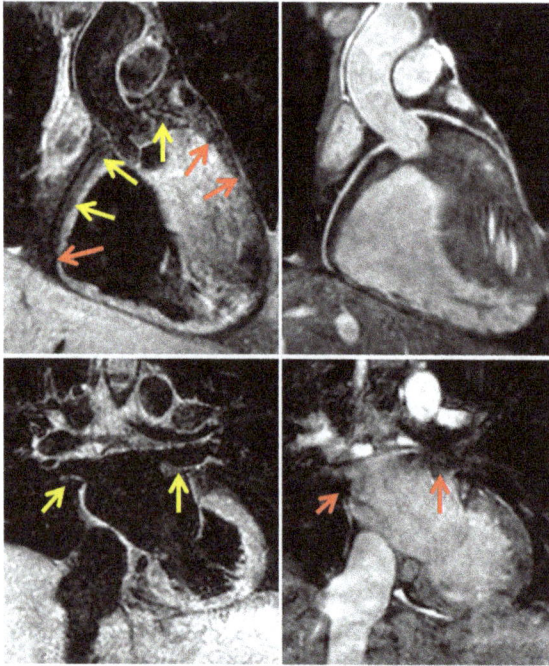

Fig. 4 3D FSE (left) and 3D bSSFP (right) of a healthy subject, reformatted to visualise the right coronary artery and left anterior descending arteries (top images), and right and left pulmonary veins (bottom images). The proximal coronaries can be visualised with 3D FSE (yellow arrows) while distal arteries are not distinguishable. However, the pulmonary veins are clearly seen in the 3D FSE, unlike 3D bSSFP where flow artifacts hamper visualization

in the PVs. Three patients had poor image quality of head and neck vessels (3 right subclavian arteries, 2 right common carotid arteries, 1 left common carotid and 1 left subclavian artery were not seen adequately). Pulmonary arteries showed more than mild blurring in 3 cases (all with stenotic lesions causing dephasing artifacts). In two cases, the SVC had more than mild blurring.

In contrast, 3D FSE achieved full segmental diagnoses in 5 cases (23.8% success rate). All failed cases were due to inadequate image quality of coronary origins while PV visualization was successful in all cases. Additionally, the coronary sinus had more than mild blurring in 2 cases and the left subclavian artery visualization failed in 2 cases. The combination of 3D bSSFP and 3D FSE was able to provide the full segmental morphological diagnosis for all cases. A patient with a coronary fistula, which could be visualized with 3D FSE but not 3D bSSFP, is shown in Fig. 5. A case where pulmonary arteries were visualized with 3D FSE but not 3D bSSFP (due to dephasing artifact from a pulmonary artery band) is shown in Fig. 6. Example images from 4 CHD patients with improved visualization of PVs are shown in Fig. 7.

Segmental anatomy, based on the 3D FSE and 3D bSSFP sequences, was considered accurate in all cases where visualization was possible. Thirteen cases had known anatomy from previous surgery and imaging, in all cases segmental diagnosis was accurate based on 3D FSE and 3D bSSFP sequences. Two cases required CMR as the PV anatomy was not known. In both cases the segmental diagnosis was accurate based on the 3D FSE and 3D bSSFP sequences as confirmed on subsequent surgery. Three cases had normal segmental anatomy (1

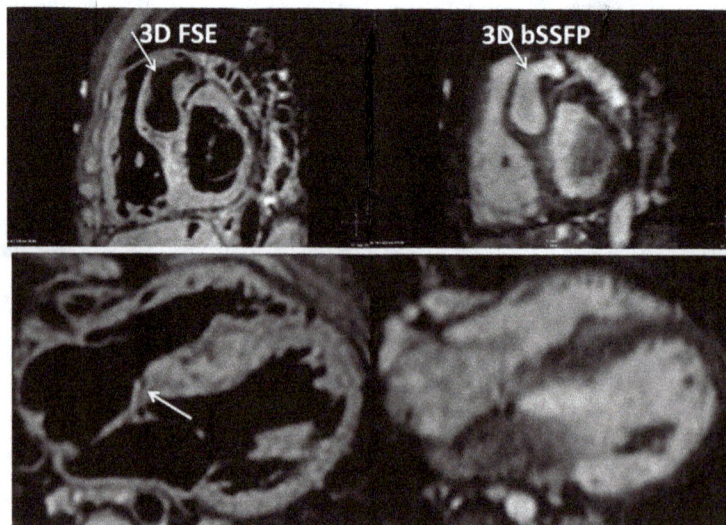

Fig. 5 3D FSE (left) and 3D bSSFP (right) images of a 4 year old patient with a large interventricular septal coronary pouch adjacent to the left anterior descending artery (arrows, top images). The patient also had a coronary fistula from the right coronary artery which could be visualized with 3D FSE (arrow, bottom left) but not 3D bSSFP (bottom right)

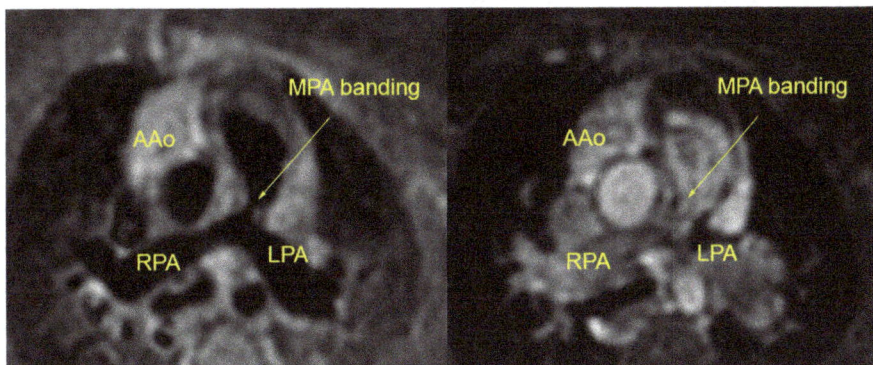

Fig. 6 3D FSE (left) and 3D bSSFP (right) images of a 6 month old patient with a pulmonary artery band (as palliation for an unbalanced atrioventricular septal defect). The pulmonary artery anatomy (which is vital for subsequent surgical planning) is clearly seen with 3D FSE (arrow) but not 3D bSSFP (right) due to dephasing artifact from turbulent flow after the band. The patient went on to have an uneventful cavopulmonary anastomosis. AAo = ascending aorta; MPA = main pulmonary artery; RPA = right pulmonary artery; LPA = left pulmonary artery

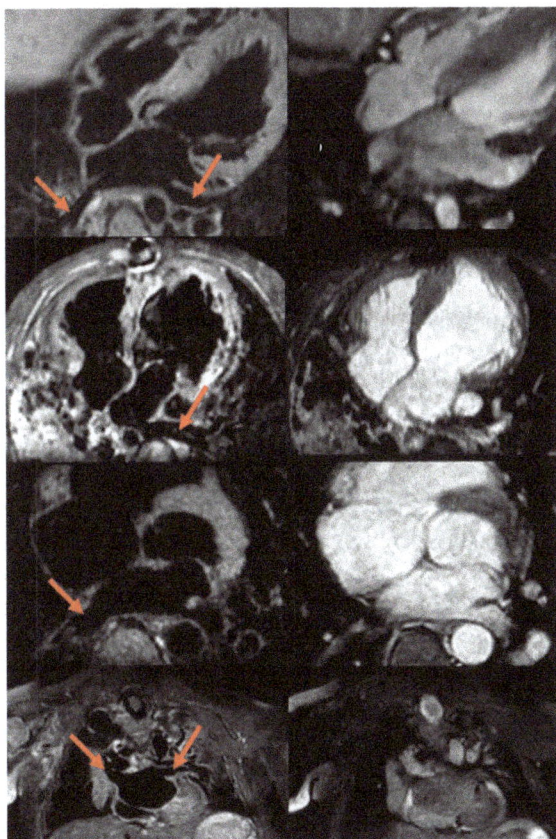

Fig. 7 Example images from four patients with congenital heart disease. 3D FSE images are shown on the left, 3D bSSFP images on the right hand side for each patient. Red arrows mark the pulmonary veins which are well visualized on 3D FSE, but not sufficiently or not at all on 3D bSSFP

fistula, 1 Kawasaki disease and 1 bicuspid aortic valve) on echocardiographic imaging and this was also shown on independent analysis using the 3D FSE and 3D bSSFP sequences. These 3 cases did not have surgical confirmation. A further 3 cases required CMR for uncertain coronary origins based on echocardiography. In all these 3 cases, coronary anatomy was demonstrated by CMR based on the 3D bSSFP sequences. Two of these cases had abnormal coronary artery origins that are known to be benign variants and thus do not have surgical confirmation. The remaining case had normal coronary origins based on the 3D FSE and 3D bSSFP sequences. All 3 patients who underwent CMR to determine coronary origins and course were discharged from further follow-up based on this assessment.

Both the SNR_l (42.9 ± 12.0 vs 23.1 ± 9.8; $P < 0.001$) and the CNR_l (26.6 ± 7.6 vs 19.3 ± 8.5; $P = 0.006$) were higher for 3D SSFP vs 3D FSE.

Discussion

In this study, we have demonstrated the feasibility of 3D FSE for black-blood imaging of the whole heart and great vessels. In particular, 3D FSE is better at visualizing the PVs compared to conventional anatomical 3D CMR using bright-blood bSSFP. However, 3D FSE is inferior compared to 3D bSSFP for coronary artery imaging.

3D FSE has been widely used for brain [25–28] or musculoskeletal imaging [29–31]. Recent pulse sequence improvements, using non-selective refocusing pulses with variable flip angles allow rapid data acquisition with improved point-spread functions. However, despite its many advantages, 3D FSE for CMR has remained limited to aortic vessel wall imaging [7, 8]. Aortic imaging is technically less challenging than whole-heart imaging because both respiratory and cardiac motion conditions are more benign in the aorta compared to cardiac structures. An important step for enabling whole-heart 3D FSE is therefore to introduce ECG-triggering and respiratory motion compensation, to minimize motion-induced de-phasing. To minimize respiratory motion, a conventional respiratory navigator approach was employed using gating and tracking. Although further improvements in image quality may be achieved using more advanced respiratory motion compensation techniques such as self-navigation [32] or image-based navigation [33, 34], in this study only pulse sequence features which are available on all major vendors' scanners were employed.

In the phantom study, we demonstrate that good flow suppression can be achieved for blood flow aligned with the readout gradient for velocities of 30 mm/s. This velocity spoils approximately 75% of the blood signal, as shown in Fig. 2b. Comparable flow sensitivity is achieved with 2D DIR, which relies on flow perpendicular to the slice direction, assuming 16 mm slice re-inversion width and 400 inversion time. For 3D FSE the de-phasing of the blood signal occurs during the startup echoes which take approximately 30 ms, and in the simulations we have only considered constant velocity flow during this time. Higher order motion will yield further de-phasing. Improved flow suppression performance may be achieved by using additional startup echoes, extending the startup period, at the expense of reducing time during the cardiac rest period available for image acquisition.

Due to the need for close temporal proximity between respiratory motion estimation and acquisition of centre of k-space, a centric profile order is almost exclusively used for navigator gated, high-resolution CMR [35]. A centric profile order could potentially cause FID artifacts from tissue outside 90° excitation volume that only experiences the refocussing pulses which, apart from the first refocussing pulse, are all smaller than 180°. To mitigate FID artifacts 3D FSE protocol employ signal averaging, or conservative slice oversampling (increased number of slice encoding steps) which leads to increased scan time [13]. However, as demonstrated in the phantom and in vivo experiment with slice excitation width half of the encoded ROV, practically no signal was observed in tissue experiencing only non-selective refocusing pulses. This justifies the use of a low slice oversampling factor (1.2 was used to account for imperfections in slice excitation profile) and the absence of signal averaging. As a result, the scan time of the 3D FSE was comparable to the 3D bSSFP scan in both healthy subjects and patients. Additional scan time reduction could be achieved using outer volume suppression [36, 37]. With this approach further suppression of peripheral tissue may be achieved by incorporating a slab-selective RF pulse for the first refocusing pulse, orthogonal to the excitation pulse, resulting in only a 2D selective "inner volume" experiencing both excitation and refocusing [12, 38].

As demonstrated in the patient study, 3D FSE offers very clear advantages in pulmonary vein imaging compared to 3D bSSFP, while 3D bSSFP provides superior coronary artery imaging. The combination of 3D bSSFP and 3D FSE was very successful in achieving a full sequential segmental diagnosis in CHD. In particular, structures that are prone to dephasing artifact in 3D bSSFP, such as stenotic lesions and pulmonary veins, tended to show good blood suppression and superior image quality in the 3D FSE images. This made the acquisition of both sequences complementary in achieving a full segmental diagnosis. Other studies reviewing the rate of full segmental diagnosis of 3D bSSFP show a higher rate of success [39, 40], but these studies define success merely as operator confidence in segmental connections.

Our study defined success as only mild blurring or no blurring but showed high success rate overall using the combination of non-contrast 3D ECG-triggered sequences. However, proximal coronary artery visualization in the 3D FSE images was poor in most cases. This is likely due to the orientation of the coronary arteries relative to the readout direction. Due to the complex geometry of the coronary arteries, and the importance of aligning the readout direction with the direction of flow to achieve blood suppression, there is unlikely to be an orientation which allows good depiction of all three arteries in a single whole-heart acquisition. Gradients may be inserted during the startup echoes along the phase- and slice-encoding directions to achieve flow suppression in all three dimensions. However, the gradients should be balanced within each echo-spacing to ensure constructively aligned spin echoes and stimulated echoes. As the readout gradient strength is defined as the maximum possible to minimize echo-spacing and acquisition time, the use of additional gradients may result in lowered achievable readout gradient strength and longer echo-spacing, and susceptibility to eddy currents. Alternatively, magnetisation preparation pulses such as motion sensitized driven-equilibrium [41, 42] or delay alternating with nutation for tailored excitation [43] could be used to de-phase flowing blood in any direction. Motion sensitized driven-equilibrium achieves black-blood contrast by adding strong de-phasing gradients within a T2-preparation module. However, due to the short T2 of the myocardium and vessel wall this will introduce a significant SNR penalty. Delay alternating with nutation for tailored excitation achieves blood suppression by performing a series of phase-altering, small flip angle RF pulses with gradients in between, exploiting the large steady state signal difference between static and moving spin. Although this results in less T2-weighting, a large number of RF pulses are required to reach steady-state. As a result, the pre-pulse is relatively long (approximately 100–200 ms) which reduces the time available for imaging within the cardiac cycle. In general, any flow dependent pre-pulses have to be performed during the cardiac rest period to avoid motion-induced signal loss which is a limitation of such approaches. An alternative to using pre-pulses may be to use a targeted oblique thin-slab 3D FSE acquisition for each coronary artery [44], and ensure that readout-direction is aligned with the main course of the coronary artery to ensure maximum blood suppression. Improved coronary conspicuity may also be achieved by disabling the fat suppression pulse which could yield high contrast between the epicardial fat embedding the coronary arteries and the suppressed signal from the coronary lumen. Recently, an intravascular iron-based contrast agent, ferumoxytol, has been demonstrated to improve blood suppression for 2D black-blood FSE [45]. A similar approach may prove beneficial to improve blood suppression for 3D FSE as well, due to the significantly shortened T2 of the blood pool.

Previous studies using 3D bSSFP have demonstrated excellent image quality for pulmonary vein imaging [46, 47], which differs significantly from the findings of this study. Both previous studies include patients with atrial fibrillation which typically have lower flow through the pulmonary veins, leading to more favourable conditions for 3D bSSFP compared to our paediatric and healthy subject cohort. Secondly, both previous studies use non-standard 3D bSSFP protocol with non-selective RF pulses, which has the favourable property of allowing for shorter echo time and repetition time. This in turn leads to less de-phasing between RF pulse and echo, as well as less de-phasing between RF pulses, and subsequently higher signal in the presence of flow compared to conventional slab-selective RF-pulses. The drawback of non-selective pulses is that the field-of-view must be large enough to encompass the entire torso to avoid wrap from excited chest wall and back signal. This can lead to an increased scan time which is undesirable. In this study we have used standard 3D bSSFP protocol with slab selective RF pulses, which appears to yield flow artifacts in the pulmonary veins in this patient cohort and the healthy volunteers.

Although 3D FSE may not be used as a direct replacement for 3D bSSFP due to the unreliability for coronary artery visualisation, the combination of 3D bSSFP and 3D FSE can be used to achieve a full segmental diagnosis, and subsequently may avoid the use of contrast-enhanced CMRA. This may justify the additional scan time incurred by including 3D FSE alongside 3D bSSFP in the CMR protocol. With the advent of increased vigilance regarding the use of gadolinium-based contrast agents in children, clinicians may reduce the need for contrast agents by performing both 3D FSE and 3D bSSFP. However, further studies are required to compare the diagnostic performance of 3D bSSFP and 3D FSE compared to CE CMRA.

In the healthy subject study without gadolinium administration, the SNR_l of 3D bSSFP which aims to yield high signal from blood, was higher than the SNR of 3D FSE where a constant echo signal across the echo train for myocardiium (or vessel wall) is sought. However, the CNR_l between blood and myocardium was similar between 3D bSSFP and FSE, which indicates that the methods can yield similar differentiation of blood and myocardium, provided that slowly flowing blood signal is adequately suppressed for 3D FSE or that rapidly flowing blood signal is not de-phased for 3D bSSFP. Although the patient data shows improved SNR_l and CNR_l for the 3D bSSFP sequence, this is likely due to the administration of gadolinium in these clinically indicated examinations. However, the proposed 3D FSE may suffer from lower SNR in patients with high heart-rates as this would lead to more frequently applied excitation pulses. Triggering on alternate heart-beats may improve SNR in these cases at the expense of prolonging scan time.

A limitation of this study is that no comparison with alternative whole-heart 3D black-blood techniques was performed such as T2 prepared phase sensitive inversion recovery [48] or interleaved T2prep acquisition [15]. This was primarily due to time constraints as the gradient echo based black blood scans have a significantly longer scan time as previously described. Further studies are required to compare the merits of 3D FSE to other techniques for volumetric black-blood CMR, such as interleaved T2prep [15], T2 prepared inversion recovery [48, 49], or motion sensitized driven equilibrium [17]. The ability of 3D FSE to suppress flowing blood is limited to primarily the readout direction. This makes the orientation of the FOV relative to the blood flow an important consideration for 3D FSE. Although this was observed in the preliminary pilot study, a limitation of this study was that no systematic evaluation was performed of the ideal orientation to visualise a particular cardiac anatomy.

Conclusion

The feasibility of 3D FSE for whole-heart black-blood CMR imaging has been demonstrated. The proposed approach enables high-resolution black-blood whole-heart CMR imaging in a scan time similar to that of the comparable bright-blood technique 3D bSSFP. In patients with CHD, 3D FSE was found to be particularly effective at visualizing the PVs but failed to visualize the coronary arteries in many cases. However, the combination of 3D bSSFP and 3D FSE whole-heart imaging improves the success rate of cardiac morphological diagnosis compared to either technique in isolation may be an attractive alternative to gadolinium contrast enhanced morphological CMR.

Additional file

> **Additional file 1: Figure S1.** The orientation of the field-of-view determines effectiveness of blood suppression as gradients are only performed in readout direction during startup echoes. As a result, for coronal orientation with readout in foot-head direction, blood signal is well-supressed in the descending aorta while residual signal is present in the aortic arch (arrows). Similarly, for a transverse orientation with readout along the anterior-posterior direction, the blood signal in the aortic arch is better suppressed while significant blood signal can be seen in the descending aorta (arrows). **Figure S2.** Scan planning of 3D FSE, using a narrower excitation volume than encoding volume in the slice direction (a) to spatially encode potential artifacts arising from the non-selective refocusing pulses. Resulting 3D FSE image shown in slice-encoding direction demonstrating excellent suppression of outer volume signal (b). In-plane images through the inner volume (c) and outer volume (d) shows the effectiveness of outer volume suppression. The signal in the outer volume image is magnified by a factor of 50 to highlight the signal suppression in these vials which ranged in T1 from 250 ms to 1500 ms.

Abbreviations

2D: Two-dimensional; 3D: Three-dimensional; bSSFP: Balances steady-state free precession; CE: Contrast enhanced; CHD: Congenital heart disease; CMR: Cardiovascular magnetic resonance; CMRA: Cardiovascular magnetic resonance angiography; CNR_l: Local contrast-to-noise ratio; DIR: Double inversion recovery; ECG: Electrocardiogram; ESP: Echo spacing; FID: Free induction decay; FOV: Field-of-view; FSE: Fast spin echo; LAD: Left anterior descending coronary artery; PV: Pulmonary vein; RCA: Right coronary artery; RF: Radiofrequency; ROI: Region of interest; SENSE: Sensitivity encoding; SNR_l: Local signal-to-noise ratio

Funding

This work was supported by the Department of Health through the National Institute for Health Research (NIHR) comprehensive Biomedical Research Centre award to Guy's & St Thomas' NHS Foundation Trust in partnership with King's College London and King's College Hospital NHS Foundation Trust. The Division of Imaging Sciences receives also support as the Centre of Excellence in Medical Engineering (funded by the Wellcome Trust and EPSRC; grant number WT 088641/Z/09/Z).

Authors' contributions

MH conceived of the study, developed the sequence, acquired data, performed processing and analysis and drafted the manuscript. TH contributed to study design, data analysis and patient data collection. RAZ contributed to study design, data analysis and patient data collection. AT contributed to study design, data analysis and patient data collection. BB contributed to study design, and patient data collection. GG contributed to study design, data analysis and patient data collection. AD contributed to patient data collection and data analysis. All authors participated in revising the manuscript, read and approved the final manuscript.

Consent for publication

Written informed consent was obtained from patients for publication of their individual details and accompanying images in this manuscript. The consent form is held in the patients' clinical notes and is available for review by the Editor-in-Chief.

Competing interests

The authors declare that they have no competing interests.

Author details

¹School of Biomedical Engineering and Imaging Sciences, King's College London, London, UK. ²Departments of Pediatrics and Radiology, University of Texas Southwestern/Children's Health, Dallas, TX, USA.

References

1. Fratz S, Chung T, Greil GF, Samyn MM, Taylor AM, Valsangiacomo Buechel ER, Yoo SJ, Powell AJ. Guidelines and protocols for cardiovascular magnetic resonance in children and adults with congenital heart disease: SCMR expert consensus group on congenital heart disease. J Cardiovasc Magn Reson. 2013;15:51.
2. Weber OM, Martin AJ, Higgins CB. Whole-heart steady-state free precession coronary artery magnetic resonance angiography. Magn Reson Med. 2003; 50(6):1223–8.
3. Beerbaum P, Sarikouch S, Laser KT, Greil G, Burchert W, Korperich H. Coronary anomalies assessed by whole-heart isotropic 3D magnetic resonance imaging for cardiac morphology in congenital heart disease. J Magn Reson Imaging. 2009;29(2):320–7.
4. Bieri O, Scheffler K. Flow compensation in balanced SSFP sequences. Magn Reson Med. 2005;54(4):901–7.
5. Vyas HV, Greenberg SB, Krishnamurthy R. MR imaging and CT evaluation of congenital pulmonary vein abnormalities in neonates and infants. Radiographics. 2012;32(1):87–98.
6. Edelman RR, Chien D, Kim D. Fast selective black blood MR imaging. Radiology. 1991;181(3):655–60.
7. Eikendal AL, Blomberg BA, Haaring C, Saam T, van der Geest RJ, Visser F, Bots ML, den Ruijter HM, Hoefer IE, Leiner T. 3D black blood VISTA vessel wall cardiovascular magnetic resonance of the thoracic aorta wall in young, healthy adults: reproducibility and implications for efficacy trial sample sizes: a cross-sectional study. J Cardiovasc Magn Reson. 2016;18:20.
8. Mihai G, Varghese J, Lu B, Zhu H, Simonetti OP, Rajagopalan S. Reproducibility of thoracic and abdominal aortic wall measurements with three-dimensional, variable flip angle (SPACE) MRI. J Magn Reson Imaging. 2015;41(1):202–12.
9. Wehrum T, Dragonu I, Strecker C, Schuchardt F, Hennemuth A, Drexl J, Reinhard T, Bohringer D, Vach W, Hennig J, et al. Aortic atheroma as a source of stroke - assessment of embolization risk using 3D CMR in stroke patients and controls. J Cardiovasc Magn Reson. 2017;19(1):67.
10. Busse RF, Hariharan H, Vu A, Brittain JH. Fast spin echo sequences with very long echo trains: design of variable refocusing flip angle schedules and generation of clinical T2 contrast. Magn Reson Med. 2006;55(5):1030–7.
11. Busse RF, Brau AC, Vu A, Michelich CR, Bayram E, Kijowski R, Reeder SB, Rowley HA. Effects of refocusing flip angle modulation and view ordering in 3D fast spin echo. Magn Reson Med. 2008;60(3):640–9.
12. Mitsouras D, Mulkern RV, Owens CD, Conte MS, Ersoy H, Luu TM, Whitmore AG, Creager MA, Rybicki FJ. High-resolution peripheral vein bypass graft wall studies using high sampling efficiency inner volume 3D FSE. Magn Reson Med. 2008;59(3):650–4.
13. Mugler JP 3rd. Optimized three-dimensional fast-spin-echo MRI. J Magn Reson Imaging. 2014;39(4):745–67.
14. Magland JF, Rajapakse CS, Wright AC, Acciavatti R, Wehrli FW. 3D fast spin echo with out-of-slab cancellation: a technique for high-resolution structural imaging of trabecular bone at 7 tesla. Magn Reson Med. 2010;63(3):719–27.
15. Andia ME, Henningsson M, Hussain T, Phinikaridou A, Protti A, Greil G, Botnar RM. Flow-independent 3D whole-heart vessel wall imaging using an interleaved T2-preparation acquisition. Magn Reson Med. 2013;69(1):150–7.
16. Varela M, Morgan R, Theron A, Dillon-Murphy D, Chubb H, Whitaker J, Henningsson M, Aljabar P, Schaeffter T, Kolbitsch C, et al. Novel MRI technique enables non-invasive measurement of Atrial Wall thickness. IEEE Trans Med Imaging. 2017;36(8):1607–14.
17. Srinivasan S, Hu P, Kissinger KV, Goddu B, Goepfert L, Schmidt EJ, Kozerke S, Nezafat R. Free-breathing 3D whole-heart black-blood imaging with motion sensitized driven equilibrium. J Magn Reson Imaging. 2012;36(2):379–86.
18. Hinks RS, Constable RT. Gradient moment nulling in fast spin echo. Magn Reson Med. 1994;32(6):698–706.
19. Storey P, Atanasova IP, Lim RP, Xu J, Kim D, Chen Q, Lee VS. Tailoring the flow sensitivity of fast spin-echo sequences for noncontrast peripheral MR angiography. Magn Reson Med. 2010;64(4):1098–108.
20. Coolen BF, Poot DH, Liem MI, Smits LP, Gao S, Kotek G, Klein S, Nederveen AJ. Three-dimensional quantitative T1 and T2 mapping of the carotid artery: sequence design and in vivo feasibility. Magn Reson Med. 2016;75(3):1008–17.
21. Weigel M. Extended phase graphs: dephasing, RF pulses, and echoes - pure and simple. J Magn Reson Imaging. 2015;41(2):266–95.
22. Captur G, Gatehouse P, Keenan KE, Heslinga FG, Bruehl R, Prothmann M, Graves MJ, Eames RJ, Torlasco C, Benedetti G, et al. A medical device-grade T1 and ECV phantom for global T1 mapping quality assurance-the T1

mapping and ECV standardization in cardiovascular magnetic resonance (T1MES) program. J Cardiovasc Magn Reson. 2016;18(1):58.

23. McConnell MV, Khasgiwala VC, Savord BJ, Chen MH, Chuang ML, Edelman RR, Manning WJ. Comparison of respiratory suppression methods and navigator locations for MR coronary angiography. AJR Am J Roentgenol. 1997;168(5):1369–75.

24. Yu J, Agarwal H, Stuber M, Schar M. Practical signal-to-noise ratio quantification for sensitivity encoding: application to coronary MR angiography. J Magn Reson Imaging. 2011;33(6):1330–40.

25. Mugler JP 3rd, Bao S, Mulkern RV, Guttmann CR, Robertson RL, Jolesz FA, Brookeman JR. Optimized single-slab three-dimensional spin-echo MR imaging of the brain. Radiology. 2000;216(3):891–9.

26. Pouwels PJ, Kuijer JP, Mugler JP 3rd, Guttmann CR, Barkhof F. Human gray matter: feasibility of single-slab 3D double inversion-recovery high-spatial-resolution MR imaging. Radiology. 2006;241(3):873–9.

27. Kallmes DF, Hui FK, Mugler JP 3rd. Suppression of cerebrospinal fluid and blood flow artifacts in FLAIR MR imaging with a single-slab three-dimensional pulse sequence: initial experience. Radiology. 2001;221(1):251–5.

28. Chagla GH, Busse RF, Sydnor R, Rowley HA, Turski PA. Three-dimensional fluid attenuated inversion recovery imaging with isotropic resolution and nonselective adiabatic inversion provides improved three-dimensional visualization and cerebrospinal fluid suppression compared to two-dimensional flair at 3 tesla. Investig Radiol. 2008;43(8):547–51.

29. Kijowski R, Gold GE. Routine 3D magnetic resonance imaging of joints. J Magn Reson Imaging. 2011;33(4):758–71.

30. Gold GE, Busse RF, Beehler C, Han E, Brau AC, Beatty PJ, Beaulieu CF. Isotropic MRI of the knee with 3D fast spin-echo extended echo-train acquisition (XETA): initial experience. AJR Am J Roentgenol. 2007;188(5):1287–93.

31. Welsch GH, Zak L, Mamisch TC, Paul D, Lauer L, Mauerer A, Marlovits S, Trattnig S. Advanced morphological 3D magnetic resonance observation of cartilage repair tissue (MOCART) scoring using a new isotropic 3D proton-density, turbo spin echo sequence with variable flip angle distribution (PD-SPACE) compared to an isotropic 3D steady-state free precession sequence (true-FISP) and standard 2D sequences. J Magn Reson Imaging. 2011;33(1):180–8.

32. Piccini D, Littmann A, Nielles-Vallespin S, Zenge MO. Respiratory self-navigation for whole-heart bright-blood coronary MRI: methods for robust isolation and automatic segmentation of the blood pool. Magn Reson Med. 2012;68(2):571–9.

33. Pang J, Bhat H, Sharif B, Fan Z, Thomson LE, LaBounty T, Friedman JD, Min J, Berman DS, Li D. Whole-heart coronary MRA with 100% respiratory gating efficiency: self-navigated three-dimensional retrospective image-based motion correction (TRIM). Magn Reson Med. 2014;71(1):67–74.

34. Henningsson M, Smink J, van Ensbergen G, Botnar R. Coronary MR angiography using image-based respiratory motion compensation with inline correction and fixed gating efficiency. Magn Reson Med. 2018;79(1):416–22.

35. Spuentrup E, Manning WJ, Botnar RM, Kissinger KV, Stuber M. Impact of navigator timing on free-breathing submillimeter 3D coronary magnetic resonance angiography. Magn Reson Med. 2002;47(1):196–201.

36. Mitsouras D, Mulkern RV, Rybicki FJ. Strategies for inner volume 3D fast spin echo magnetic resonance imaging using nonselective refocusing radio frequency pulses. Med Phys. 2006;33(1):173–86.

37. Feinberg DA, Hoenninger JC, Crooks LE, Kaufman L, Watts JC, Arakawa M. Inner volume MR imaging: technical concepts and their application. Radiology. 1985;156(3):743–7.

38. Hussain T, Clough RE, Cecelja M, Makowski M, Peel S, Chowienczyk P, Schaeffter T, Greil G, Botnar R. Zoom imaging for rapid aortic vessel wall imaging and cardiovascular risk assessment. J Magn Reson Imaging. 2011;34(2):279–85.

39. Hussain T, Lossnitzer D, Bellsham-Revell H, Valverde I, Beerbaum P, Razavi R, Bell AJ, Schaeffter T, Botnar RM, Uribe SA, et al. Three-dimensional dual-phase whole-heart MR imaging: clinical implications for congenital heart disease. Radiology. 2012;263(2):547–54.

40. Sorensen TS, Korperich H, Greil GF, Eichhorn J, Barth P, Meyer H, Pedersen EM, Beerbaum P. Operator-independent isotropic three-dimensional magnetic resonance imaging for morphology in congenital heart disease: a validation study. Circulation. 2004;110(2):163–9.

41. Wang J, Yarnykh VL, Hatsukami T, Chu B, Balu N, Yuan C. Improved suppression of plaque-mimicking artifacts in black-blood carotid atherosclerosis imaging using a multislice motion-sensitized driven-equilibrium (MSDE) turbo spin-echo (TSE) sequence. Magn Reson Med. 2007;58(5):973–81.

42. Zhu C, Graves MJ, Yuan J, Sadat U, Gillard JH, Patterson AJ. Optimization of improved motion-sensitized driven-equilibrium (iMSDE) blood suppression for carotid artery wall imaging. J Cardiovasc Magn Reson. 2014;16:61.

43. Viessmann O, Li L, Benjamin P, Jezzard P. T2-weighted intracranial vessel wall imaging at 7 tesla using a DANTE-prepared variable flip angle turbo spin echo readout (DANTE-SPACE). Magn Reson Med. 2017;77(2):655–63.

44. Stuber M, Botnar RM, Danias PG, Sodickson DK, Kissinger KV, Van Cauteren M, De Becker J, Manning WJ. Double-oblique free-breathing high resolution three-dimensional coronary magnetic resonance angiography. J Am Coll Cardiol. 1999;34(2):524–31.

45. Nguyen KL, Park EA, Yoshida T, Hu P, Finn JP. Ferumoxytol enhanced black-blood cardiovascular magnetic resonance imaging. J Cardiovasc Magn Reson. 2017;19(1):106.

46. François CJ, Tuite D, Deshpande V, Jerecic R, Weale P, Carr JC. Pulmonary vein imaging with unenhanced three-dimensional balanced steady-state free precession MR angiography: initial clinical evaluation. Radiology. 2009;250(3):932–9.

47. Krishnam MS, Tomasian A, Malik S, Singhal A, Sassani A, Laub G, Finn JP, Ruehm S. Three-dimensional imaging of pulmonary veins by a novel steady-state free-precession magnetic resonance angiography technique without the use of intravenous contrast agent: initial experience. Investig Radiol. 2009;44(8):447–53.

48. Liu CY, Bley TA, Wieben O, Brittain JH, Reeder SB. Flow-independent T (2)-prepared inversion recovery black-blood MR imaging. J Magn Reson Imaging. 2010;31(1):248–54.

49. Ginami G, Neji R, Phinikaridou A, Whitaker J, Botnar RM, Prieto C. Simultaneous bright- and black-blood whole-heart MRI for noncontrast enhanced coronary lumen and thrombus visualization. Magn Reson Med. 2018;79(3):1460–72.

15

Nonenhanced hybridized arterial spin labeled magnetic resonance angiography of the extracranial carotid arteries using a fast low angle shot readout at 3 Tesla

Ioannis Koktzoglou[1,2*], Matthew T. Walker[1,2], Joel R. Meyer[1,2], Ian G. Murphy[1,3] and Robert R. Edelman[1,3]

Abstract

Background: To evaluate ungated nonenhanced hybridized arterial spin labeling (hASL) magnetic resonance angiography (MRA) of the extracranial carotid arteries using a fast low angle shot (FLASH) readout at 3 Tesla.

Methods: In this retrospective, institutional review board-approved and HIPAA-compliant study, we evaluated the image quality (4-point scale) of nonenhanced hASL MRA using a FLASH readout with respect to contrast-enhanced MRA (CEMRA) in 37 patients presenting with neurologic symptoms. Two certified neuroradiologists independently evaluated 407 arterial segments (11 per patient) for image quality. The presence of vascular pathology was determined by consensus reading. Gwet's AC1 was used to assess inter-rater agreement in image quality scores, and image quality scores were correlated with age and body mass index. Objective measurements of arterial lumen area and sharpness in the carotid arteries were compared to values obtained with CEMRA. Comparisons were also made with conventional nonenhanced 2D time-of-flight (TOF) MRA.

Results: CEMRA provided the best image quality, while nonenhanced hASL FLASH MRA provided image quality that exceeded 2D TOF at the carotid bifurcation and in the internal and external carotid arteries. All nine vascular abnormalities of the carotid and intracranial arteries detected by CEMRA were depicted with hASL MRA, with no false positives. Inter-rater agreement of image quality scores was highest for CEMRA (AC1 = 0.87), followed by hASL (AC1 = 0.61) and TOF (AC1 = 0.43) ($P < 0.001$, all comparisons). With respect to CEMRA, agreement in cross-sectional lumen area was significantly better with hASL than TOF in the common carotid artery (intraclass correlation (ICC) = 0.90 versus 0.66; $P < 0.05$) and at the carotid bifurcation (ICC = 0.87 versus 0.54; $P < 0.05$). Nonenhanced hASL MRA provided superior arterial sharpness with respect to CEMRA and 2D TOF ($P < 0.001$).

Conclusion: Although inferior to CEMRA in terms of image quality and inter-rater agreement, hASL FLASH MRA offers an alternative to 2D TOF for the nonenhanced evaluation of the extracranial carotid arteries at 3 Tesla. Compared with 2D TOF, nonenhanced hASL FLASH MRA provides improved quantification of arterial cross-sectional area, vessel sharpness, inter-rater agreement and image quality.

Keywords: Magnetic resonance angiography, Carotid, Intracranial, Arterial spin labeling, Nonenhanced

* Correspondence: ikoktzoglou@gmail.com
[1]Department of Radiology, NorthShore University HealthSystem, Evanston, USA
[2]University of Chicago Pritzker School of Medicine, Chicago, USA
Full list of author information is available at the end of the article

Background

Disorders of the extracranial carotid arteries including stenoses, dissections and aneurysms are frequently evaluated using contrast-enhanced magnetic resonance angiography (CEMRA). However, CEMRA is contraindicated in patients with moderate to severe renal insufficiency, which can be present in over 25 % of patients with stroke [1–4]. Furthermore, in patients with suspected stroke, contrast agents may be reserved for the assessment of cerebral perfusion [5].

Nonenhanced MRA may address the above drawbacks of CEMRA. Time-of-flight (TOF) magnetic resonance angiography (MRA) is a well-established and easy-to-use method for diagnosing disorders of the extracranial carotid arteries without the use of contrast agents [6–10]. Although it is often used in clinical practice, TOF has well-known drawbacks including artifacts from saturation and dephasing of flowing spins, as well as limited vascular coverage with respect to CEMRA [11]. To address the shortcomings of TOF, as well as to potentially better serve patients with renal insufficiency, alternate nonenhanced MRA techniques have been reported, including inversion-recovery fast spin-echo or balanced steady-state free precession (bSSFP) angiography [12–14], and quiescent-interval slice-selective (QISS) angiography using a fast low-angle shot (FLASH) readout [15]. Raoult and colleagues [13] postulated that better suppression of static background tissue would likely improve the clinical utility of nonenhanced MRA of the extracranial carotid arteries, and mentioned that arterial spin labeling (ASL) methods, initially described long ago [16, 17], might achieve this.

Recent work has reported the potential of advanced ASL-based MRA for imaging arteries of the head and neck with complete suppression of static background signal [18–20]. In particular, a hybrid of pseudo-continuous and pulsed ASL (hASL) has been shown to efficiently portray long lengths of the extracranial carotid arteries at 1.5 Tesla without the need for cardiac gating [21], with a FLASH variant providing the most accurate portrayal of stenoses in vitro [22]. On the basis of these reports, our department incorporated an ungated 3D FLASH variant of hASL MRA into the standard-of-care neck MRA exam at 3 Tesla to serve as a pre-contrast scout for clinical purposes only. The purpose of this retrospective study was to evaluate the image quality of this clinical scout protocol for portraying the extracranial carotid arteries at 3 Tesla in patients undergoing 2D TOF and CEMRA protocols.

Methods

In this retrospective, Health Insurance Portability and Accountability Act-compliant study, a waiver of the requirement for patient consent was approved by the institutional review board of NorthShore University HealthSystem. Nonenhanced 3D hASL MRA was acquired as a clinical scout scan prior to injection of contrast media in consecutive patients who were referred for neck MRA with and without contrast material.

Study inclusion criteria were age ≥18 years and referral based on the clinical suspicion of stenosis or stroke and evaluation with TOF, hASL MRA, and CEMRA. Study exclusion criteria included the following: contraindications to cardiovascular magnetic resonance (CMR), renal impairment that precluded CEMRA (defined by glomerular filtration rate lower than 30 mL/min/1.73 m^2), inability to complete or non-diagnostic image quality on any of the three MRA acquisitions (hASL, TOF, CEMRA), and previous arterial revascularization including stent placement. No scans were re-acquired in the case of non-diagnostic image quality.

Imaging system and protocols

Imaging was performed on a 3 Tesla CMR system (MAGNETOM Skyra, Siemens Healthcare, Erlangen, Germany) having a maximum gradient strength of 45mT/m and a maximum slew rate of 200mT/m/ms. The CMR signal was received by a 20-channel head and neck coil (Head/Neck 20, Siemens Healthcare, Erlangen, Germany). Imaging was performed with 2D TOF MRA, 3D hASL MRA, and 3D CEMRA. TOF and CEMRA were acquired using institutional standard-of-care protocols. CEMRA was performed using 0.1 mmol/kg of gadobutrol (Gadavist, Bayer HealthCare, Whippany, NJ) injected in an antecubital vein at 2 mL/s. Imaging parameters for all protocols are listed in Table 1.

hASL MRA consisted of a prototype ungated 3D coronal FLASH readout (Fig. 1) that was preceded by pseudo-continuous [23] and pulsed [16] radiofrequency (RF) labeling; the timing of the sequence was similar to that of a prior report [21] with minor differences to account for the use of a FLASH readout (see Fig. 1 caption for details). Locations of RF labeling planes were transparent to the CMR operator; the operator positioned the coronal slab over the carotid arteries (centering at the approximate level of the carotid bifurcations) and executed the scan.

Qualitative analysis

After data acquisition, image processing was performed on a workstation (Leonardo; Siemens Healthcare, Erlangen, Germany) by a CMR scientist (I.K.) who did not participate in image scoring. After non-vascular background tissue was cropped using a 3D volume visualization and editing tool, rotating maximum intensity projection (MIP) image sets (72 projections separated by 5°) were created from each MR angiographic volume. These image sets were anonymized, randomized

Table 1 Imaging Parameters

	hASL	TOF	CEMRA
Orientation	coronal	axial	coronal
Acquisition type	3D	2D	3D
TR (ms)	5.8	19.0	3.2
TE (ms)	3.9	3.7	1.2
Flip angle (degrees)	5	60	25
Field of view (mm)[a]	256 × 256 [256-320 × 256-320]	220 × 220	320 × 260
Matrix	256 × 256	256 × 256	352 × 286
Slices[a]	60 [60–80]	100 [60-120]	80
In-plane resolution (mm)[a]	1.0 × 1.0 [1.0-1.25 × 1.0-1.25]	0.9 × 0.9	0.9 × 0.9
Slice thickness (mm)	1.0	2.0	1.2
Partial Fourier (phase)	none	none	6/8th
Partial Fourier (slice)	6/8th	none	6/8th
Scan time[a]	4.6 [4.6–6.1] min	4.7 [2.8–5.6] min	19 s
Flow Compensation	yes	yes	no
Slice Oversampling	none	–	20 %
Bandwidth (Hz/pixel)	349	465	590

[a]values given as median [range]; all protocols used a generalized auto-calibrating partially parallel acquisition (GRAPPA) factor of 2

and then independently reviewed by two certified neuroradiologists (M.W. and J.M.). The neuroradiologists were blinded to the patient name, the clinical history of the patient, and the results of other diagnostic procedures.

Image quality was scored for the following 11 locations: 1 and 2 - bilateral common carotid arteries; 3 and 4 - bilateral carotid bulb and proximal internal carotid arteries; 5 and 6 - bilateral mid-cervical internal carotid arteries; 7 and 8 - bilateral petrous internal carotid arteries; 9 and 10 - bilateral external carotid arteries; and 11 - intracranial arteries. The following 4-point scoring system was used: 1 = non-diagnostic, barely visible lumen rendering the segment non-diagnostic; 2 = fair, ill-defined vessel borders with suboptimal image quality

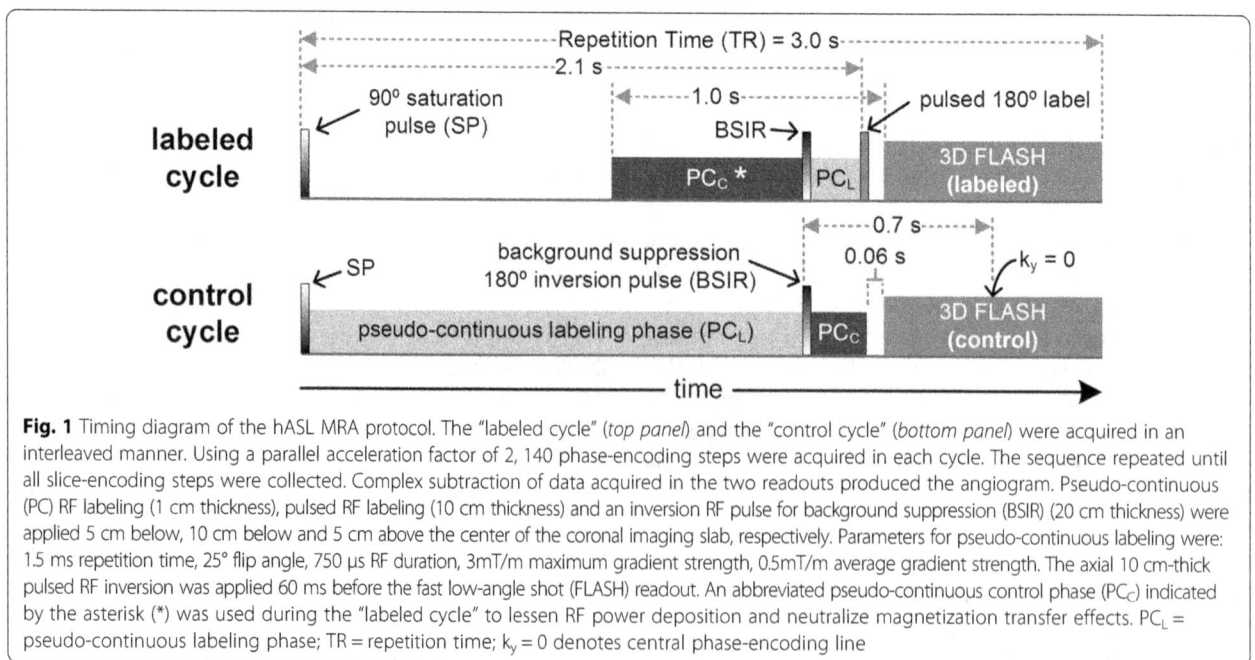

Fig. 1 Timing diagram of the hASL MRA protocol. The "labeled cycle" (*top panel*) and the "control cycle" (*bottom panel*) were acquired in an interleaved manner. Using a parallel acceleration factor of 2, 140 phase-encoding steps were acquired in each cycle. The sequence repeated until all slice-encoding steps were collected. Complex subtraction of data acquired in the two readouts produced the angiogram. Pseudo-continuous (PC) RF labeling (1 cm thickness), pulsed RF labeling (10 cm thickness) and an inversion RF pulse for background suppression (BSIR) (20 cm thickness) were applied 5 cm below, 10 cm below and 5 cm above the center of the coronal imaging slab, respectively. Parameters for pseudo-continuous labeling were: 1.5 ms repetition time, 25° flip angle, 750 µs RF duration, 3mT/m maximum gradient strength, 0.5mT/m average gradient strength. The axial 10 cm-thick pulsed RF inversion was applied 60 ms before the fast low-angle shot (FLASH) readout. An abbreviated pseudo-continuous control phase (PC$_C$) indicated by the asterisk (*) was used during the "labeled cycle" to lessen RF power deposition and neutralize magnetization transfer effects. PC$_L$ = pseudo-continuous labeling phase; TR = repetition time; k$_y$ = 0 denotes central phase-encoding line

for diagnosis; 3 = good, with some minor inhomogeneities not influencing vessel delineation; and 4 = excellent, sharply defined arterial borders with excellent image quality for highly confident diagnosis.

The presence of arterial pathology was noted independently by both reviewers; discrepancies were settled by consensus review.

Quantitative analysis

In each patient, measurements of arterial cross-sectional area and arterial sharpness were obtained in one randomly selected artery per subject, similar to the approach of Kramer et al. [12]. Source images were loaded into 3D image analysis software (Leonardo, Siemens Healthcare, Erlangen, Germany) where axial source reformations were created at three locations (Fig. 2a): location 1 - at the level of the flow divider of the carotid bifurcation, location 2 - common carotid artery two centimeters below location 1, and location 3 - two centimeters above location 1 through the proximal internal carotid artery. Cross-sectional measurements of arterial lumen area for hASL and TOF were compared to CEMRA, which served as the reference standard. Arterial lumen area measurements were obtained in an objective manner by computing the area enclosed by the full-width-at-half-maximum signal points of 60 radial

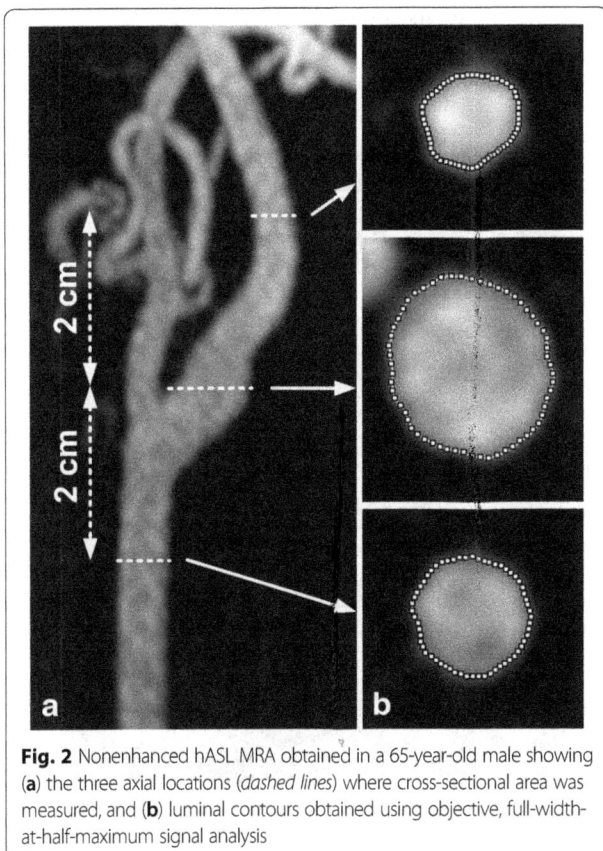

Fig. 2 Nonenhanced hASL MRA obtained in a 65-year-old male showing (**a**) the three axial locations (*dashed lines*) where cross-sectional area was measured, and (**b**) luminal contours obtained using objective, full-width-at-half-maximum signal analysis

spokes emanating from the center of the vessel (Fig. 2b) [24]. Arterial sharpness at the carotid bifurcation (location 1) was measured as the inverse of the distance between the 20th and 80th percentile points in the 60 spokes [25]; the median sharpness value across the 60 spokes was used.

Statistical analysis of data

Statistical analysis was performed using R software (version 3.2.1, The R Foundation for Statistical Computing, Vienna, Austria). In handling missing scoring data which occurred if an arterial location was outside the imaged field of view, list-wise deletion was used for comparisons involving three groups while pair-wise deletion was used for comparisons involving two groups.

Due to the inability to conduct the quantitative and diagnostic analyses above, and because no attempts were made to re-acquire scans with non-diagnostic image quality, patients with at least one imaging scan having non-diagnostic image quality (as assessed by median image quality of <2 across 11 segments by at least one reviewer) were excluded from further analysis. Excluded cases were reviewed by a CMR scientist (I.K.) to determine the cause of artifact. In the remaining data, differences in image quality scores between techniques were identified using non-parametric Friedman tests and post-hoc Wilcoxon signed-rank tests. Interrater agreement was computed using Gwet's AC1, which is more reliable than Cohen's κ when there is a high level of agreement [26]. AC1 was interpreted as follows: 0.01–0.20, slight agreement; 0.21–0.40, fair agreement, 0.41–0.60, moderate agreement; 0.61–0.80, substantial agreement; and 0.81–0.99, almost perfect agreement [27]. The spearman rank correlation coefficient (ρ) was used to evaluate whether image quality (as summarized by the median image quality score across 11 arterial locations and both reviewers) was correlated with age and body mass index (BMI). Agreement of quantitative cross-sectional arterial area measurements was assessed by intraclass correlation coefficient (ICC) and Bland-Altman analysis [28]. Differences in arterial sharpness between techniques were determined using repeated measures analysis of variance with post-hoc Tukey testing. Differences in proportions of diagnostic scans were assessed using a 3-sample test for equality of proportions. P-values less than 0.05 indicated statistical significance.

Results

Between October 2014 and January 2015, 45 patients underwent MRA of their carotid arteries using hASL, TOF and CEMRA in the same scan session. Eight patients were excluded from analysis due to non-diagnostic studies (median image quality of <2) on either hASL ($n = 5$) and TOF ($n = 3$) exams, leaving data from 37 patients (13 men, 24 women; mean age, 67.5 ± 15.7 years) which were included in our analysis. The percentage of scans with diagnostic image quality (i.e. median image quality scores of ≥2 by both reviewers) was 88.9 % (40/45) for hASL, 93.3 % (42/45) for TOF, and 100 % (45/45) for CEMRA ($P = $ NS between techniques). All eight non-diagnostic scans were attributed to motion artifact. Indications for imaging in the remaining 37 patients included dysphasia ($n = 8$), dizziness ($n = 6$), weakness ($n = 4$), transient ischemic attack ($n = 3$), headaches ($n = 2$), visual field deficit ($n = 2$), amnesia ($n = 2$), confusion ($n = 2$), diplopia ($n = 2$), pulsatile tinnitus ($n = 2$), suspected carotid dissection ($n = 1$), aneurysm ($n = 1$), infarct ($n = 1$) and vertigo ($n = 1$).

Qualitative analysis: summary and segmental analysis

A total of 407 arterial locations (37 subjects, 11 locations/subject) were analyzed. Excluding arterial locations outside the field of view (3 of 407 for CEMRA, 14 of 407 for hASL MRA, and 89 of 407 for TOF MRA), a total of 318 locations were portrayed by all three techniques. Each of these 318 locations was interpreted by two reviewers, resulting in a total of 636 evaluations.

Representative angiograms obtained with hASL MRA at 3 Tesla are shown in Figs. 3 and 4. With hASL, the intracranial arteries were visualized if the field of view was sufficiently large in the head-foot direction (Fig. 5). Image quality scores and inter-rater agreement values for each technique with respect to location are summarized in Table 2. CEMRA provided significantly better image quality than the nonenhanced techniques across all arterial locations for both reviewers, except in the left and right carotid siphons ($P < 0.05$), where image quality between CEMRA and nonenhanced hASL MRA did not significantly differ for reviewer 2. When scores were aggregated across all locations, CEMRA provided the best image quality, with median scores of 4 for both reviewers ($P < 0.001$), followed by hASL MRA (median scores of 4 and 3 for reviewers 1 and 2) and 2D TOF (median scores of 3 and 2 for reviewers 1 and 2).

For both reviewers, hASL MRA provided better image quality than TOF in the following 8 locations of the extracranial carotid arteries: bilateral proximal internal carotid arteries (ICAs), bilateral mid-cervical ICAs, bilateral petrous ICAs, and bilateral external carotid arteries ($P < 0.05$). Reviewers 1 and 2 scored the left and right common carotid arteries better with hASL than with TOF, respectively. For the intracranial arteries (which were not assessable by 2D TOF because of limited axial coverage), image quality scores for noncontrast hASL MRA (median/mean values of 2.0/2.4 and 2.0/2.5 for reviewers 1 and 2, respectively) and CEMRA (median/mean values of 3.0/2.7 and 3.0/2.9) significantly differed ($P < 0.05$) for reviewer 2 but not reviewer 1.

Qualitative analysis: inter-rater agreement

Inter-rater agreement in the carotid arteries was substantial for hASL MRA (AC1 = 0.61, 95 % confidence

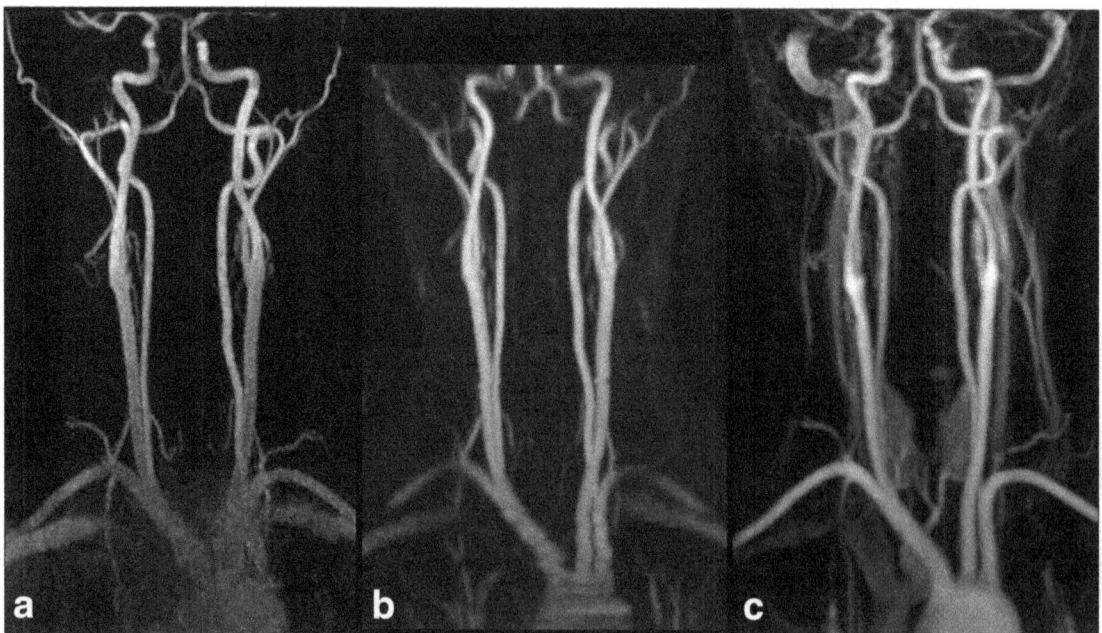

Fig. 3 Representative coronal maximum intensity projection images obtained in a 42-year-old female with (**a**) nonenhanced hASL MRA, (**b**) nonenhanced TOF MRA and (**c**) CEMRA

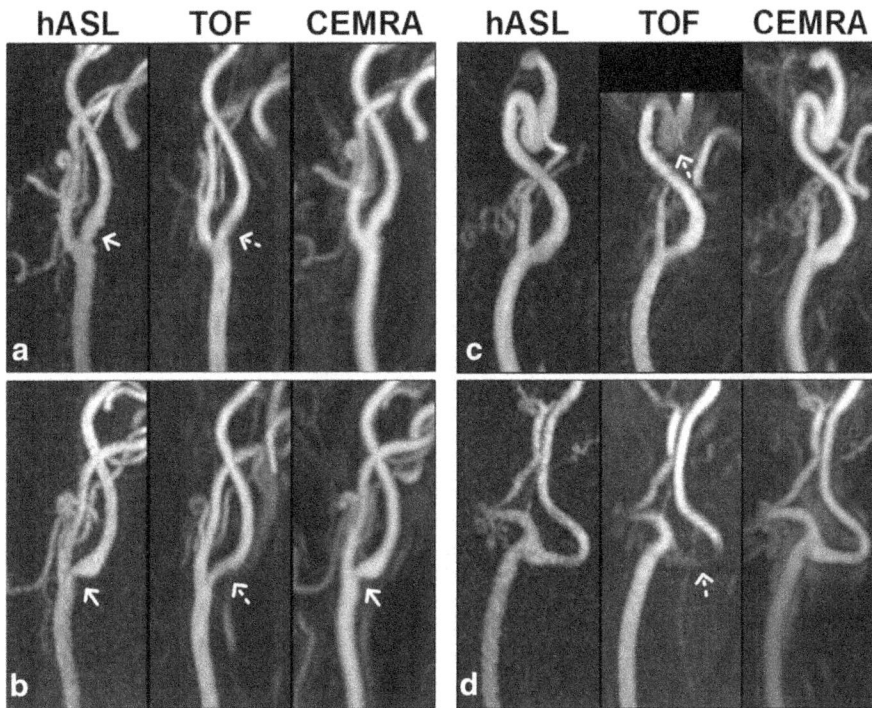

Fig. 4 Representative maximum intensity projection images (30 mm thickness) of four carotid bifurcations obtained with hASL, TOF and CEMRA. **a** Luminal irregularity in the proximal internal carotid artery (ICA) of a 78-year-old male is well depicted by hASL (*arrow*), obscured by TOF (*dashed arrow*), and corroborated by CEMRA. **b** Moderate stenosis of the contralateral ICA in the same patient (*arrows*). Note the agreement between hASL and CEMRA in terms of arterial morphology and severity of disease; saturation of the carotid bulb, however, is evident with TOF (*dashed arrow*). Carotid bifurcations in (**c**) an 84-year-old female and (**d**) a 55-year-old male. Signal saturation effects observed with TOF (*dashed arrows*) are not observed with hASL. There is excellent correspondence of arterial morphology between hASL and CEMRA

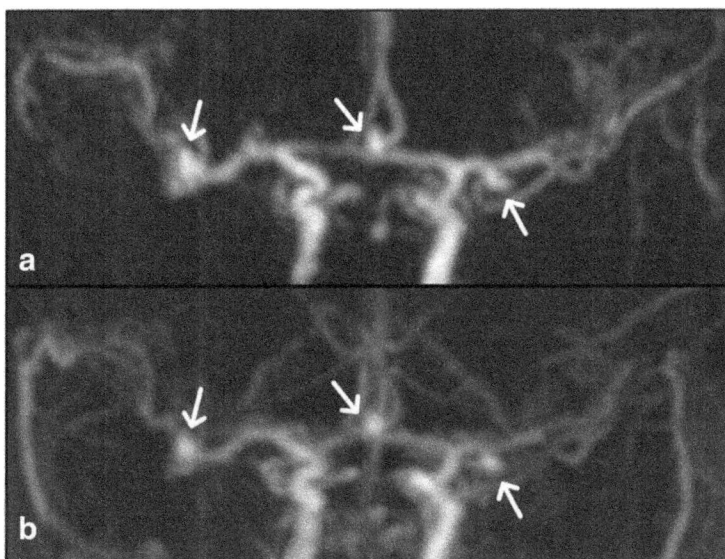

Fig. 5 Coronal maximum intensity projection images of 65-year-old female with intracranial aneurysms (*arrows*) obtained with (**a**) nonenhanced hASL MRA and (**b**) CEMRA. Note the excellent depiction of the aneurysms and with hASL MRA and correspondence with CEMRA. TOF results not shown due to insufficient coverage

Table 2 Image Quality Scores and Inter-rater Agreement

Arterial Location	Image Quality						Inter-rater Agreement (AC1)		
	hASL		TOF		CEMRA				
	R1	R2	R1	R2	R1	R2	hASL	TOF	CEMRA
1. left CCA [*]	2.0(2.7) [**]	2.0(1.9)	2.0(2.3)	2.0(1.9)	4.0(4.0) [***]	4.0(3.7) [***]	0.39	0.37	0.71
2. right CCA [*]	2.0(2.6)	2.0(2.1) [**]	2.0(2.3)	2.0(1.8)	4.0(4.0) [***]	4.0(3.8) [***]	0.46	0.34	0.78
3. left bulb and prox. ICA [*]	4.0(3.7) [**]	4.0(3.4) [**]	3.0(2.8)	3.0(2.6)	4.0(3.9) [***]	4.0(3.9) [***]	0.67	0.42	0.91
4. right bulb and prox. ICA [*]	4.0(3.6) [**]	4.0(3.5) [**]	3.0(2.8)	3.0(2.6)	4.0(3.9) [***]	4.0(3.9) [***]	0.75	0.39	0.91
5. left mid-cervical ICA [*]	4.0(3.6) [**]	4.0(3.6) [**]	3.0(2.9)	3.0(2.6)	4.0(4.0) [***]	4.0(3.9) [***]	0.71	0.38	0.94
6. right mid-cervical ICA [*]	4.0(3.6) [**]	4.0(3.6) [**]	3.0(2.8)	3.0(2.6)	4.0(3.9) [***]	4.0(3.9) [***]	0.79	0.45	0.97
7. left petrous ICA [*]	3.5(2.8) [**]	4.0(3.4) [**]	1.5(1.9)	2.0(1.7)	4.0(4.0) [***]	4.0(4.0) [**]	0.47	0.36	0.94
8. right petrous ICA [*]	4.0(3.0)	4.0(3.4) [**]	2.0(2.2)	2.0(1.8)	4.0(4.0) [***]	4.0(4.0) [**]	0.62	0.30	0.91
9. left ECA [*]	4.0(3.5) [**]	4.0(3.4) [**]	3.0(2.6)	2.0(2.4)	4.0(3.9) [***]	4.0(3.7) [***]	0.47	0.56	0.81
10. right ECA [*]	4.0(3.4) [**]	4.0(3.4) [**]	3.0(2.6)	2.0(2.5)	4.0(3.9) [***]	4.0(3.8) [***]	0.60	0.60	0.78
All Locations [*]	4.0(3.3) [**]	3.0(3.1) [**]	3.0(2.6)	2.0(2.3)	4.0(3.9) [***]	4.0(3.8) [***]	0.61	0.43 [****]	0.87 [****]

Image quality data are presented as median (mean); 1: non-diagnostic, 4: excellent
Data summarize findings from locations depicted by all three techniques
R1 reviewer 1, *R2* reviewer 2, *CCA* common carotid artery, *ICA* internal carotid artery, *ECA* external carotid artery
[*] $P < 0.05$, Bonferroni-corrected Friedman test across techniques
[**] $P < 0.05$ vs. TOF for the same reviewer
[***] $P < 0.05$ vs. hASL and TOF for the same reviewer
[****] $P < 0.05$ vs. hASL for AC1 value

interval (CI): 0.54–0.67; $P < 0.001$), moderate for TOF MRA (AC1 = 0.43, 95 % CI: 0.36–0.50; $P < 0.001$) and almost perfect for CEMRA (AC1 = 0.87, 95 % CI: 0.83–0.91; $P < 0.001$). In the intracranial arteries, inter-rater agreement was fair for both hASL MRA (AC1 = 0.60, $P < 0.001$) and CEMRA (AC1 = 0.55, $P < 0.001$).

Qualitative analysis: impact of age and body mass index
There were no significant correlations between image quality and age for hASL ($\rho = 0.08$, $P = 0.62$), TOF ($\rho = -0.31$, $P = 0.07$) and CEMRA ($\rho = -0.09$, $P = 0.59$). Similarly, there were no significant correlations between image quality and body mass index for hASL ($\rho = -0.06$, $P = 0.73$), TOF ($\rho = 0.01$, $P = 0.96$) and CEMRA ($\rho = -0.01$, $P = 0.95$).

Detection of arterial pathology
Using CEMRA as the reference standard, hASL MRA detected 5 of 5 instances of internal carotid arterial pathology (4 stenoses, 1 fibromuscular dysplasia) with no false positives, and 4 of 4 instances of intracranial arterial pathology (3 aneurysms, 1 middle cerebral artery stenosis) with no false positives. Due to limitations in image quality, only 2 of the 5 instances of carotid pathology (2 stenoses) were detected using TOF MRA; there were no false positive findings with TOF. Intracranial pathology was not evaluable by TOF due to insufficient coverage.

Quantitative analysis
Measurements of cross-sectional lumen area are summarized in Fig. 6. Compared to CEMRA, better

agreement of cross-sectional lumen area was obtained with hASL MRA than with TOF at the common carotid artery (ICC = 0.90 for hASL versus 0.66 for TOF, $P < 0.05$), carotid bifurcation (ICC = 0.87 versus 0.53, $P < 0.05$), and internal carotid artery (ICC = 0.65 versus 0.57). Results of the Bland-Altman analyses are shown in Table 3. hASL MRA had smaller absolute biases and smaller to comparable 95 % limits of agreement for cross-sectional lumen area as compared with TOF MRA. The three techniques differed in arterial sharpness ($P < 0.001$). Arterial sharpness was best with hASL MRA (0.74 ± 0.12 mm^{-1}) ($P < 0.001$ versus TOF and CEMRA), followed by TOF (0.63 ± 0.13 mm^{-1}) and CEMRA (0.57 ± 0.10 mm^{-1}), which did not statistically differ.

Discussion
In this retrospective study, we investigated whether ungated hASL MRA using a FLASH readout and Cartesian k-sampling trajectory could faithfully display the extracranial carotid arteries at 3 Tesla without the use of contrast agents. Our results indicate the affirmative. Although inferior to CEMRA, image quality obtained with hASL MRA was found to be superior to 2D TOF for displaying the carotid bifurcation, internal carotid arteries and external carotid arteries. In addition, inter-rater agreement was improved with hASL MRA as compared with TOF MRA. Furthermore, compared with values obtained with TOF, measurements of cross-sectional arterial area obtained with hASL better agreed with values obtained from first-pass CEMRA. Finally, arterial

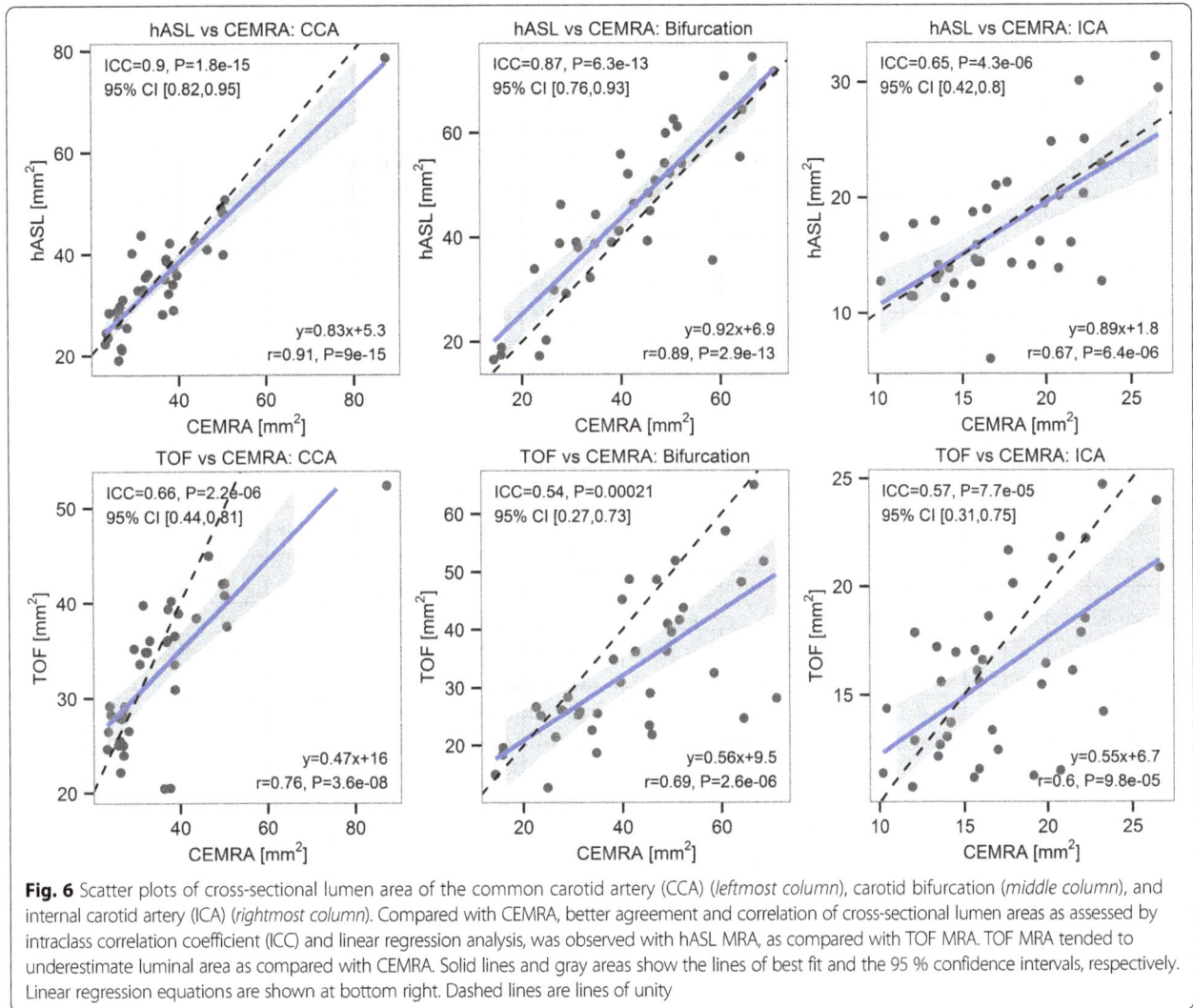

Fig. 6 Scatter plots of cross-sectional lumen area of the common carotid artery (CCA) (*leftmost column*), carotid bifurcation (*middle column*), and internal carotid artery (ICA) (*rightmost column*). Compared with CEMRA, better agreement and correlation of cross-sectional lumen areas as assessed by intraclass correlation coefficient (ICC) and linear regression analysis, was observed with hASL MRA, as compared with TOF MRA. TOF MRA tended to underestimate luminal area as compared with CEMRA. Solid lines and gray areas show the lines of best fit and the 95 % confidence intervals, respectively. Linear regression equations are shown at bottom right. Dashed lines are lines of unity

sharpness provided by hASL MRA was improved with respect to TOF and CEMRA.

Of the three techniques available for comparison in this study, CEMRA provided the best image quality and inter-rater agreement in the extracranial carotid arteries.

Table 3 Bland-Altman Analyses of Cross-Sectional Lumen Area with Respect to CEMRA

Technique	Location	Bias (mm^2)	95 % Limits of agreement (mm^2)
hASL	CCA	−0.8	(−10.7, 9.1)
TOF	CCA	−2.6	(−18.2, 13.0)
hASL	Bifurcation	3.5	(−11.2, 18.2)
TOF	Bifurcation	−8.6	(−31.0, 13.8)
hASL	ICA	0.2	(−8.5, 8.2)
TOF	ICA	−1.1	(−8.4, 6.1)

Nonenhanced technique minus CEMRA

CCA common carotid artery, *ICA* internal carotid artery

This finding is not unexpected given that CEMRA is a fast, reliable and accurate technique for evaluating the extracranial carotid arteries at 1.5 and 3 Tesla [29–34]. For patients in whom Gd-based contrast is contraindicated or when it is useful to save contrast for other purposes (such as the assessment of cerebral perfusion in patients with suspected stroke), however, nonenhanced MRA remains an important diagnostic option. Nonenhanced MRA is also useful backup in circumstances when CEMRA is mistimed with respect to first-pass of contrast bolus and there is insufficient delineation of the carotid arteries due to an early acquisition, or considerable venous contamination due to a late acquisition. Also, given the growing concern of Gd accumulation in the brain following contrast-enhanced CMR studies with unknown long-term consequences [35, 36], review of high-quality nonenhanced MRA may afford one the option of skipping CEMRA.

Nonenhanced 2D TOF is routinely used for depicting the extracranial carotid arteries prior to CEMRA and in patients who cannot receive Gd-based contrast agents. In this study, hASL MRA provided better image quality than 2D TOF MRA at the carotid bulb and in the internal and external carotid arteries. The improved image quality of hASL for depicting the carotid arteries relative to 2D TOF is consistent with prior reports at 1.5 Tesla using bSSFP readouts [20, 21], and is ascribed to the method's elimination of background signal, reduced sensitivity to saturation of the CMR signal from in-plane and recirculating blood flow, and higher spatial resolution in the head-foot direction. These results are also consistent with an in-vitro study that found that hASL FLASH MRA more accurately portrayed carotid arterial morphology than 2D and 3D TOF over a wide range of physiological flow rates [22]. In this work, we did not compare hASL to 3D TOF, which more accurately displays stenoses of the carotid bifurcation than 2D TOF [10, 37]. Nevertheless, it would have been impractical to acquire 3D TOF spanning the entire length of the extracranial carotid arteries due to scan time considerations and respiratory motion in the upper chest.

To our knowledge, this is the first study reporting the feasibility of using ASL-based MRA for portraying the extracranial carotid arteries in consecutive patients imaged in a clinical environment. Prior works have reported the feasibility of ASL-based MRA for depicting the carotid arteries of non-consecutive patients imaged in a non-clinical research environment [16, 17, 20, 21]. The results of our study therefore indicate that hASL MRA of the extracranial carotid arteries is feasible and can be performed by CMR technologists without the need for special training or expertise.

Recent works have reported the following nonenhanced alternatives to TOF for the evaluation of the extracranial carotid arteries at 3 Tesla: inversion-recovery bSSFP [12, 13]; inversion-recovery fast spin-echo [14]; and QISS using a FLASH readout [15]. Direct comparisons of hASL MRA with these recent methods were outside the scope of this retrospective study. Nonetheless, the following statements can be made after careful examination of the literature. Compared with hASL MRA, inversion-recovery bSSFP methods are expected to provide reduced scan times and motion sensitivity, due to the lack of signal subtraction. On the other hand, inversion-recovery protocols only partially suppress signal from background tissues such as muscle, fat and cerebrospinal fluid. This is in stark contrast to hASL MRA which eliminates background signal and therefore allows for the creation of rotating MIP images similar to what is done with CEMRA, without requiring one to first remove background signal prior to MIP generation (of note, background signal was removed for all image sets in this study to facilitate the fairest comparisons, but such processing was not necessary for hASL MRA). Furthermore, the FLASH readout used with hASL MRA is less sensitive than bSSFP imaging to B0 and B1 inhomogeneity, which are worsened at 3 Tesla [38]. To date, cardiac-gated inversion-recovery fast spin-echo angiography has provided promising initial results in volunteers, but the approach has used larger voxel sizes of 3.5 mm^3 (versus 1.0 mm^3 voxels for hASL MRA) and has been unable to visualize intracranial arteries due to dephasing of the CMR signal at the skull base [14]. In comparison, intracranial vessels were depicted with fair to good image quality with hASL MRA in the present study.

We did not evaluate the thoracic inlet in this study because of the lack of respiratory motion compensation. The recently described approach of cardiac-gated QISS FLASH MRA [15], which uses tilted overlapping thin slices, is expected to provide for better display the thoracic inlet and carotid origins than hASL MRA. Conversely, drawbacks of QISS FLASH MRA include the need for cardiac gating and the slice resolution constraints associated with 2D imaging. With respect to prior implementations of hASL MRA at 1.5 Tesla that have used radial sampling trajectories and bSSFP readouts [21, 22], the presented variant of hASL MRA (which applies a Cartesian sampling trajectory and a FLASH readout) is simpler to implement and is less sensitive to artifacts from gradient timing errors and main magnetic field inhomogeneity, especially at 3 Tesla, the preferred field strength for clinical neurovascular MRA [39–41]. Finally, compared with variants using bSSFP readouts, the use of a FLASH readout is expected to improve the display of turbulent flow near severe carotid stenoses [22].

This study had some limitations. One limitation is that there was a relatively low incidence of carotid arterial pathology in our cohort (13.5 %, 5 of 37 patients), reflecting the breadth of patients with neurologic symptoms undergoing carotid MRA. Nonetheless, nonenhanced hASL MRA detected all instances of carotid disease observed at CEMRA without any false positives; by comparison, limitations in image quality for 2D TOF resulted in 3 false negative findings. Another limitation is the exclusion of 8 of 45 patients because of non-diagnostic image quality caused by motion artifact. Even though the proportion of diagnostic scans between the three techniques (hASL, TOF, CEMRA) did not reach statistical significance, all non-diagnostic MRA scans were nonenhanced. In our experience, motion-corrupted nonenhanced MRA can often be salvaged by reminding the patient to hold still and re-acquiring the scan; of note, re-acquisition was not attempted for any scan included in this retrospective study.

In the display of intracranial vessels, subtractive arterial spin-labeled MRA has previously demonstrated the ability to depict flow alterations, collateral flow patterns and arterio-venous malformations within the brain [19, 42–47]. The display of intracranial arteries and CEMRA-confirmed intracranial aneurysms and stenoses in our study is in general agreement with these prior works and suggests that hASL MRA at 3 Tesla using a FLASH readout may have a role in the simultaneous evaluation of extracranial and intracranial arteries in a single nonenhanced acquisition.

Conclusions
hASL FLASH MRA offers an appealing alternative to 2D TOF MRA for nonenhanced MRA of the extracranial carotid arteries at 3 Tesla. The hASL FLASH MRA protocol may have utility as a pre-contrast scout, in the assessment of the carotid arteries in patients with renal insufficiency, and when it is desirable to save contrast agents for cerebral perfusion imaging.

Abbreviations
ASL: Arterial spin labeling; bSSFP: balanced steady-state free precession; CI: confidence interval; CCA: common carotid artery; CEMRA: contrast-enhanced magnetic resonance angiography; CMR: cardiovascular magnetic resonance; ECA: external carotid artery; FLASH: fast low-angle shot; hASL: hybridized arterial spin labeling; ICA: internal carotid artery; ICC: intraclass correlation; MRA: magnetic resonance angiography; QISS: quiescent interval slice-selective; RF: radiofrequency; TOF: time of flight.

Competing interests
IK is an inventor on a patent application describing the hybridized arterial spin labeling CMR pulse sequence. No non-financial conflicts of interest exist for any of the authors.

Authors' contributions
IK conceived the study, developed the CMR pulse sequence, performed the statistical analyses, and drafted and revised the manuscript. MTW and JRM participated in image review and scoring of pathology and revised the manuscript. IGM performed quantitative measurements and drafted the manuscript. RRE conceived the study, participated in the overall design of the study, and drafted and revised the manuscript. All authors read and approved the final manuscript.

Author details
[1]Department of Radiology, NorthShore University HealthSystem, Evanston, USA. [2]University of Chicago Pritzker School of Medicine, Chicago, USA. [3]Northwestern University Feinberg School of Medicine, Chicago, USA.

References
1. Kuo PH, Kanal E, Abu-Alfa AK, Cowper SE. Gadolinium-based MR contrast agents and nephrogenic systemic fibrosis. Radiology. 2007;242(3):647–9.
2. Saeed F, Kousar N, Qureshi K, Laurence TN. A review of risk factors for stroke in patients with chronic kidney disease. J Vasc Interv Neurol. 2009;2(1):126–31.
3. Kidney Disease Statistics for the United States. 2012. http://www.niddk.nih.gov/health-information/health-statistics/Pages/kidney-disease-statistics-united-states.aspx. Accessed 15 Jan 2016.
4. Mozaffarian D, Benjamin EJ, Go AS, et al. Heart disease and stroke statistics-2015 update: a report from the american heart association. Circulation. 2015;131(4):e29–e322.
5. Jahng GH, Li KL, Ostergaard L, Calamante F. Perfusion magnetic resonance imaging: a comprehensive update on principles and techniques. Korean J Radiol. 2014;15(5):554–77.
6. Keller PJ, Drayer BP, Fram EK, Williams KD, Dumoulin CL, Souza SP. MR angiography with two-dimensional acquisition and three-dimensional display. Work in progress. Radiology. 1989;173(2):527–32.
7. Masaryk AM, Ross JS, DiCello MC, Modic MT, Paranandi L, Masaryk TJ. 3DFT MR angiography of the carotid bifurcation: potential and limitations as a screening examination. Radiology. 1991;179(3):797–804.
8. Blatter DD, Bahr AL, Parker DL, Robison RO, Kimball JA, Perry DM, Horn S. Cervical carotid MR angiography with multiple overlapping thin-slab acquisition: comparison with conventional angiography. AJR Am J Roentgenol. 1993;161(6):1269–77.
9. Huston 3rd J, Lewis BD, Wiebers DO, Meyer FB, Riederer SJ, Weaver AL. Carotid artery: prospective blinded comparison of two-dimensional time-of-flight MR angiography with conventional angiography and duplex US. Radiology. 1993;186(2):339–44.
10. De Marco JK, Nesbit GM, Wesbey GE, Richardson D. Prospective evaluation of extracranial carotid stenosis: MR angiography with maximum-intensity projections and multiplanar reformation compared with conventional angiography. AJR Am J Roentgenol. 1994;163(5):1205–12.
11. Yucel EK, Anderson CM, Edelman RR, Grist TM, Baum RA, Manning WJ, Culebras A, Pearce W. AHA scientific statement. Magnetic resonance angiography : update on applications for extracranial arteries. Circulation. 1999;100(22):2284–301.
12. Kramer H, Runge VM, Morelli JN, Williams KD, Naul LG, Nikolaou K, Reiser MF, Wintersperger BJ. Magnetic resonance angiography of the carotid arteries: comparison of unenhanced and contrast enhanced techniques. Eur Radiol. 2011;21(8):1667–76.
13. Raoult H, Gauvrit JY, Schmitt P, Le Couls V, Bannier E. Non-ECG-gated unenhanced MRA of the carotids: optimization and clinical feasibility. Eur Radiol. 2013;23(11):3020–8.
14. Takei N, Miyoshi M, Kabasawa H. Noncontrast MR angiography for supraaortic arteries using inflow enhanced inversion recovery fast spin echo imaging. J Magn Reson Imaging. 2012;35(4):957–62.
15. Koktzoglou I, Murphy IG, Giri S, Edelman RR. Quiescent interval low angle shot magnetic resonance angiography of the extracranial carotid arteries. Magn Reson Med 2015.
16. Nishimura DG, Macovski A, Pauly JM, Conolly SM. MR angiography by selective inversion recovery. Magn Reson Med. 1987;4(2):193–202.
17. Edelman RR, Siewert B, Adamis M, Gaa J, Laub G, Wielopolski P. Signal targeting with alternating radiofrequency (STAR) sequences: application to MR angiography. Magn Reson Med. 1994;31(2):233–8.
18. Robson PM, Dai W, Shankaranarayanan A, Rofsky NM, Alsop DC. Time-resolved vessel-selective digital subtraction MR angiography of the cerebral vasculature with arterial spin labeling. Radiology. 2010;257(2):507–15.
19. Yan L, Wang S, Zhuo Y, Wolf RL, Stiefel MF, An J, Ye Y, Zhang Q, Melhem ER, Wang DJ. Unenhanced dynamic MR angiography: high spatial and temporal resolution by using true FISP-based spin tagging with alternating radiofrequency. Radiology. 2010;256(1):270–9.
20. Koktzoglou I, Gupta N, Edelman RR. Nonenhanced extracranial carotid MR angiography using arterial spin labeling: improved performance with pseudocontinuous tagging. J Magn Reson Imaging. 2011;34(2):384–94.
21. Koktzoglou I, Meyer JR, Ankenbrandt WJ, Giri S, Piccini D, Zenge MO, Ianagan O, Desai T, Gupta N, Edelman RR. Nonenhanced arterial spin labeled carotid MR angiography using three-dimensional radial balanced steady-state free precession imaging. J Magn Reson Imaging. 2015;41(4):1150–6.
22. Koktzoglou I, Giri S, Piccini D, Grodzki DM, Flanagan O, Murphy IG, Gupta N, Collins JD, Edelman RR. Arterial spin labeled carotid MR angiography: A phantom study examining the impact of technical and hemodynamic factors. Magn Reson Med. 2016;75(1):295–301.
23. Dai W, Garcia D, de Bazelaire C, Alsop DC. Continuous flow-driven inversion for arterial spin labeling using pulsed radio frequency and gradient fields. Magn Reson Med. 2008;60(6):1488–97.
24. Merkx MA, Bescos JO, Geerts L, Bosboom EM, van de Vosse FN, Breeuwer M. Accuracy and precision of vessel area assessment: manual versus automatic lumen delineation based on full-width at half-maximum. J Magn Reson Imaging. 2012;36(5):1186–93.
25. Li D, Carr JC, Shea SM, Zheng J, Deshpande VS, Wielopolski PA, Finn JP. Coronary arteries: magnetization-prepared contrast-enhanced three-dimensional volume-targeted breath-hold MR angiography. Radiology. 2001;219(1):270–7.

26. Gwet KL. Computing inter-rater reliability and its variance in the presence of high agreement. Br J Math Stat Psychol. 2008;61(Pt 1):29–48.

27. Viera AJ, Garrett JM. Understanding interobserver agreement: the kappa statistic. Fam Med. 2005;37(5):360–3.

28. Bland JM, Altman DG. Statistical methods for assessing agreement between two methods of clinical measurement. Lancet. 1986;1(8476):307–10.

29. Phan T, Huston 3rd J, Bernstein MA, Riederer SJ, Brown Jr RD. Contrast-enhanced magnetic resonance angiography of the cervical vessels: experience with 422 patients. Stroke. 2001;32(10):2282–6.

30. Carr JC, Ma J, Desphande V, Pereles S, Laub G, Finn JP. High-resolution breath-hold contrast-enhanced MR angiography of the entire carotid circulation. AJR Am J Roentgenol. 2002;178(3):543–9.

31. Willinek WA, von Falkenhausen M, Born M, Gieseke J, Holler T, Klockgether T, extor HJ, Schild HH, Urbach H. Noninvasive detection of steno-occlusive disease of the supra-aortic arteries with three-dimensional contrast-enhanced magnetic resonance angiography: a prospective, intra-individual comparative analysis with digital subtraction angiography. Stroke. 2005; 36(1):38–43.

32. Nael K, Villablanca JP, Pope WB, McNamara TO, Laub G, Finn JP. Supraaortic arteries: contrast-enhanced MR angiography at 3.0 T–highly accelerated parallel acquisition for improved spatial resolution over an extended field of view. Radiology. 2007;242(2):600–9.

33. Willinek WA, Bayer T, Gieseke J, von Falkenhausen M, Sommer T, Hoogeveen R, Wilhelm K, Urbach H, Schild HH. High spatial resolution contrast-enhanced MR angiography of the supraaortic arteries using the quadrature body coil at 3.0 T: a feasibility study. Eur Radiol. 2007;17(3): 618–25.

34. Menke J. Diagnostic accuracy of contrast-enhanced MR angiography in severe carotid stenosis: meta-analysis with metaregression of different techniques. Eur Radiol. 2009;19(9):2204–16.

35. Kanda T, Ishii K, Kawaguchi H, Kitajima K, Takenaka D. High signal intensity in the dentate nucleus and globus pallidus on unenhanced T1-weighted MR images: relationship with increasing cumulative dose of a gadolinium-based contrast material. Radiology. 2014;270(3):834–41.

36. McDonald RJ, McDonald JS, Kallmes DF, Jentoft ME, Murray DL, Thielen KR, Williamson EE, Eckel LJ. Intracranial Gadolinium Deposition after Contrast-enhanced MR Imaging. Radiology. 2015;275(3):772–82.

37. Scarabino T, Carriero A, Magarelli N, Florio F, Giannatempo GM, Bonomo L, Salvolini U. MR angiography in carotid stenosis: a comparison of three techniques. Eur J Radiol. 1998;28(2):117–25.

38. Sekihara K. Steady-state magnetizations in rapid NMR imaging using small flip angles and short repetition intervals. IEEE Trans Med Imaging. 1987;6(2): 157–64.

39. Bernstein MA, Huston 3rd J, Lin C, Gibbs GF, Felmlee JP. High-resolution intracranial and cervical MRA at 3.0 T: technical considerations and initial experience. Magn Reson Med. 2001;46(5):955–62.

40. Al-Kwifi O, Emery DJ, Wilman AH. Vessel contrast at three Tesla in time-of-flight magnetic resonance angiography of the intracranial and carotid arteries. Magn Reson Imaging. 2002;20(2):181–7.

41. Willinek WA, Born M, Simon B, Tschampa HJ, Krautmacher C, Gieseke J, Urbach H, Textor HJ, Schild HH. Time-of-flight MR angiography: comparison of 3.0-T imaging and 1.5-T imaging–initial experience. Radiology. 2003;229(3):913–20.

42. Essig M, Engenhart R, Knopp MV, Bock M, Scharf J, Debus J, Wenz F, Hawighorst H, Schad LR, van Kaick G. Cerebral arteriovenous malformations: improved nidus demarcation by means of dynamic tagging MR-angiography. Magn Reson Imaging. 1996;14(3):227–33.

43. Warmuth C, Ruping M, Forschler A, Koennecke HC, Valdueza JM, Kauert A, Schreiber SJ, Siekmann R, Zimmer C. Dynamic spin labeling angiography in extracranial carotid artery stenosis. AJNR Am J Neuroradiol. 2005;26(5):1035–43.

44. Xu J, Shi D, Chen C, Li Y, Wang M, Han X, Jin L, Bi X. Noncontrast-enhanced four-dimensional MR angiography for the evaluation of cerebral arteriovenous malformation: a preliminary trial. J Magn Reson Imaging. 2011;34(5):1199–205.

45. Lanzman RS, Kropil P, Schmitt P, et al. Nonenhanced ECG-gated time-resolved 4D steady-state free precession (SSFP) MR angiography (MRA) for assessment of cerebral collateral flow: comparison with digital subtraction angiography (DSA). Eur Radiol. 2011;21(6):1329–38.

46. Lanzman RS, Kropil P, Schmitt P, Wittsack HJ, Orzechowski D, Kuhlemann J, Buchbender C, Miese FR, Antoch G, Blondin D. Nonenhanced ECG-gated

time-resolved 4D steady-state free precession (SSFP) MR angiography (MRA) of cerebral arteries: comparison at 1.5 T and 3 T. Eur J Radiol. 2012;81(4):e531–535.

47. Raoult H, Bannier E, Robert B, Barillot C, Schmitt P, Gauvrit JY. Time-resolved spin-labeled MR angiography for the depiction of cerebral arteriovenous malformations: a comparison of techniques. Radiology. 2014;271(2):524–33.

16

Individual component analysis of the multi-parametric cardiovascular magnetic resonance protocol in the CE-MARC trial

David P Ripley[1], Manish Motwani[1], Julia M. Brown[2], Jane Nixon[2], Colin C. Everett[2], Petra Bijsterveld[1], Neil Maredia[1], Sven Plein[1] and John P. Greenwood[1*]

Abstract

Background: The CE-MARC study assessed the diagnostic performance investigated the use of cardiovascular magnetic resonance (CMR) in patients with suspected coronary artery disease (CAD). The study used a multi-parametric CMR protocol assessing 4 components: i) left ventricular function; ii) myocardial perfusion; iii) viability (late gadolinium enhancement (LGE)) and iv) coronary magnetic resonance angiography (MRA). In this pre-specified CE-MARC sub-study we assessed the diagnostic accuracy of the individual CMR components and their combinations.

Methods: All patients from the CE-MARC population ($n = 752$) were included using data from the original blinded-read. The four individual core components of the CMR protocol was determined separately and then in paired and triplet combinations. Results were then compared to the full multi-parametric protocol.

Results: CMR and X-ray angiography results were available in 676 patients. The maximum sensitivity for the detection of significant CAD by CMR was achieved when all four components were used (86.5 %). Specificity of perfusion (91.8 %), function (93.7 %) and LGE (95.8 %) on its own was significantly better than specificity of the multi-parametric protocol (83.4 %) (all $P < 0.0001$) but with the penalty of decreased sensitivity (86.5 % vs. 76.9 %, 47.4 % and 40.8 % respectively). The full multi-parametric protocol was the optimum to rule-out significant CAD (Likelihood Ratio negative (LR-) 0.16) and the LGE component alone was the best to rue-in CAD (LR+ 9.81). Overall diagnostic accuracy was similar with the full multi-parametric protocol (85.9 %) compared to paired and triplet combinations. The use of coronary MRA within the full multi-parametric protocol had no additional diagnostic benefit compared to the perfusion/function/LGE combination (overall accuracy 84.6 % vs. 84.2 % ($P = 0.5316$); LR- 0.16 vs. 0.21; LR+ 5.21 vs. 5.77).

Conclusions: From this pre-specified sub-analysis of the CE-MARC study, the full multi-parametric protocol had the highest sensitivity and was the optimal approach to rule-out significant CAD. The LGE component alone was the optimal rule-in strategy. Finally the inclusion of coronary MRA provided no additional benefit when compared to the combination of perfusion/function/LGE.

Keywords: Magnetic resonance, Perfusion magnetic resonance imaging, Sensitivity, Specificity

---

* Correspondence: j.greenwood@leeds.ac.uk
[1]Multidisciplinary Cardiovascular Research Centre (MCRC) & Leeds Institute of Cardiovascular and Metabolic Medicine, University of Leeds, Leeds, UK
Full list of author information is available at the end of the article

Background

Coronary artery disease (CAD) is a leading cause of death and disability worldwide. Cardiovascular magnetic resonance (CMR) is recognised in international guidelines as a non-invasive imaging option for the investigation of suspected CAD [1–3]. The CE-MARC study was the largest prospective evaluation of the diagnostic accuracy of CMR in stable CAD to date [4, 5]. The trial adopted a multi-parametric CMR protocol assessing left ventricular (LV) function, myocardial perfusion, viability and coronary artery anatomy in a single study. A rigorous study design avoided referral bias by mandating that all patients underwent X-ray coronary angiography (XRA) as the reference test independent of the result of the CMR or single-photon emission computed tomography (SPECT) scans. The results from CE-MARC and its sub-analyses have shown that CMR had high diagnostic accuracy for suspected CAD in males and females, in single and multi-vessel disease, had higher overall diagnostic accuracy and was also cost effective compared to SPECT [6, 7].

Previous studies designed to determine the diagnostic accuracy of the individual components of the CMR examination have been small and revealed contrasting results. Some have shown the full multi-parametric approach had higher diagnostic accuracy over the individual components of the combined examination, although these were performed in selected populations [8–11]. Furthermore the clinical utility of imaging coronary artery anatomy for the detection of stenosis by magnetic resonance angiography (MRA) within already lengthy protocols remains to be established. Klein *et al.* demonstrated that MRA at 1.5 Tesla (T) did not add to the diagnostic accuracy over perfusion and late gadolinium enhancement (LGE) [11]. Other investigators have evaluated the effect of adding coronary MRA to stress perfusion and LGE on diagnostic performance in the intermediate to high risk group; when compared to invasive pressure-wire derived fractional flow reserve (FFR) at 1.5 T there was no significant improvement in diagnostic accuracy [12].

This predefined sub-study of CE-MARC compared the diagnostic accuracy of the full multi-parametric CMR protocol with the individual components, and their paired and triplet combinations. The aim was to determine the diagnostic accuracy of the individual components and their combinations in a large, prospective, real-world population of patients with suspected CAD requiring further investigation.

Methods

Study design

CE-MARC was a prospective study of 752 consecutive patients with suspected angina and at least one cardiovascular risk factor. Screening and recruitment occurred between March 2006 and August 2009 [4, 5]. All patients were scheduled to undergo SPECT and CMR (in randomized order), followed by XRA within 4 weeks. Inclusion and exclusion criteria have been previously published [4, 5]. Patients provided informed written consent and the study was approved by the local Research Ethics Committee and complied with the Declaration of Helsinki (2000).

All patients from the CE-MARC population were included in this pre-specified sub-analysis. CMR results were from the original, blinded visual read. The diagnostic accuracy of each individual core component of the multi-parametric CMR protocol (perfusion, LV function, MRA and LGE) was determined separately and then in paired or triplet combinations. The results were compared with the full multi-parametric protocol.

CMR and analysis

The multi-parametric CMR (1.5-Tesla Intera CV, Philips, Best, The Netherlands) protocol and pulse sequence parameters have previously been described [4, 5]. The primary analysis used all four components of the multi-parametric CMR study. Criteria for a positive CMR result was any of the following: a) regional wall motion abnormality (RWMA) on cine imaging; b) hypoperfusion on stress/rest perfusion imaging; c) significant stenosis on MRA; d) infarct on LGE images (Table 1) following a 'believe the positive rule'. Individual component image quality scores for CMR (cines, perfusion, LGE, MRA) were graded 1 (unusable) to 4 (excellent).

X-ray angiography

XRA images were analysed by two experienced cardiologists blinded to the CMR and SPECT results. Significant CAD was defined as ≥70 % stenosis of a first order coronary artery measuring ≥2 mm in diameter, or left main stem stenosis ≥50 % by quantitative coronary angiography (QCA) (QCAPlus, Sanders Data Systems, Palo Alto, California, USA).

Statistical analysis

Statistical analyses were performed by the Clinical Trials Research Unit, University of Leeds. Confidence intervals for the sensitivity, specificity, overall accuracy and positive (PPV) and negative predictive values (NPV) were calculated with the Wilson score method. Sensitivities and specificities were compared by the McNemar's test, and predictive values were compared using the generalised score statistic. The positive (LR+) and negative likelihood ratios (LR-) were calculated using standard methods [13]. Assessment of the value of each component as "add on tests" were made with relative likelihood

Table 1 Criteria for a positive CMR result in the CE-MARC study

Parameter	Method	Positive criteria
RWMA	Wall motion in each segment (17-segment model) was visually graded on post-stress cine imaging [0 = normal, 1 = mild-moderate hypokinesis, 2 = severe hypokinesis, 3 = akinesis, 4 = dyskinesis]	Wall motion Score ≥1 in two or more adjacent segments, or ≥2 in one or more segments
Ischemia	Perfusion in each segment (17-segment model)[a] was visually graded at rest and then stress [0 = normal, 1 = equivocal, 2 = subendocardial defect, 3 = transmural defect, 4 = transmural defect and wall thinned]	Decrease in perfusion score ≥2 between rest and stress in any segment, or ≥1 in each of two adjacent segments[b]
Stenosis	Percentage of coronary artery luminal narrowing visually assessed on MRA	≥70 % stenosis or ≥50 % left main stem stenosis
Infarction	LGE images were visually assessed for hyper-enhancement in each segment (17-segment model) [0 = none, 1 = 1–25 %, 2 = 26–50 %, 3 = 51–75 %, 4= > 75 %]	Any score ≥1 in a pattern consistent with myocardial infarction

RWMA regional wall motion abnormality, MRA magnetic resonance coronary angiography, LGE late-gadolinium enhancement

[a]17-segment model excluding apical cap

[b]With the exception of change between 'normal' and 'equivocal', which was coded as 'normal'

ratios [13]. Statistical analysis performed using with SAS software, version 9.2 at a two-sided 5 % significance level.

Results

Study population

Both CMR and XRA were available in 676 patients (mean 60 ± 9.5 years, 62 % male). For the individual components LGE was available in 674 (99.7 %), perfusion in 661 (97.8 %), ventricular function in 676 (100 %) and MRA in 597 (88.3 %). The prevalence of XRA defined significant CAD was 39 % and further demographic details are shown in Table 2.

Diagnostic accuracy

The sensitivity of the combined CMR protocol was 86.5 % (95 % CI: 81.9–90.1), specificity 83.4 % (79.5–86.7), PPV 77.2 % (72.1–81.6 %), NPV 90.5 % (87.1–93.0) and overall diagnostic accuracy 84.6 % (81.7–87.1). The diagnostic accuracy of the individual components, paired and triplet combinations compared to the full multi-parametric protocol are presented in Table 3 and Fig. 1.

We have shown that of the individual components, perfusion had numerically the highest sensitivity (76.9 %), NPV (86.0 %) and overall diagnostic accuracy (85.9 %), whilst LGE had the highest specificity (95.8 %) and PPV (86.4 %) for the detection of significant CAD.

The maximum sensitivity (86.5 %) and NPV (90.5 %) for the detection of significant CAD by CMR was achieved when the full multi-parametric protocol was used, no individual component, paired or triplet combination outperformed the full multi-parametric protocol. However its lower specificity and PPV, meant that its

overall diagnostic accuracy (84.6 %) was broadly similar to the majority of paired and triplet combinations (Table 3).

In terms of specificity, the individual components of perfusion (91.8 %), ventricular function (93.7 %) and LGE (95.8 %) all performed significantly better than the multi-parametric protocol (83.4 %) ($P < 0.0001$ for all). In addition, combining LGE with either ventricular function (91.7 %) or MRA (90.0 %) significantly improved the test specificity compared to the multi-parametric protocol ($P < 0.0001$ for each). For overall diagnostic performance, no individual component or combination was better statistically than the full multi-parametric protocol (Table 3). The use of coronary MRA had no additional diagnostic benefit in terms of overall diagnostic accuracy when performed within a multi-parametric protocol (84.6 % Vs. 84.2 %) ($X^2 = 0.3913, 1 \mathrm{df}, P = 0.5316$).

The value of components as individual and add on tests: likelihood ratios

The highest likelihood ratio positive (LR+) was achieved when using LGE imaging alone (LR+ 9.81) signifying this individual component as the best approach for ruling in a diagnosis. All individual, paired and triplet combinations had higher LR+ than the full multi-parametric protocol (Table 4). However the full multi-parametric protocol had the lowest LR- (0.16) than all of the individual components and their combinations, signifying this as the best approach to rule out significant CAD. The absolute likelihood ratios for all of the components and their combinations are displayed in Table 4. Table 5 illustrates relative likelihood ratios using selected components as "add-on" tests to

Table 2 Summary of demographic and angiographic characteristics

		$n = 676$
Age (years)		60.3 ± 9.5
Male gender		421 (62 %)
Body Mass Index (kg/m^2)		29.0 ± 4.3
Ethnicity	White	643 (95 %)
	Black	5 (1 %)
	Asian	24 (4 %)
	Other	4 (1 %)
Smoking status	Never smoked	236 (35 %)
	Ex-smoker	315 (47 %)
	Current smoker	125 (18 %)
Systolic Blood Pressure (mmHg)		138.1 ± 20.9
Diastolic Blood Pressure (mmHg)		79.0 ± 11.3
Previous admission for AMI or ACS		54 (8.0 %)
Previous PCI		37 (5 %)
Hypertension		347 (51 %)
Diabetes mellitus		85 (13 %)
	Type I	4 (5 %)
	Type II	81 (95 %)
Family history of premature CAD	Yes	392 (58 %)
	No	237 (35 %)
	Unknown	47 (7 %)
Total cholesterol (mmol/L)		5.2 (1.2)
Medication		
Aspirin and/or Clopidogrel		404 (60 %)
Statin		301 (45 %)
ACEi/A2 Receptor Blockers		229 (37.2 %)
Beta-blocker		203 (33.0 %)
Patients undergoing X-ray angiography		
Any significant stenosis		266 (39 %)
Triple Vessel Disease		40 (6 %)
Double Vessel Disease		83 (12 %)
Single Vessel Disease		143 (21 %)
LMS Disease		22 (3 %)
LAD Disease		169 (25 %)
LCx Disease		126 (19 %)
RCA Disease		105 (16 %)

Mean ± standard deviation. Number (percentage)
AMI acute myocardial infarction, *ACS* acute coronary syndrome, *PCI* percutaneous coronary intervention, *CAD* coronary artery disease, *ACEi* angiotensin converting enzyme inhibitor, *A2* angiotensin 2, *LMS* left main stem, *LAD* left anterior descending, *LCx* left circumflex, *RCA* right coronary artery

stress perfusion imaging alone, and the absolute number of new true and false positives cases produced with each combination.

Discussion

This pre-specified sub-study of the CE-MARC study has demonstrated the diagnostic accuracy of the individual components and the paired and triplet combinations from the multi-parametric CMR examination. The three main findings were that i) no individual component or combination of components outperformed the full multi-parametric protocol to rule out significant coronary artery disease; ii) the LGE component has the best performance to rule-in significant CAD; and iii) the addition of MRA to function/perfusion/LGE does not offer any incremental benefit.

Likelihood ratios

We have shown the absolute likelihood ratio (LR) for each component and their combinations (Table 4) and demonstrated how many more (or less) times a particular component or combination result is likely in patients with CAD compared to those without the disease. LR is defined as the ratio of the expected test results in subjects with a certain disease to the subjects without disease, and they directly link the pre-test and post-test probability of the disease. A likelihood ratio of greater than 1 is associated with the presence of disease, whereas a ratio of less than 1 would indicate the test result is associated with the absence of disease. Importantly, as likelihood ratios are based on the ratio of sensitivity and specificity of an individual test, they are independent of disease prevalence, and can therefore be applied to different populations. The presented LRs can therefore be applied directly at the individual level and used to calculate how the probability of having CAD changes after the result of an individual component or combination of components of the CMR examination. Positive and negative likelihood ratios are therefore useful to understand the role of a test result in changing a clinician's estimate of the probability of disease in a patient.

The LR for positive tests (LR+) is the likelihood that a given test result would be expected in a patient with the disease (i.e., how much more likely the positive test result is to occur in subjects with the disease compared to those without the disease). LR+ is the best indicator for a rule-in diagnosis and the higher the LR+ the more indicative of disease. LR+ is calculated as follows: LR+ = sensitivity/(1 − specificity). Therefore high sensitivity and specificity result in high LR+. The individual components of LGE (LR+ 9.81) and perfusion (9.35) had the highest LR+ amongst all the individual components and combinations with LGE benefitting from very high specificity to overcome poor sensitivity, and perfusion benefitting from both high sensitivity and specificity. For both components tested in isolation, a positive test finding increased the

Table 3 Diagnostic accuracy of a multi-parametric CMR exam and its individual components, paired and triplet combinations compared to the reference test X-ray angiography

	Sensitivity (95 % CI)	Specificity (95 % CI)	PPV (95 % CI)	NPV (95 % CI)	Overall accuracy (95 % CI)
Overall multi-parametric CMR study (all components) ($n = 676$)	86.5 (81.8, 90.1)	83.4 (79.5, 86.7)	77.2 (72.1, 81.6)	90.5 (87.1, 93.0)	84.6 (81.7, 87.1)
Individual CMR components					
LGE ($n = 674$)	40.8 (35.0, 46.8)	95.8 (93.4, 97.4)	86.4 (79.3, 91.3)	71.4 (67.5, 75.0)	74.2 (70.7, 77.3)
Perfusion ($n = 661$)	76.9 (71.4, 81.6)	91.8 (88.7, 94.1)	85.8 (80.8, 89.7)	86.0 (82.4, 89.0)	85.9 (83.1, 88.4)
Ventricular function ($n = 676$)	47.4 (41.4, 53.4)	93.7 (90.9, 95.6)	82.9 (76.1, 88.1)	73.3 (69.3, 76.9)	75.4 (72.1, 78.5)
MRA ($n = 597$)	71.2 (65.1, 76.7)	89.8 (86.3, 92.5)	81.8 (75.9, 86.5)	83.0 (79.0, 86.4)	82.6 (79.3, 85.4)
Paired combinations					
Perfusion/LGE ($n = 676$)	78.6 (73.3, 83.1)	89.3 (85.9, 91.9)	82.6 (77.5, 86.8)	86.5 (82.9, 89.5)	85.1 (82.2, 87.5)
Perfusion/function ($n = 676$)	80.1 (74.9, 84.4)	87.3 (83.7, 90.2)	80.4 (75.2, 84.7)	87.1 (83.5, 90.0)	84.5 (81.5, 87.0)
Perfusion/MRA ($n = 676$)	82.3 (77.3, 86.4)	89.0 (85.6, 91.7)	83.0 (78.0, 87.0)	88.6 (85.2, 91.3)	86.4 (83.6, 88.8)
Function/LGE ($n = 676$)	52.6 (46.6, 58.6)	91.7 (88.6, 94.0)	80.5 (73.9, 85.7)	74.9 (70.9, 78.5)	76.3 (73.0, 79.4)
Function/MRA ($n = 676$)	72.9 (67.3, 77.9)	87.8 (84.3, 90.6)	79.5 (74.0, 84.1)	83.3 (79.5, 86.6)	82.0 (78.9, 84.7)
LGE/MRA ($n = 676$)	69.2 (63.4, 74.4)	90.0 (86.7, 92.5)	81.8 (76.2, 86.3)	81.8 (78.0, 85.1)	81.8 (78.7, 84.5)
Triplet combinations					
Perfusion/LGE/function ($n = 676$)	81.6 (76.5, 85.8)	85.9 (82.1, 88.9)	78.9 (73.7, 83.3)	87.8 (84.2, 90.6)	84.2 (81.2, 86.7)
Perfusion/LGE/MRA ($n = 676$)	84.6 (79.8, 88.4)	86.6 (82.9, 89.5)	80.4 (75.3, 84.6)	89.6 (86.3, 92.3)	85.8 (83.0, 88.2)
Perfusion/function/MRA ($n = 676$)	85.3 (80.6, 89.1)	84.9 (81.1, 88.0)	78.5 (73.5, 82.9)	89.9 (86.5, 92.5)	85.1 (82.2, 87.5)
LGE/function/MRA ($n = 676$)	75.2 (69.7, 80.0)	86.1 (82.4, 89.1)	77.8 (72.4, 82.5)	84.2 (80.5, 87.4)	81.8 (78.7, 84.5)

CMR cardiovascular magnetic resonance, *LGE* late gadolinium enhancement, *LR-* Likelihood Ratio Negative, *LR+* Likelihood Ratio Positive, *MRA* magnetic resonance coronary angiography

odds of the patient having CAD more than 9 fold. Therefore a positive LGE or perfusion test is a good test for ruling in the diagnosis of CAD.

Likelihood ratios for negative tests (LR-) demonstrate how much less likely the negative result will occur in subjects with the disease to the probability that the same result will occur without the disease. LR- is calculated as follows: LR- = (1 − specificity)/sensitivity and is a good indicator for ruling-out the diagnosis. For a single component, perfusion imaging produced the smallest likelihood ratio of disease for a negative finding (LR- 0.25): i.e., the odds of a patient having CAD were reduced by 75 % to one quarter of the pre-test odds with a normal perfusion result. By comparison, the odds of having CAD were only reduced by around 40 % with a negative LGE finding (LR- 0.62). Therefore for a single component, perfusion resulted in the greatest change in post-test odds of having coronary disease, and an overall diagnostic accuracy of 85.9 %. In terms of both positive and negative likelihood ratios, no paired or triplet combination offered a significant benefit over the best performing component of perfusion alone.

When combining the information from the four components in the full multi-parametric protocol using the "believe the positive" rule, the consequent reductions in specificity were not met by similar increases in sensitivity,

which resulted in a comparatively low LR+ of 5.21. The full multi-parametric CMR examination, however, with all 4 components combined had the lowest LR- (0.16) indicating that the combination of all 4 components was best for ruling out CAD.

The high LR+, low LR- and high overall diagnostic accuracy of the single perfusion component demonstrates that perfusion imaging ought to have most influence on a physician's risk stratification of the patients' likelihood of having significant underlying CAD. We have therefore shown the relative likelihood ratios of the perfusion component as the starting point, and building on this using selected combinations as "add on" tests, highlighting the number of new true and false positive cases produced by each combination (Table 5). This analysis showed that no add on test to perfusion imaging is preferable for ruling in the diagnosis (since all add on tests reduce the relative LR+), but adding on components can improve the rule-out value of the CMR examination (all add on tests reduce the LR-).

Comparative literature

There have been a number of other studies analysing the diagnostic performance of the components of the CMR examination, although none of this magnitude and many of which being performed in highly selected populations.

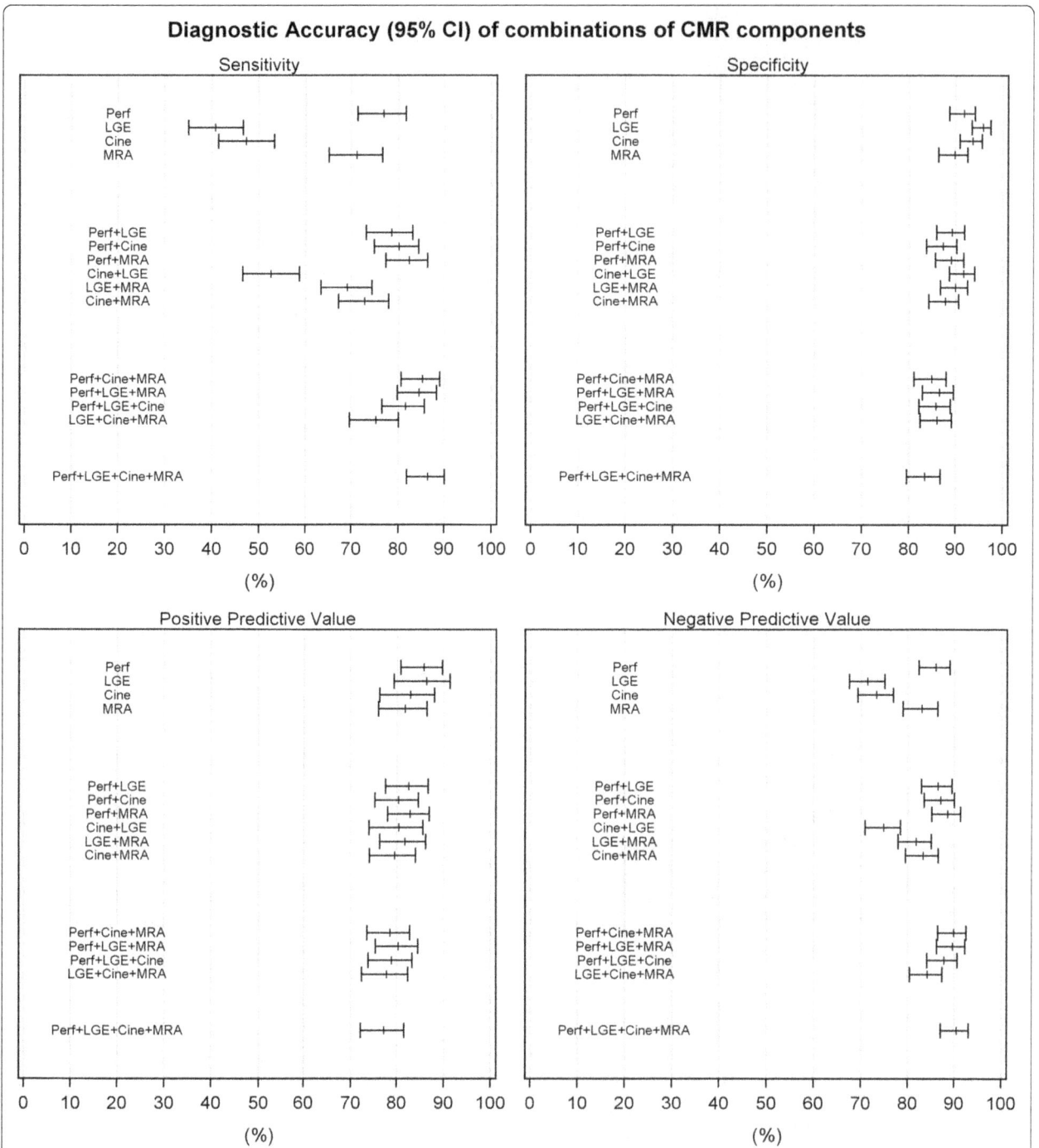

Fig 1 Diagnostic accuracy of the individual components and their combinations compared to the full multi-parametric CMR examination. Cine – Cine imaging; LGE – late gadolinium enhancement; Perf –perfusion imaging; MRA – magnetic resonance coronary angiography

One study analysed the diagnostic accuracy of CMR components in 100 patients preselected for X-ray coronary angiography (≥70 % stenosis as the reference standard) [8]. The CMR protocol included wall motion, stress and rest perfusion and LGE. The analysis algorithm considered LGE images first with presence of severe CAD diagnosed if LGE was positive in an ischaemic pattern. If LGE was negative the perfusion images were analysed and a reversible defect used to diagnose CAD. This analysis algorithm had a sensitivity (89 %) and specificity (87 %) - which was similar to the CE-MARC study. In terms of individual components compared to CE-MARC, the perfusion component in this previous study had the highest sensitivity (84 % vs. 77 % in our

Table 4 Likelihood ratios positive and negative for the multi-parametric CMR exam and its individual components, paired and triplet combinations compared to the reference test X-ray angiography

	Likelihood ratio + ve (95 % CI)	Likelihood ratio –ve (95 % CI)
Overall multi-parametric CMR study (all components) (n = 676)	5.21 (4.17, 6.51)	0.16 (0.12, 0.22)
Individual CMR components		
LGE (n = 674)	9.81 (6.02, 15.97)	0.62 (0.56, 0.68)
Perfusion (n = 661)	9.35 (6.70, 13.05)	0.25 (0.20, 0.31)
Ventricular function (n = 676)	7.47 (5.04, 11.07)	0.56 (0.50, 0.63)
MRA (n = 597)	7.01 (5.11, 9.61)	0.32 (0.26, 0.39)
Paired combinations		
Perfusion/LGE (n = 676)	7.32 (5.50, 9.75)	0.24 (0.19, 0.30)
Perfusion/function (n = 676)	6.31 (4.86, 8.20)	0.23 (0.18, 0.29)
Perfusion/MRA (n = 676)	7.50 (5.66, 9.94)	0.20 (0.15, 0.26)
Function/LGE (n = 676)	6.35 (4.51, 8.93)	0.52 (0.45, 0.59)
Function/MRA (n = 676)	5.98 (4.57, 7.83)	0.31 (0.25, 0.38)
LGE/MRA (n = 676)	6.92 (5.12, 9.35)	0.34 (0.29, 0.41)
Triplet combinations		
Perfusion/LGE/function (n = 676)	5.77 (4.51, 7.37)	0.21 (0.17, 0.28)
Perfusion/LGE/MRA (n = 676)	6.31 (4.90, 8.11)	0.18 (0.13, 0.24)
Perfusion/function/MRA (n = 676)	5.64 (4.46, 7.14)	0.17 (0.13, 0.23)
LGE/function/MRA (n = 676)	5.41 (4.21, 6.95)	0.29 (0.23, 0.36)

population) although with a significantly lower specificity (58 % vs. 92 %). Wall motion scoring was not considered in their analysis algorithm; cine images were acquired and had a similar sensitivity (49 % vs. 47 %) but lower specificity (73 % vs. 94 %) than in our study.

In patients with non ST-segment elevation myocardial infarction our group has previously evaluated the diagnostic accuracy of all 4 components of the CMR examination, performed within 72 h of presentation, with an overall sensitivity of 96 %, specificity 83 %, PPV 96 % and NPV 83 % [9]. Once again the perfusion component of the examination yielded the highest sensitivity (88 %),

although in this study it was higher than when compared to our stable elective population (77 %).

Cury *et al.* studied a mixed cohort of 47 patients (14 with previous MI) and also demonstrated that stress perfusion imaging had the highest sensitivity (81 %) and LGE the highest specificity (94 %) [10]. The maximum diagnostic accuracy was achieved with the combination of stress perfusion and LGE, and unsurprisingly this was again higher in the sub-group of patients with previous myocardial infarction than those with suspected CAD and no prior infarction (93 % vs. 86 %).

The clinical utility of imaging coronary artery anatomy with dedicated coronary MRA protocols in expert centres has been demonstrated to have good diagnostic accuracy for the detection of proximal CAD [14]. Technical advances at 3.0 Tesla and using a 32 channel coil have been shown to further improve signal to noise ratio and overall accuracy compared with initial reports, yielding sensitivities of 92-96 % [15, 16]. However, the efficacy of coronary imaging within a combined CMR protocol remains to be established. Klein *et al.* performed coronary MRA, stress and rest perfusion and LGE imaging on 54 patients with suspected CAD, again showing the perfusion component was the most accurate alone (sensitivity 87 %, specificity 88 %). They showed that the addition of LGE to stress perfusion imaging did not improve the overall diagnostic accuracy (sensitivity 88 %, specificity 88 %). In terms of coronary imaging, 15 % of overall MRA had non-diagnostic image quality; whole heart MRA had significantly inferior diagnostic accuracy due to poor specificity (sensitivity 92 %, specificity 56 %) unless only those with excellent MRA image quality (n = 18, 33 %) were analysed, whereupon it remained similar to the perfusion component alone (sensitivity 86 %, specificity 91 %) [11]. Other investigators have evaluated the effect of adding coronary MRA to stress perfusion CMR on diagnostic performance; when compared to invasive pressure-wire derived fractional flow reserve (FFR) at 1.5 T there was no significant improvement in diagnostic accuracy [12].

Table 5 Relative likelihood ratios and the numbers of new true positive and false positive cases produced by adding on further components sequentially to stress perfusion imaging in isolation

	Relative LR+	Relative LR-	New true positive cases produced	New false positives cases produced
Perfusion (+LGE)	0.78	0.91	7	11
Perfusion (+function)	0.68	0.89	9	18
Perfusion (+MRA)	0.79	0.76	16	12
Perfusion + LGE (+function)	0.79	0.89	8	14
Perfusion + LGE (+MRA)	0.86	0.74	16	11
Perfusion + function (+MRA)	0.89	0.76	14	10
Perfusion + function (+LGE)	0.91	0.94	4	6

LGE late gadolinium enhancement, *LR* likelihood ratio, *MRA* magnetic resonance coronary angiography

Coronary MRA remains a time consuming acquisition, which often is non-diagnostic when performed within an already long multi-parametric protocol. In our study 79 patients (11.7 %) had non-diagnostic coronary MRA images. Furthermore, in those with adequate or excellent image quality (*n* = 597), the addition of the coronary MRA made no difference statistically on the overall diagnostic accuracy of the CMR examination. Equally, whilst some triplet combinations with MRA offer similar diagnostic accuracy, the components of cine, LGE and perfusion imaging offer clinical information above and beyond detection of coronary disease (i.e., left ventricular volumes/ejection fraction, myocardial viability and ischaemic burden) which may have additional prognostic importance.

Conclusions

From this pre-specified sub-analysis of the CE-MARC study, using the original blinded visual-read, we have demonstrated the diagnostic accuracy of the individual components and their combinations from the full multi-parametric CMR exam. In patients presenting with stable chest pain, the stress perfusion component of the multi-parametric CMR exam was the single most important component for overall diagnostic accuracy. However, the full combined multi-parametric protocol was the optimal approach for disease rule-out, and the LGE component best for rule-in. The inclusion of coronary MRA had no additional overall diagnostic benefit within a multi-parametric protocol.

Abbreviations
CAD: Coronary Artery Disease; CMR: Cardiovascular Magnetic Resonance; FFR: Fractional Flow Reserve; LGE: Late Gadolinium Enhancement; LR: Likelihood Ratio; LR+: Likelihood Ratio for Positive Tests; LR-: Likelihood Ratio for Negative Tests; LV: Left Ventricle; MRA: Magnetic Resonance Angiography; NPV: Negative Predictive Value; PPV: Positive Predictive Value; RWMA: Regional Wall Motion Abnormality; SPECT: Single Photon Emission Computed Tomography; XRA: X-Ray Angiography.

Competing interests
The authors declare that they have no competing interests.

Authors' contributions
DPR: Analysis, interpretation of data, drafting of the manuscript. MM: Critical & intellectual revision of the manuscript. JMB planned the study, provided advice of the statistics, analysed the data and interpreted the results. JN planned the study and analysed the data. CCE did the statistical analyses and interpreted the results. NM and PB collected and analysed the data. SP planned the study, analysed the data, interpreted the results and co-led the study. JPG planned the study, led the clinical trial, analysed the data, interpreted the results. All authors read and approved the final manuscript.

Acknowledgements
None.

Funding
CE-MARC was funded by the British Heart Foundation (RG/05/004). SP is funded by a British Heart Foundation Senior Fellowship (FS/10/62/28409).

Author details
[1]Multidisciplinary Cardiovascular Research Centre (MCRC) & Leeds Institute of Cardiovascular and Metabolic Medicine, University of Leeds, Leeds, UK. [2]Clinical Trials Research Unit, University of Leeds, Clinical Trials Research House, 71-75 Clarendon Rd, Leeds, UK.

References
1. Hundley WG, Bluemke DA, Finn JP, Flamm SD, Fogel MA, Friedrich MG, et al. ACCF/ACR/AHA/NASCI/SCMR 2010 expert consensus document on cardiovascular magnetic resonance: a report of the American College of Cardiology Foundation Task Force on Expert Consensus Documents. Circulation. 2010;121(22):2462–508.
2. Hendel RC, Patel MR, Kramer CM, Poon M, Carr JC, Gerstad NA, et al. ACCF/ACR/SCCT/SCMR/ASNC/NASCI/SCAI/SIR 2006 appropriateness criteria for cardiac computed tomography and cardiac magnetic resonance imaging: a report of the American College of Cardiology Foundation Quality Strategic Directions Committee Appropriateness Criteria Working Group, American College of Radiology, Society of Cardiovascular Computed Tomography, Society for Cardiovascular Magnetic Resonance, American Society of Nuclear Cardiology, North American Society for Cardiac Imaging, Society for Cardiovascular Angiography and Interventions, and Society of Interventional Radiology. J Am Coll Cardiol. 2006;48(7):1475–97.
3. Montalescot G, Sechtem U, Achenbach S, Andreotti F, Arden C, Budaj A, et al. 2013 ESC guidelines on the management of stable coronary artery disease: The Task Force on the management of stable coronary artery disease of the European Society of Cardiology. Eur Heart J. 2013;34(38):2949–3003.
4. Greenwood JP, Maredia N, Younger JF, Brown JM, Nixon J, Everett CC, et al. Cardiovascular magnetic resonance and single-photon emission computed tomography for diagnosis of coronary heart disease (CE-MARC): a prospective trial. Lancet. 2012;379(9814):453–60.
5. Greenwood JP, Maredia N, Radjenovic A, Brown JM, Nixon J, Farrin AJ, et al. Clinical evaluation of magnetic resonance imaging in coronary heart disease: the CE-MARC study. Trials. 2009;10:62.
6. Greenwood JP, Motwani M, Maredia N, Brown JM, Everett CC, Nixon J, et al. Comparison of cardiovascular magnetic resonance and single-photon emission computed tomography in women with suspected coronary artery disease from the Clinical Evaluation of Magnetic Resonance Imaging in Coronary Heart Disease (CE-MARC) Trial. Circulation. 2014;129(10):1129–38.
7. Walker S, Girardin F, McKenna C, Ball SG, Nixon J, Plein S, et al. Cost-effectiveness of cardiovascular magnetic resonance in the diagnosis of coronary heart disease: an economic evaluation using data from the CE-MARC study. Heart. 2013;99(12):873–81.
8. Klem I, Heitner JF, Shah DJ, Sketch Jr MH, Behar V, Weinsaft J, et al. Improved detection of coronary artery disease by stress perfusion cardiovascular magnetic resonance with the use of delayed enhancement infarction imaging. J Am Coll Cardiol. 2006;47(8):1630–8.
9. Plein S, Greenwood JP, Ridgway JP, Cranny G, Ball SG, Sivananthan MU. Assessment of non-ST-segment elevation acute coronary syndromes with cardiac magnetic resonance imaging. J Am Coll Cardiol. 2004;44(11):2173–81.
10. Cury RC, Cattani CA, Gabure LA, Racy DJ, de Gois JM, Siebert U, et al. Diagnostic performance of stress perfusion and delayed-enhancement MR imaging in patients with coronary artery disease. Radiology. 2006;240(1):39–45.
11. Klein C, Gebker R, Kokocinski T, Dreysse S, Schnackenburg B, Fleck E, et al. Combined magnetic resonance coronary artery imaging, myocardial perfusion and late gadolinium enhancement in patients with suspected coronary artery disease. J Cardiovasc Magn Reson. 2008;10:45.
12. Bettencourt N, Ferreira N, Chiribiri A, Schuster A, Sampaio F, Santos L, et al. Additive value of magnetic resonance coronary angiography in a comprehensive cardiac magnetic resonance stress-rest protocol for detection of functionally significant coronary artery disease: a pilot study. Circ Cardiovasc Imaging. 2013;6(5):730–8.
13. Hayen A, Macaskill P, Irwig L, Bossuyt P. Appropriate statistical methods are required to assess diagnostic tests for replacement, add-on, and triage. J Clin Epidemiol. 2010;63(8):883–91.
14. Kim WY, Danias PG, Stuber M, Flamm SD, Plein S, Nagel E, et al. Coronary magnetic resonance angiography for the detection of coronary stenoses. N Engl J Med. 2001;345(26):1863–9.

17

Free breathing contrast-enhanced time-resolved magnetic resonance angiography in pediatric and adult congenital heart disease

Jennifer A Steeden[1*], Bejal Pandya[1,2], Oliver Tann[3] and Vivek Muthurangu[1,3]

Abstract

Background: Contrast enhanced magnetic resonance angiography (MRA) is generally performed during a long breath-hold (BH), limiting its utility in infants and small children. This study proposes a free-breathing (FB) time resolved MRA (TRA) technique for use in pediatric and adult congenital heart disease (CHD).

Methods: A TRA sequence was developed by combining spiral trajectories with sensitivity encoding (SENSE, x4 kx-ky and x2 kz) and partial Fourier (75% in kz). As no temporal data sharing is used, an independent 3D data set was acquired every ~1.3s, with acceptable spatial resolution (~2.3x2.3x2.3mm). The technique was tested during FB over 50 consecutive volumes. Conventional BH-MRA and FB-TRA data was acquired in 45 adults and children with CHD. We calculated quantitative image quality for both sequences. Diagnostic accuracy was assessed in all patients from both sequences. Additionally, vessel measurements were made at the sinotubular junction ($N = 43$), proximal descending aorta ($N = 43$), descending aorta at the level of the diaphragm ($N = 43$), main pulmonary artery ($N = 35$), left pulmonary artery ($N = 35$) and the right pulmonary artery ($N = 35$). Intra and inter observer variability was assessed in a subset of 10 patients.

Results: BH-MRA had significantly higher homogeneity in non-contrast enhancing tissue (coefficient of variance, $P < 0.0001$), signal-to-noise ratio ($P < 0.0001$), contrast-to-noise ratio ($P < 0.0001$) and relative contrast ($P = 0.02$) compared to the FB-TRA images. However, homogeneity in the vessels was similar in both techniques ($P = 0.52$) and edge sharpness was significantly ($P < 0.0001$) higher in FB-TRA compared to BH-MRA. BH-MRA provided overall diagnostic accuracy of 82%, and FB-TRA of 87%, with no statistical difference between the two sequences ($P = 0.77$). Vessel diameter measurements showed excellent agreement between the two techniques ($r = 0.98$, $P < 0.05$), with no bias (0.0mm, $P = 0.71$), and clinically acceptable limits of agreement (-2.7 to +2.8mm). Inter and intra observer reproducibility showed good agreement of vessel diameters ($r > 0.988$, $P < 0.0001$), with negligible biases (between -0.2 and +0.1mm) and small limits of agreement (between -2.4 and +2.5mm).

Conclusions: We have described a FB-TRA technique that is shown to enable accurate diagnosis and vessel measures compared to conventional BH-MRA. This simplifies the MRA technique and will enable angiography to be performed in children and adults whom find breath-holding difficult.

Keywords: Free-breathing, Time-resolved MR angiography, 3D stack-of-spirals, Congenital heart disease

* Correspondence: jennifer.steeden@ucl.ac.uk
[1]UCL Centre for Cardiovascular Imaging, University College London, 30 Guildford Street, London WC1N 1EH, UK
Full list of author information is available at the end of the article

Background

Assessment of thoracic (or cardiac) anatomy is important in patients with congenital heart disease (CHD) and is one of the main indications for cardiovascular magnetic resonance (CMR) in this population [1]. Contrast enhanced MR angiography (CE-MRA) has a proven ability to detect vascular stenoses, dilation and other abnormalities [25] and is often used for this purpose. However, acquisition of high resolution, three-dimensional (3D) data is time consuming, normally taking between 10–25 s. Thus, to prevent image degradation as a result of respiratory motion, CE-MRA is generally performed during a breath-hold. Unfortunately, this limits the use of CE-MRA in small children (who are unable to comply with breath-hold instructions) and severely dyspnoeic adults. In these groups, a better approach might be to acquire each volume so quickly that respiratory motion has limited effect on image quality. This would enable CE-MRA to be performed during free-breathing and would open up this technique to a wider group of patients.

Such an approach has been partially realized by time resolved MR angiography (TRA), in which a series of volume angiograms are acquired in quick succession [7]. This technique is mainly used to provide information about perfusion kinetics [8,9], as well as to simplify scan timing in relation to the passage of the contrast bolus [10]. However, the majority of time-resolved MRA sequences use some form of data sharing across time (e.g. contrast-enhanced timing-robust angiography; CENTRA keyhole [11], sliding window [12], or time-resolved echo-shared angiographic technique; TREAT [13]), making them sensitive to respiratory motion artifacts. Thus, conventional TRA sequences are often performed during a breath-hold to ensure sufficient image quality.

In this study, we propose an alternative method of accelerating time resolved angiography; namely by combining time efficient spiral trajectories with sensitivity encoding (SENSE). The benefit of this approach is that there is no temporal data sharing. This may allow sufficient image quality to be achieved during free-breathing conditions. The specific aims of this study were; a) To demonstrate the feasibility of acquiring free-breathing time resolved MRA (FB-TRA) in pediatric and adult congenital heart disease, b) To quantitatively assess image quality of FB-TRA in comparison with a conventional breath-hold angiographic sequence (BH-MRA), c) To compare the diagnostic accuracy of FB-TRA to conventional BH-MRA, and d) To assess the accuracy and reproducibility of vessel measurements made from FB-TRA compared to BH-MRA.

Methods

Study population

Between June and July 2014, 45 consecutive children with heart disease (congenital and cardiomyopathy) and adults with congenital heart disease (32 male, 13 female) were enrolled into this study. Inclusion criteria were: a) Clinical referral for cardiac MR imaging and b) Clinically necessary CE-MRA. The exclusion criteria were general contraindications to MR, such as pregnancy or MR-incompatible implants. One further child was recruited in whom contrast administration was required for tissue characterization, but not CE-MRA. In this child it was possible to perform the conventional BH-MRA sequence during free breathing and compare with FB-TRA. The local research ethics committee approved the study and written consent was obtained from all subjects/guardians.

Imaging protocol

Imaging was performed on a 1.5 Tesla MR scanner (Avanto, Siemens Medical Solutions, Erlangen, Germany) using two spine coils and one body-matrix coil (giving a total of 12 coil elements). A 20–22 gauge plastic intravenous cannula was placed in the subject's antecubital vein for administration of contrast agent. BH-MRA was performed as part of the clinical scan and FB-TRA was performed at the end of the clinical scan. The interval between the two scans was 29 ± 10 min (range: 10 to 48 min). The same contrast injection protocol was used for each scan; 0.2 mL/kg of Gadoteric acid (Dotarem, Guerbet, Roissy, France) up to a maximum of 10 mL, being injected at a rate of 2 mL/s. The specifics of the two MRA sequences are detailed below.

Breath-hold MRA sequence

BH-MRA was performed using a 3D Cartesian spoiled gradient echo (SPGR) sequence, acquired in the sagittal orientation. This sequence was accelerated with GRAPPA in the phase encode direction (full parameter details in Table 1). Optimal timing was ensured through the use of a 2D thick slab SPGR bolus tracking sequence. This sequence allowed visualization of contrast as it passed through the heart and great vessels, allowing the BH-MRA to be triggered when the contrast entered the relevant anatomy. In most patients, both left and right heart visualization was required and two angiograms (~13.5 s breath-hold each) were acquired after a single injection of contrast agent, with a 15 s pause between them. In a minority of patients who clinically required visualization of just one vascular bed, only pulmonary or aortic angiograms were acquired.

Free-breathing TRA sequence

FB-TRA was performed using an in-house 3D stack-of-spirals SPGR sequence acquired in the transverse orientation. A uniform density spiral k-space filling strategy was used in kx-ky (readout duration ~5 ms), with 16 interleaves required to fill k-space at each of the 96 kz positions. In order to accelerate the acquisition, kx-ky data

Table 1 Sequence parameters for the BH-MRA and FB-TRA sequences

	BH-MRA	FB-TRA
TE/TR (ms)	~0.8/1.9	~1.5/9.1
Readouts	Cartesian	Spiral
Spiral interleaves for fully sampled kx-ky	-	16 Spiral
Cardiac gating	ECG	None
Acceleration factor (in kx-ky)	2 (GRAPPA)	4 (SENSE)
Partial-Fourier in ky	75 %	-
Matrix size	~144×256	196×196
Image FOV (mm)	~250×435×260	450×450×220
Orientation	Sagittal	Transverse
Number of slices	~144	96
Slice thickness (mm)	~2.0	2.3
Flip angle	25°	25°
Pixel bandwidth (Hz/pixel)	1500	2170
Acceleration factor (in kz)	-	2 (SENSE)
Partial-Fourier in kz	75 %	75 %
Breath-hold duration (s)	~13.5	Free-breathing
Measurements	2 per vasculature of interest(1 pre-contrast, 1 post-contrast)	50
Spatial resolution (mm)	~1.7×1.7×1.8	~2.3×2.3×2.3
Temporal resolution (s)	~13.5	~1.3
Total acquisition time (m:s)	~2:30	~1:25

was undersampled by a factor of four and kz was undersampled by a factor of two. In addition, partial Fourier (75 %) was applied along kz. The sampling pattern in kx-ky was rotated by one position for each acquired kz position, in order to reduce artifacts [14]. This undersampled data was reconstructed online using an iterative non-Cartesian 3D SENSE algorithm [15], combined with a homodyne reconstruction [16]. In order to calculate the coil sensitivities from the data itself, the sampling pattern had to be rotated by one position in kx-ky for each volume and shifted by one position in kz every fourth volume. Combining eight consecutive volumes resulted in a fully sampled central 50 % of k-space, from which the coil sensitivities were calculated by dividing the corresponding image data by the sum of squares of all the coil data [17]. The necessary 'reference data' for the homodyne reconstruction was taken from the central kz positions of the acquired data [16]. The total acceleration factor achieved was 10.7x and enabled acquisition of an acceptable spatial resolution volume (~2.3×2.3×2.3 mm) every ~1.3 s. All sequence parameters can be seen in Table 1.

Image analysis

All image data was analyzed using the OsiriX open source DICOM viewing platform (Osirix 5.9, OsiriX foundation, Switzerland) [18]. The BH-MRA and FB-TRA data for each patient were separately anonymized using a random

number identifier. All observers were blinded to the patient identity, the other MR data acquired as part of the clinical scan and the results of other diagnostic examinations. The specific image analysis procedures are described below.

Image quality

Quantitative image quality was assessed by measuring coefficient of variance (CoV), signal-to-noise ratio (SNR), contrast-to-noise ratio (CNR), relative contrast (RC) and edge sharpness (by J.A.S, 7 years experience). The CoV and RC required measurement of the mean and standard deviation of signal intensities (SI, σ) in the blood pool and in a non-enhancing tissue. The blood pool measures were made using vessel regions-of-interest (ROI's) placed at the sinotubular junction (Ao1) and main pulmonary artery (MPA) from the frame with the highest contrast. The spinal fluid (which is a non-contrast enhancing tissue) was used to make tissue measures. Vessel and tissue CoV and RC were then calculated as follows:

$$Cov_{vessel} = \frac{\sigma_{vessel}}{SI_{vessel}}$$
$$Cov_{tissue} = \frac{\sigma_{tissue}}{SI_{tissue}}$$
$$RC = \frac{(SI_{vessel} - SI_{tissue})}{(SI_{vessel} + SI_{tissue})}$$

True quantification of SNR and CNR in images acquired using non-Cartesian parallel imaging is non-trivial, due to the uneven distribution of noise [19]. However, noise can be was estimated as σ_{tissue} allowing SNR and CNR to be calculated using the formula below [20,21];

$$SNR = \frac{SI_{vessel}}{\sigma_{tissue}}$$
$$CNR = \frac{(SI_{vessel} - SI_{tissue})}{\sigma_{tissue}}$$

Quantitative edge sharpness (ES) was calculated (from the frame with visually the highest contrast) by measuring the maximum gradient of the normalized pixel intensities across the border of the vessel of interest as previously described [22]. ES was calculated from multiplanar reformatted cross sectional images at six equidistant positions along the thoracic Aorta, and six positions along the pulmonary vasculature (four equidistant positions along the MPA and one in each of the branch PA's).

Diagnostic accuracy

Assessment of the diagnostic accuracy of the two angiographic sequences was performed by two evaluators (V.M. with 12 years CMR experience, and B.P. with 4 years CMR experience) who were not involved in the clinical reporting of the CMR scans for the subjects in this study. Data from each angiographic sequence was separately consensus reviewed in a randomized order using multiplanar reformatting. It should be noted that all frames of the FB-TRA reformats were assessed. Six arterial segments (Aortic root (AoR), aortic arch (AoA), Descending aorta (DescAo), main pulmonary artery (MPA), right pulmonary artery (RPA) and left pulmonary artery (LPA)) were specifically assessed for the presence of stenosis and dilation. In addition, any other positive diagnoses were noted. The diagnosis from the angiographic data was compared to the diagnosis as stated in the clinical CMR report (as assessed from the whole CMR examination, including 3D whole heart imaging and selected cine, black blood and flow imaging).

Vessel measurements

One observer (V.M.) measured aortic and pulmonary artery diameters from multiplanar reformats, derived from the BH-MRA and FB-TRA. The FB-TRA multiplanar reformats had an additional temporal dimension and diameters were measured in the frame in which the vessel of interest had the greatest contrast and were displayed most sharply. Aortic diameter was assessed in three positions; the sinotubular junction (Ao1), the proximal descending aorta (Ao2) and descending aorta at the level of the diaphragm (Ao3). Pulmonary artery diameters were assessed in the MPA, the mid LPA and the mid RPA. Where a stenosis

was present, the vessel diameter measurements were made at the position of the narrowing. Intraobserver variability (by V.M., > 7 days between measurements) of vessel diameter measurements from both sequences was assessed in a subset of 10 patients, who had both aortic and pulmonary BH-MRA. Additionally, interobserver variability of vessel diameter measurements was performed in these 10 patients (by V.M. and a second observer, B.P.).

Statistical analysis

All statistical analysis was performed using GraphPad Prism (GraphPad Software Inc., San Diego, CA). The results are expressed as the mean ± standard-deviation. Paired t-tests were used to compare BH-MRA and FB-TRA, in terms image quality and vessel diameter measurements. Additionally, correlation coefficients were calculated.

Diagnostic accuracy was assessed by calculation of the sensitivity and specificity of the BH-MRA and FB-TRA sequences, for the detection of stenosis and dilation. A Fisher's exact test was used to assess if there were any significant differences in the diagnostic accuracy of the two techniques. The McNemar chi-squared statistical test was used to assess if there were any significance differences in the sensitivity or specificity of the two techniques.

Bland-Altman analysis was performed to give measures of agreement between the vessel diameter measurements from the two sequences, as well as inter and intra observer agreement [23]. One-way ANOVA tests were used to compare the difference in vessel diameter measurements from the two techniques, between all vessel segments. A P-value of less than .05 indicated a significant difference.

Results

The median age of the patients enrolled in the comparative arm of this study was 23.1 ± 15.7 years (range: 8 to 80 years, 13 of whom were less than 18 years old). The cardiovascular diagnoses in these patients were; repaired tetralogy of Fallot ($n = 7$); hypertrophic cardiomyopathy ($n = 6$); Marfan syndrome ($n = 6$); transposition of the great arteries, post arterial switch ($n = 3$), post atrial switch ($n = 3$); repaired coarctation of the aorta ($n = 5$); pulmonary stenosis ($n = 3$); repaired ventricular septal defect ($n = 3$); dilated aortic root ($n = 2$); repaired anomalous pulmonary venous drainage ($n = 1$); repaired atrial septal defect ($n = 1$); repaired truncus arteriosus ($n = 1$); cor triatriatum ($n = 1$); Ebstein's anomaly ($n = 1$); subaortic stenosis ($n = 1$); and dilated right ventricle ($n = 1$).

FB-TRA data was successfully acquired in all 45 patients. In 33 patients both pulmonary and aortic BH-MRA's were acquired, in 10 patients only an aortic BH-MRA was clinically indicated, and in the remaining two patients only a pulmonary BH-MRA was indicated. All subjects were able to follow breath-holding instructions.

The child in whom a free breathing BH-MRA (in both the pulmonary and aortic vasculature) was acquired was 10 years old and had a diagnosis of dilated cardiomyopathy.

Image quality

Figure 1 shows images acquired using the BH-MRA sequence but during free breathing. It should be noted that there is a loss of vessel edge sharpness and increased artifact due to respiratory motion. This is compared to the FB-TRA in the same patient, which has better edge definition and very little respiratory artifact (Fig. 1).

In the comparative arm of the study, the image quality of both MRA sequences was good. The FB-TRA images contained some residual aliasing resulting from the high acceleration factor used, however these artifacts were mostly in the outer portions of the images. Figure 2 shows examples of the multiplanar reformatted image quality from the two sequences, in one 16 year old patient with an LPA stenosis. Figure 3 shows multiple frames from the FB-TRA sequence, compared to the BH-MRA sequence, in one 29 year old patient, who has an atrial switch – the full FB-TRA movie can be seen online in Additional file 1. Figure 4 shows multiple frames from a 3D reconstruction of the FB-TRA images, compared to the BH-MRA sequence, in one 41 year old patient showing kinking of the LPA – the full FB-TRA movie can be seen online in Additional file 2.

Quantitative image quality results are shown in Table 2. Signal homogeneity (as measured using CoV) in the non-enhancing tissue was found to be significantly higher in the BH-MRA images compared to the FB-TRA images ($P < 0.0001$), however the vessels were found to have a similar homogeneity in both techniques ($P = 0.52$). The BH-MRA images had significantly higher SNR ($P < 0.0001$), CNR ($P < 0.0001$) and RC ($P = 0.02$) compared to the FB-TRA images. However, average edge sharpness was significantly ($P < 0.0001$) higher in the FB-TRA images compared to the BH-MRA images, although the standard deviation of ES was significantly higher in the FB-TRA images ($P < 0.0001$).

Diagnostic accuracy

Anatomical lesions detected by assessment of the whole CMR as stated in the CMR report are listed in Table 3. The BH-MRA sequence provided the correct overall diagnosis in 37/45 patients (diagnostic accuracy = 82 %), and the FB-TRA sequence in 39/45 patients (diagnostic accuracy = 87 %), with no statistical difference between the two sequences ($P = 0.77$). The diagnostic failures are listed in Table 4. It should be noted that in four patients, both reviewers found the same, incorrect diagnosis in the BH-MRA and FB-TRA sequences. In two cases, dynamic kinking/obstruction were poorly appreciated on both ungated MRA sequences. In the third case, isolated valvar stenosis of a pulmonary homograft was not visible on either angiogram. In the remaining case a baffle leak post atrial switch was missed by the BH-MRA and FB-TRA sequences.

The specific ability of the two sequences to assess stenosis ($N = 13$) or dilation ($N = 53$) in the imaged vessel segments ($N = 234$) was also assessed. Overall, the BH-MRA sequence provided the correct diagnosis in 228/234 segments (diagnostic accuracy = 97 %) and the FB-TRA in 230/234 segments (diagnostic accuracy = 98 %), with no statistical difference between the groups ($P = 0.75$). The sensitivity of BH-MRA for specifically identifying stenosis was 62 % compared to 69 % for FB-TRA, with both having a specificity of 100 %. The sensitivity of BH-MRA for identifying dilation was 98 % and of FB-TRA was 100 %, with specificities of 100 % for both sequences. There were no statistical differences between the sequences in terms of sensitivity and specificity to stenosis ($P = 0.56$, $P = 1.0$ respectively) or dilation ($P = 0.32$, $P = 1.0$ respectively).

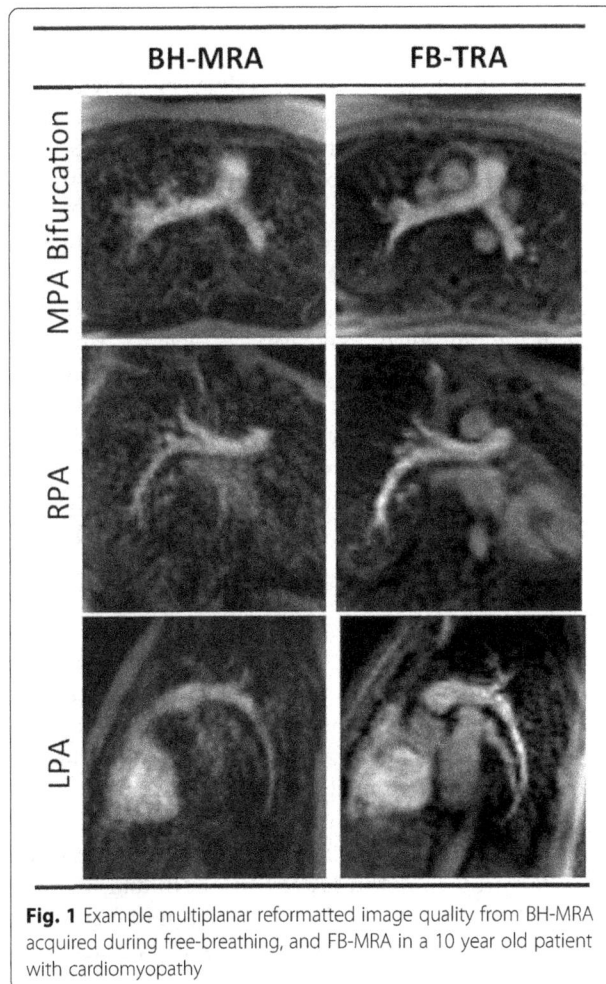

Fig. 1 Example multiplanar reformatted image quality from BH-MRA acquired during free-breathing, and FB-MRA in a 10 year old patient with cardiomyopathy

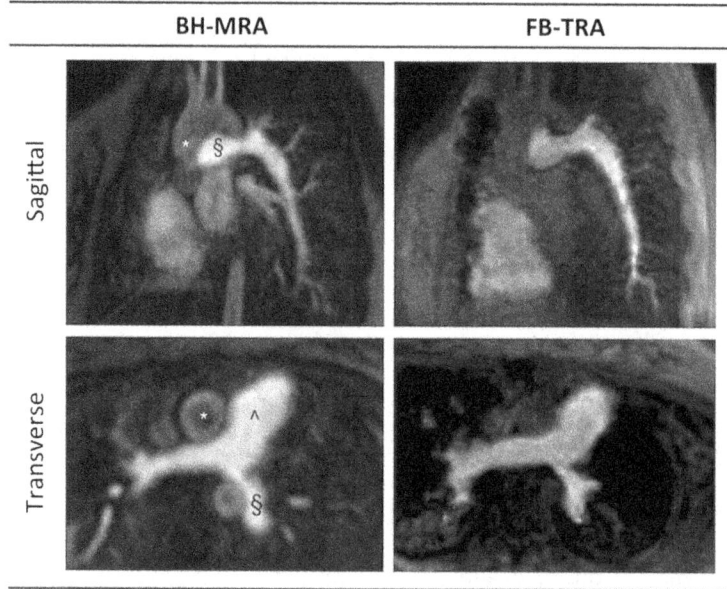

Fig. 2 Example multiplanar reformatted image quality from one 16 year old patient with an LPA stenosis, from both BH-MRA and FB-TRA.
* Ascending Aorta, § Left Pulmonary Artery, ^ Main Pulmonary Artery

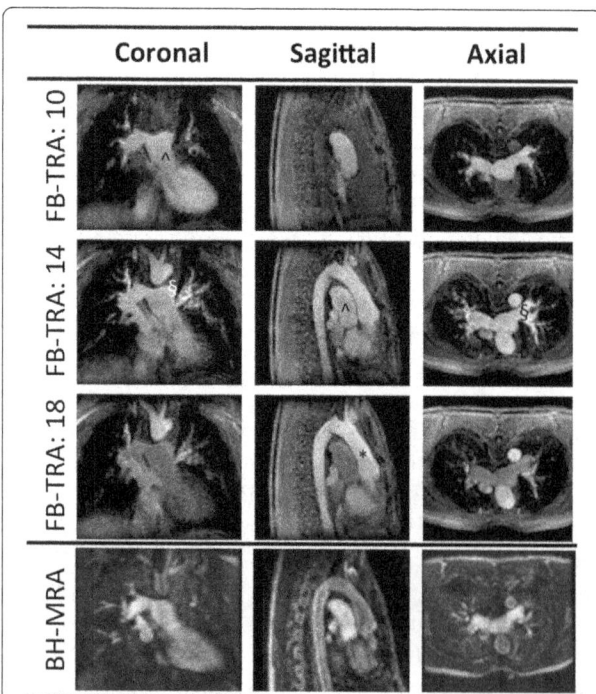

Fig. 3 Example image quality in multiple frames (denoted by the numbers in the table header) from the FB-TRA sequence compared to the BH-MRA sequence, in one 29 year old patient whom has undergone an atrial switch. The full movie can be seen online in Additional file 1. * Ascending Aorta, § Left Pulmonary Artery, ^ Main Pulmonary Artery

Vessel measurements

The vessel diameters were successfully measured in all 234 imaged vessel segments (Ao1, Ao2 and Ao3 in 43 patients, and MPA, RPA and LPA in 35 patients). Scatter and Bland Altman plots for all 234 segments are shown in Fig. 5 with excellent agreement ($r = 0.98$, $P < 0.05$), no bias (0.0 mm, $P = 0.71$), and clinically acceptable limits of agreement (-2.7 to $+2.8$ mm). There was similarly good agreement between BH-MRA and FB-TRA for each of the individual segments (see Table 5), with one-way ANOVA finding no statistical difference between segments ($P = 0.1013$).

Inter and intra observer reproducibility showed good agreement of vessel diameters ($r > 0.988$, $P < 0.0001$), with negligible biases (between -0.2 and $+0.1$ mm) and small limits of agreement (between -2.4 and $+2.5$ mm). See Table 6 for results.

Discussion

We have shown that it is possible to perform free-breathing high spatio-temporal resolution time resolved angiography, in a population of 45 patients with paediatric and adult congenital heart disease. This was achieved through the use of a highly accelerated 3D stack of spirals acquisition with no data sharing between frames. The main findings were; i) FB-TRA was feasible in all patients, ii) FB-TRA had lower SNR, CNR and RC than BH-MRA, iii) FB-TRA had a similar diagnostic accuracy to BH-MRA, and iv) Vessel measurements made with the two sequences were comparable.

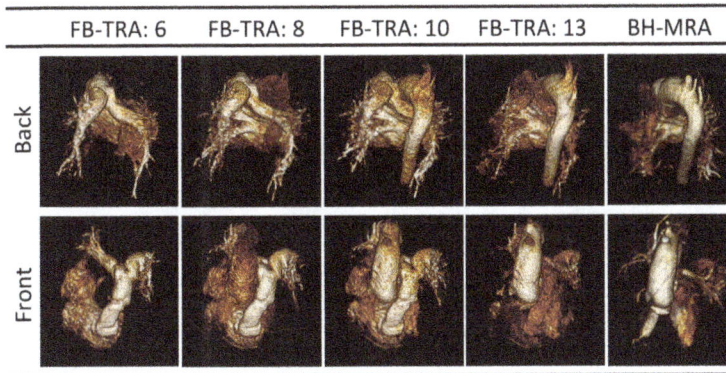

Fig. 4 Multiple frames from a 3D reconstruction of the FB-TRA images (denoted by the numbers in the table header) compared to the BH-MRA sequence, in one patient showing kinking of the LPA. The full movie can be seen online in Additional file 2

Time resolved angiography

The main aim of this study was to demonstrate that rapid acquisition allows angiographic data to be acquired during free-breathing. Rapid acquisition is the hallmark of time resolved angiography and we employed this approach in the current study. However, unlike the majority of TRA sequences, our implementation did not rely on data sharing techniques such as sliding window reconstruction [12], CENTRA keyhole [11] or TREAT [13]. Instead, we used a combination of efficient k-space filling with spiral trajectories, sensitivity encoding and partial Fourier to achieve rapid acquisition (~1.3 s/volume). The benefit of this approach is that data used for reconstruction of each volume only contains a limited amount of respiratory motion. We were able to show that this resulted in better image quality compared to conventional MR angiography performed during free breathing

(duration ~13 s). Slightly unexpectedly, we also found that FB-TRA images had significantly higher average edge sharpness than BH-MRA images. This is probably due to BH-MRA including more cardiac motion (10–15 heart beats) than FB-TRA (1–2 heart beats) resulting in more edge blurring, despite the breath-hold.

Highly undersampled spiral imaging does have some disadvantages. The main drawback is increased signal inhomogeneity due to spiral off-resonance effects, trajectories errors and data undersampling [27]. In our study, FB-TRA images had significantly lower SNR, CNR and tissue signal

Table 2 Quantitative image quality results for the BH-MRA and FB-TRA sequences

	BH-MRA	FB-TRA	P-value
Signal Intensity: Vessel	156.5 ± 66.4	67.7 ± 14.5*	$P < 0.0001$
Standard Deviation: Vessel	36.9 ± 21.0	15.4 ± 5.2*	$P < 0.0001$
Coefficient of Variation: Vessel (%)	23.1 ± 5.7	22.6 ± 5.0	$P = 0.52$
Signal Intensity: Tissue	20.5 ± 7.9	11.7 ± 3.4*	$P < 0.0001$
Standard Deviation: Tissue	7.2 ± 2.6	7.1 ± 2.2	$P = 0.85$
Coefficient of Variation: Tissue (%)	36.0 ± 6.6	62.7 ± 19.5*	$P < 0.0001$
SNR	24.0 ± 11.6	10.5 ± 4.2*	$P < 0.0001$
CNR	21.1 ± 11.7	8.8 ± 3.8*	$P < 0.0001$
Relative Contrast	0.74 ± 0.13	0.70 ± 0.08*	$P = 0.02$
Edge Sharpness (mm^{-1})			
Average	0.88 ± 0.39	2.33 ± 1.03*	$P < 0.0001$
Standard deviation	0.14 ± 0.08	0.25 ± 0.19*	$P < 0.0001$

*Value is statistically significantly different from BH-MRA

Table 3 Patient diagnosis

	No. of patients
Dilated AoR	12
Dilated MPA	10
Dilated DescAo	9
Dilated RPA	9
Dilated LPA	7
Dilated AoA	6
LPA stenosis	6
Atrial switch	3
Arterial switch (Lecompte)	3
DescAo stenosis	2
RPA stenosis	2
AoA stenosis	2
MPA stenosis	1
Ebsteins	1
Cor Triatrium	1
Muscular VSD	1
SV defect corrected with LA baffle	1
PDA	1
Absent LSCA	1
Aberrant RCA	1

Table 4 Misdiagnosis

BH-MRA	FB-TRA	Actual diagnosis
Proximal DescAo stenosis	Normal	Proximal DescAo stenosis
Normal	Stenosis in arch	Stenosis in arch
Cor Triatrium	None	Cor Triatrium
Normal	SVC baffle stenosis	SVC baffle stenosis
Normal	Mild Proximal LPA stenosis	Mild Proximal LPA stenosis
Normal	Dilated MPA	Dilated MPA
None	None	SVC baffle leak
Normal	Normal	Homograft stenosis
Normal	Normal	LPA stenosis
Normal	Normal	RPA stenosis

homogeneity compared to BH-MRA images. However, vessel signal homogeneity was similar for both sequences. This was probably due to less variation in contrast concentration during the rapid FB-TRA acquisition (~1.3 s) compared to the longer BH-MRA acquisition (~13.5 s), which would compensate for the increased noise. In addition, RC was only marginally higher in BH-MRA, demonstrating that there are only small differences in the tissue contrast provided by these two sequences. As will be discussed later, the similarity of these metrics may explain the comparable diagnostic accuracy. Alternative reconstruction algorithms could also be investigated to improve the image quality of the FB-TRA sequence. The most promising is compressed sensing (CS), which is well suited to angiography due to the inherent sparseness of the data [24]. However, CS reconstructions are more computationally intensive than our proposed approach and could only be justified if they significantly improved image quality.

Another problem with spiral imaging relates to the orientation of the imaging slab. In Cartesian imaging, readout oversampling reduces artifact from signal outside the FOV in the frequency encode direction. This allows the BH-MRA to be acquired in the sagittal orientation for optimization of coverage, acquisition time and coil placement for parallel imaging. In spiral imaging there is no single 'readout direction', preventing oversampling being used to reduce artifact. Thus, FB-TRA data had to be acquired in the transverse orientation to reduce the amount of signal outside the FOV. Although this may not be the optimal orientation in terms of coverage, this limitation is offset by the greater efficiency and possible undersampling available with spiral imaging.

Diagnostic accuracy

The FB-TRA and BH-MRA were found to have statistically comparable overall diagnostic accuracy, as well as similar sensitivity and specificity for detection of stenosis and dilatation. This demonstrates that although SNR and CNR were lower in FB-TRA images, diagnostic accuracy was not significantly affected. However, it should be noted that both MRA sequences missed lesions in four out of 45 patients. In all these cases, MRA failed because the lesions were dynamic, membranous or intra-cardiac, situations where ungated imaging is known to struggle [25]. This justifies the use of multiple CMR sequences when attempting to make a comprehensive diagnosis in CHD.

In terms of vessel measurements, there was also excellent agreement between FB-TRA and BH-MRA, with no

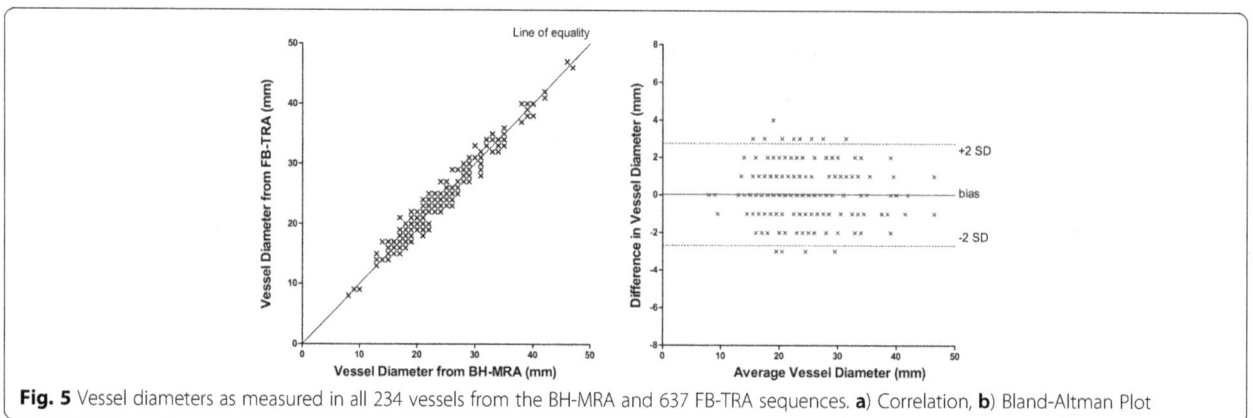

Fig. 5 Vessel diameters as measured in all 234 vessels from the BH-MRA and 637 FB-TRA sequences. **a**) Correlation, **b**) Bland-Altman Plot

Table 5 Vessel measurements

Vessel	N	BH-MRA (mm)	FB-TRA (mm)	Bias* (mm)	Limits of agreement* (mm)	Correlation coefficient* (r)	P-value*
Ao1	43	29 ± 6 (range: 21 to 46)	29 ± 6 (range: 19 to 47)	-0.2	-2.7 to 2.3	0.98	P = 0.40
Ao2	43	21 ± 5 (range: 14 to 38)	21 ± 6 (range: 14 to 40)	0.4	-3.0 to 3.7	0.96	P = 0.18
Ao3	43	19 ± 4 (range: 13 to 32)	19 ± 4 (range: 14 to 34)	0.4	-2.0 to 2.7	0.96	P = 0.06
MPA	35	29 ± 7 (range: 17 to 47)	29 ± 7 (range: 16 to 46)	0.1	-2.9 to 3.0	0.98	P = 0.82
RPA	35	22 ± 6 (range: 13 to 35)	21 ± 5 (range: 13 to 34)	-0.3	-3.1 to 2.5	0.97	P = 0.24
LPA	35	20 ± 5 (range: 8 to 31)	20 ± 5 (range: 8 to 31)	-0.3	-2.5 to 2.0	0.98	P = 0.14
Total	234	23 ± 7 (range: 8 to 47)	23 ± 7 (range: 8 to 47)	0	-2.7 to 2.8	0.98	P = 0.71

*Calculated with BH-MRA sequence

bias and clinically acceptable limits of agreement. Furthermore, there was no difference in intra and inter observer variability. This suggests that despite the reduction in image quality, FB-TRA allows accurate and reproducible quantitative and qualitative assessment of vascular structure. This may partly be related to the fact that RC and CoV_{vessel}, which both specifically relate to vessel visualization, were similar in the FB-TRA and BH-MRA sequences. In addition, improved edge sharpness may compensate for any reduction in SNR and CNR.

Clinical utility

The main clinical advantage of our technique, is that it can be performed during free-breathing. This opens up the possibility of performing MRA in patients who are unable to breath hold. However, in this study we chose patients who were able to comply with breath-hold instructions for two reasons. Firstly, at our institution children who require vascular assessment, but cannot breath hold, undergo CMR under general anaesthetic. This makes it difficult to perform a comparative study of BH-MRA and FB-TRA in this population. Secondly, to demonstrate the comparable utility of FB-TRA, it was essential that the BH-MRA be performed in an optimal way (i.e. during a breath hold). Thus, further studies are required to investigate the utility of FB-TRA in small children (<8 years). In particular, the requirement for higher resolution imaging (with the commensurate loss of SNR and CNR) and problems with higher respiratory rates would have to be addressed.

A further benefit of time resolved MRA sequences, is that it is not necessary to calculate exact bolus timing [10]. This may significantly simplify workflow, helping to reduce

Table 6 Intra and inter observer variability

	Bias (mm)	Limits of agreement (mm)	Correlation (r)
Intraobserver variability			
BH-MRA	−0.2	−2.1 to 1.7	0.99
FB-TRA	0.1	−1.7 to 1.9	0.99
Interobserver variability			
BH-MRA	0.1	−2.4 to 2.5	0.99
FB-TRA	−0.2	−2.4 to 2.1	0.99

overall scan times and increase throughput. Finally, time resolved MRA also allows assessment of perfusion kinetics [26], which although not specifically assessed in this study, may be beneficial in certain groups of patients.

Limitations

In this study, the BH-MRA sequence was always performed before FB-TRA sequence (~29 min between the two MRA scans). This was done to ensure that the clinically indicated BH-MRA was not affected by residual contrast (mean half-life of Dotarem is ~2.0/1.4 h in male/female subjects). However, this means that the FB-TRA may have been adversely affected by the contrast given for the BH-MRA. Thus, the results presented here give a conservative estimation of the FB-TRA technique in terms of image quality and diagnostic accuracy.

It was not possible to truly anonymize the BH-MRA data from the FB-TRA data, due to the temporal dimension of the TRA data. This meant that it was not possible to compare subjective image quality measures from the two sequences, as it is likely to be influenced by observer bias.

A final limitation of this technique is that the current online reconstruction is time consuming, taking approximately one hour for all 50 frames of FB-TRA data. However, the development of new highly parallel architectures, such as graphical processing units, should be able to significantly speed this up, as the pixel-wise calculations can be parallelized [28]. Alternatively, the reconstruction time could be reduced with the use of a bolus tracking sequence to visualize the contrast arriving in vasculature of interest, and trigger the start of the FB-TRA sequence, thereby reducing the amount of data acquired.

Conclusions

To conclude, we have described a free-breathing, time-resolved 3D spiral MRA technique that has been shown to enable accurate diagnosis and vessel measures compared to conventional breath-hold, Cartesian MRA. This technique simplifies the MRA technique and will enable angiography to be performed on children and adults in whom breath-holding is difficult.

Abbreviations

2D: Two-dimensional; 3D: Three-dimensional; Ao1: Sinotubular junction; Ao2: Proximal descending aorta; Ao3: Descending aorta at the level of the diaphragm; AoA: Aortic arch; AoR: Aortic root; BH-MRA: Breath-hold magnetic resonance angiography; CE-MRA: Contrast enhanced magnetic resonance angiography; CENTRA: Contrast-enhanced timing-robust angiography; CHD: Congenital heart disease; CMR: Cardiovascular magnetic resonance; CNR: Contrast-to-noise ratio; CS: Compressed Sensing; DescAo: Descending aorta; FB-TRA: Free-breathing time resolved magnetic resonance angiography; FOV: Field-of-view; LA: Left atrium; LPA: Left pulmonary artery; LSCA: Left subclavian artery; MPA: Main pulmonary artery; PDA: Patent ductus arteriosus; RC: Relative contrast; RCA: Right coronary artery; ROI: Region-of-interest; RPA: Right pulmonary artery; SENSE: Sensitivity encoding; SI: Signal intensity; SNR: Signal-to-noise ratio; SV: Single ventricle; TRA: Time resolved magnetic resonance angiography; TREAT: Time-resolved echo-shared angiographic technique; VSD: Ventricular septal defect.

Competing interests

The authors declare that they have no competing interests

Authors' contributions

JAS: Design and programming of imaging sequence and reconstruction, acquisition of data, image quality processing, data interpretation, drafting of manuscript. BP: Vessel diameter measurements (observer 2), consensus reviewing for diagnosis. OT: Acquisition of data, preliminary data analysis/interpretation. VM: Study design, vessel diameter measurements (observer 1), consensus reviewing for diagnosis data interpretation, drafting of manuscript. All authors performed critical revision and approved the final manuscript.

Author details

[1]UCL Centre for Cardiovascular Imaging, University College London, 30 Guildford Street, London WC1N 1EH, UK. [2]The Heart Hospital, University College London Hospital Foundation Trust, London W1G 8PH, UK. [3]Cardiorespiratory Unit, Great Ormond Street Hospital for Children, London WC1N 3JH, UK.

References

1. Ntsinjana H, Hughes M, Taylor A. The role of cardiovascular magnetic resonance in pediatric congenital heart disease. J Cardiovasc Magn Reson. 2011;13:51.
2. Greil GF, Powell AJ, Gildein HP, Geva T. Gadolinium-enhanced three-dimensional magnetic resonance angiography of pulmonary and systemic venous anomalies. J Am Coll Cardiol. 2002;39:335–41.
3. Prasad SK, Soukias N, Hornung T, Khan M, Pennell DJ, Gatzoulis MA, et al. Role of magnetic resonance angiography in the diagnosis of major aortopulmonary collateral arteries and partial anomalous pulmonary venous drainage. Circ. 2004;109:207–14.
4. Ferrari VA, Scott CH, Holland GA, Axel L, St. John Sutton M. Ultrafast three-dimensional contrast-enhanced magnetic resonance angiography and imaging in the diagnosis of partial anomalous pulmonary venous drainage. J Am Coll Cardiol. 2001;37:1120–8.
5. Valsangiacomo E, Levasseur S, McCrindle B, MacDonald C, Smallhorn J, Yoo S-J. Contrast-enhanced MR angiography of pulmonary venous abnormalities in children. Ped Radiol. 2003;33:92–8.
6. Geva T, Greil GF, Marshall AC, Landzberg M, Powell AJ. Gadolinium-enhanced 3-dimensional magnetic resonance angiography of pulmonary blood supply in patients with complex pulmonary stenosis or atresia: comparison with X-Ray angiography. Circ. 2002;106:473–8.
7. Korosec FR, Frayne R, Grist TM, Mistretta CA. Time-resolved contrast-enhanced 3D MR angiography. MRM. 1996;36:345–51.
8. Krishnam MS, Tomasian A, Lohan DG, Tran L, Finn JP, Ruehm SG. Low-dose, time-resolved, contrast-enhanced 3D MR angiography in cardiac and vascular diseases: correlation to high spatial resolution 3D contrast-enhanced MRA. Clinical Radiology. 2008;63:744–755.
9. Fenchel M, Saleh R, Dinh H, Lee MH, Nael K, Krishnam M, et al. Juvenile and adult congenital heart disease: time-resolved 3D contrast-enhanced MR angiography. Radiology. 2007;244:399–410.
10. Wieben O, Grist TM, Hany TF, Thornton FJ, Glaser JK, Skuldt DH, et al. Time-resolved 3D MR angiography of the abdomen with a real-time system. MRM. 2004;52:921–6.
11. Willinek WA, Gieseke J, Conrad R, Strunk H, Hoogeveen R, von Falkenhausen M, et al. Randomly segmented central k-space ordering in high-spatial-resolution contrast-enhanced MR angiography of the supraaortic arteries: initial experience. Radiology. 2002;225:583–8.
12. Zhu H, Buck DG, Zhang Z, Zhang H, Wang P, Stenger VA, et al. High temporal and spatial resolution 4D MRA using spiral data sampling and sliding window reconstruction. MRM. 2004;52:14–8.
13. Fink C, Ley S, Kroeker R, Requardt M, Kauczor H-U, Bock M. Time-resolved contrast-enhanced three-dimensional magnetic resonance angiography of the chest: combination of parallel imaging with view sharing (TREAT). Investig Radiol. 2005;40:40–8.
14. Shin T, Nayak KS, Santos JM, Nishimura DG, Hu BS, McConnell MV. Three-dimensional first-pass myocardial perfusion MRI using a stack-of-spirals acquisition. MRM. 2013;69:839–44.
15. Pruessmann KP, Weiger M, Bornert P, Boesiger P. Advances in sensitivity encoding with arbitrary k-space trajectories. MRM. 2001;46:638–51.
16. Noll DC, Nishimura DG, Macovski A. Homodyne detection in magnetic resonance imaging. Med Imaging IEEE Trans. 1991;10:154–63.
17. Nezafat R, Kellman P, Derbyshire JA, McVeigh ER. Real time high spatial-temporal resolution flow imaging with spiral MRI using auto-calibrated SENSE. IEEE Eng Med Biol Soc. 2004;1:1914–7.
18. Rosset A, Spadola L, Ratib O. OsiriX: an open-source software for navigating in multidimensional DICOM images. J Digit Imaging. 2004;17:205–16.
19. Dietrich O, Raya JG, Reeder SB, Reiser MF, Schoenberg SO. Measurement of signal-to-noise ratios in MR images: Influence of multichannel coils, parallel imaging, and reconstruction filters. JMRI. 2007;26:375–85.
20. Buerke B, Allkemper T, Kugel H, Bremer C, Evers S, Kooijman H, et al. Qualitative and quantitative analysis of routinely postprocessed (CLEAR) CE-MRA data sets: Are SNR and CNR calculations reliable? Acad Radiol. 2008;15:1111–7.
21. Dabir D, Naehle CP, Clauberg R, Gieseke J, Schild H, Thomas D. High-resolution motion compensated MRA in patients with congenital heart disease using extracellular contrast agent at 3 Tesla. J Cardiovasc Magn Reson. 2012;14:75.
22. Steeden JA, Atkinson D, Hansen MS, Taylor AM, Muthurangu V. Rapid flow assessment of congenital heart disease with high-spatiotemporal-resolution gated spiral phase-contrast MR imaging. Radiology. 2011;260:79–87.
23. Bland JM, Altman DG. Statistical methods for assessing agreement between two methods of cliical measurement. Lancet. 1986;i:307–10.
24. Rapacchi S, Han F, Natsuaki Y, Kroeker R, Plotnik A, Lehrman E, et al. High spatial and temporal resolution dynamic contrast-enhanced magnetic resonance angiography using compressed sensing with magnitude image subtraction. MRM. 2014;71:1771–83.
25. Naehle CP, Kaestner M, Müller A, Willinek WW, Gieseke J, Schild HH, et al. First-pass and steady-state MR angiography of thoracic vasculature in children and adolescents. J Am Coll Cardiol Img. 2010;3:504–13.
26. Ingrisch M, Maxien D, Schwab F, Reiser MF, Nikolaou K, Dietrich O. Assessment of pulmonary perfusion with breath-hold and free-breathing dynamic contrast-enhanced magnetic resonance imaging: quantification and reproducibility. Investig Radiol. 2014;49:382–9. 310.1097/RLI.0000000000000020.
27. Block KT, Frahm J. Spiral imaging: a critical appraisal. J Magn Reson Imaging. 2005;21:657–68.
28. Stone SS, Haldar JP, Tsao SC, Hwu WW, Sutton BP, Liang ZP. Accelerating advanced MRI reconstructions on GPUs. J Parallel Distrib Comput. 2008;68:1307–18.

18

Accelerated free breathing ECG triggered contrast enhanced pulmonary vein magnetic resonance angiography using compressed sensing

Sébastien Roujol, Murilo Foppa, Tamer A Basha, Mehmet Akçakaya, Kraig V Kissinger, Beth Goddu, Sophie Berg and Reza Nezafat[*]

Abstract

Background: To investigate the feasibility of accelerated electrocardiogram (ECG)-triggered contrast enhanced pulmonary vein magnetic resonance angiography (CE-PV MRA) with isotropic spatial resolution using compressed sensing (CS).

Methods: Nineteen patients (59 ± 13 y, 11 M) referred for MR were scanned using the proposed accelerated free breathing ECG-triggered 3D CE-PV MRA sequence (FOV = $340 \times 340 \times 110$ mm^3, spatial resolution = $1.5 \times 1.5 \times 1.5$ mm^3, acquisition window = 140 ms at mid diastole and CS acceleration factor = 5) and a conventional first-pass breath-hold non ECG-triggered 3D CE-PV MRA sequence. CS data were reconstructed offline using low-dimensional-structure self-learning and thresholding reconstruction (LOST) CS reconstruction. Quantitative analysis of PV sharpness and subjective qualitative analysis of overall image quality were performed using a 4-point scale (1: poor; 4: excellent).

Results: Quantitative PV sharpness was increased using the proposed approach (0.73 ± 0.09 vs. 0.51 ± 0.07 for the conventional CE-PV MRA protocol, $p < 0.001$). There were no significant differences in the subjective image quality scores between the techniques (3.32 ± 0.94 vs. 3.53 ± 0.77 using the proposed technique).

Conclusions: CS-accelerated free-breathing ECG-triggered CE-PV MRA allows evaluation of PV anatomy with improved sharpness compared to conventional non-ECG gated first-pass CE-PV MRA. This technique may be a valuable alternative for patients in which the first pass CE-PV MRA fails due to inaccurate first pass timing or inability of the patient to perform a 20–25 seconds breath-hold.

Keywords: Magnetic resonance angiography, Pulmonary vein, 3D acquisition, Acceleration techniques, Compressed sensing

Background

Atrial fibrillation (AF) is the most common type of cardiac arrhythmia [1]. Triggers arising from pulmonary veins have been shown to be responsible for most AF [2]. Pulmonary vein (PV) isolation (PVI) using catheter ablation [2] is now considered as an accepted treatment of paroxysmal AF [3]. During this procedure, circumferential ablation regions are created at the PV ostia to electrically isolate the PVs. PV anatomies such as the PV ostia size and the number of PVs is generally assessed prior to the PVI procedure using imaging techniques such as multidetector computed tomography (MDCT) or cardiovascular magnetic resonance (CMR) [4,5]. 3D road maps of the PVs and the left atrium are then generated from these images and are loaded into electro-anatomical mapping system for the guidance of PVI procedures [4,5]. Post PVI imaging is also performed for the detection of rare post-procedural complications such as PV stenosis or damage to the esophagus [6-8].

Both MDCT and CMR are clinically used for left atrium (LA) and PV imaging [5,9-11]. Although MDCT provides improved spatial resolution compared to CMR, it uses iodinated contrast agents and generates ionizing radiation to the patient. Furthermore, a high rate of AF recurrence

* Correspondence: rnezafat@bidmc.harvard.edu
Department of Medicine (Cardiovascular Division), Beth Israel Deaconess Medical Center and Harvard Medical School, 330 Brookline Ave, Boston, MA 02215, USA

is observed after PVI procedures, which necessitates redo PVI procedures [9]. Therefore, a non ionizing imaging approach such as CMR would be preferable for PV/LA imaging.

3D contrast-enhanced MR angiography (CE-MRA) is the current standard CMR technique to image both PVs and LA [5,10,12-15]. CE-MRA generally uses a non-ECG triggered spoiled gradient echo (GRE) sequence which is acquired within one prolonged breath-hold during the first pass of a contrast agent. To provide satisfactory contrast in the PVs, the beginning of the CE-MRA acquisition needs to be synchronized with the contrast arrival in the PVs. To this end, a real time sequence is generally acquired during the first pass of the contrast media and stopped at contrast arrival in the right ventricle. Breath-holding instructions are then given to the patients and are immediately followed by the CE-MRA acquisition. The synchronization of the breath-hold initiation with the CE-MRA acquisition and the contrast arrival in the PVs/LA is thus challenging and can fail in some patients, which results in either respiratory motion artifacts and blurring or insufficient contrast in the PVs/LA. 3D non-contrast non-ECG triggered MRA has also been proposed for imaging of the PVs/LA [16-19]. However, this approach is associated with significant loss of both SNR and CNR compared to CE-MRA [16-19] and to motion-induced blurring artifacts which leads to overestimation of the PV size [20].

Furthermore, late gadolinium enhancement (LGE) CMR [21,22] can depict the left atrial wall injury after the radiofrequency ablation for treatment of AF [23,24]. Post-PVI LGE of LA has also been used as a prognostic tool for identifying patients with AF recurrence [25]. Since 3D MR angiography (MRA) offers a good visualization of the atrial wall, an MRA-driven segmentation can be employed to facilitate the segmentation of the atrial wall and enhanced areas in 3D LA LGE [24-26]. Therefore, this approach requires fusion of MRA and LGE datasets. However, registration of non-ECG gated MRA to ECG-triggered LGE is challenging [24,25]. Therefore, an ECG-triggered 3D MRA could potentially improve the fusion of MRA and LGE datasets.

3D ECG-triggered acquisitions have been proposed in both non contrast MRA [16-19] and CE-MRA [27-30]. Since this approach prolongs the acquisition time, 3D ECG-triggered CE-MRA have been performed within one breath-hold with reduced spatial resolution [30], or under free breathing conditions [27-29] using respiratory navigation techniques [31]. Although high spatial resolution 3D CE-MRA acquisition is desirable for reliable assessment of PV/LA anatomies, it is associated to prolonged scan time which increases the sensitivity to artifact induced by the temporal variation of the contrast agent concentration. Acceleration techniques have been proposed to reduce the

scan time using parallel imaging with an acceleration rate of 2 [27,28]. Compressed-sensing (CS) [32,33] is an alternative acceleration technique that enables higher acceleration rates. CS based acceleration has been demonstrated in several applications such as non contrast free breathing PV-MRA using an acceleration factor of 4 to 6 and a retrospective undersampling of the fully-sampled data [19], as well as prospectively in LGE [34,35] using an acceleration factor of 3–4, and contrast enhanced coronary [36] using an acceleration factor of 4.

In this study, we sought to investigate the feasibility of a prospectively-accelerated free breathing, respiratory navigated, ECG-triggered 3D CE-PV MRA sequence using CS in comparison to the clinical gold-standard first-pass breath-hold non-ECG gated 3D CE-MRA.

Methods

All subjects were scanned using a 1.5 T Philips Achieva (Philips Healthcare, Best, The Netherlands) scanner and a 32-channel cardiac phased array receiver coil. In this health insurance portability and accountability act (HIPAA) compliant study, the imaging protocol was approved by our institutional review board and informed consent was obtained from all participants.

Study design

Nineteen patients (59 ± 13 years, 11 male) referred for clinical CMR in our center were recruited, including 8 pre-PVI patients and 3 post-PVI patients. All patients were in sinus rhythm at the time of CMR. The study design is shown in Figure 1. Each subject was imaged using the conventional first pass breath-hold 3D CE-PV MRA protocol and the proposed accelerated respiratory navigated ECG-triggered 3D CE-PV MRA protocol. All participants received an injection of 0.1 mmol/kg of gadobenate dimeglumine (MultiHance; Bracco Diagnostic Inc., Princeton, NJ) as a single bolus injection with rate of 2 mL/s.

As part of the clinical protocol, the conventional breath-hold 3D CE-PV MRA sequence was repeated three times, one time before contrast injection for training purpose (Dynamic #1), once during the first pass of the contrast agent (Dynamic #2), and a last time in case of incorrect timing of the first pass acquisition (Dynamic #3). For each of three acquisitions, the subjects were instructed for two maximum capacity respirations followed by a ~20 second end-expiratory breath-hold. The three acquisitions of the conventional breath-hold 3D CE-PV MRA used a gradient recalled echo (GRE) sequence with the following parameters: TR/TE/α =3.2 ms/1.12 ms/40°, FOV =320 × 320 × 90 mm^3, voxel size = 1.5 × 1.5 × 1.5 mm^3, SENSE acceleration factor = 2.5 (FH direction), scan duration = 20 s, and frequency, phase, and slice encoding directions = (RL, FH, AP, respectively). To obtain maximum contrast in the PVs and LA, the sequence used a centric profile reordering. In

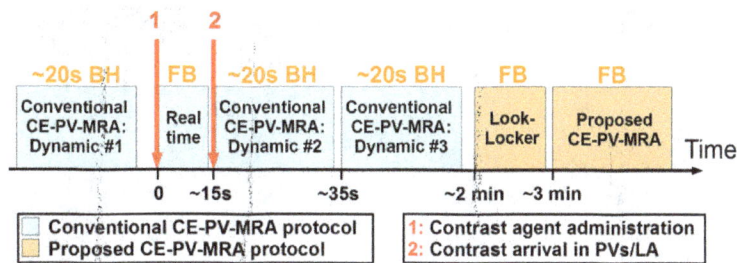

Figure 1 Study design of the patient study. The conventional CE-PV-MRA protocol is acquired during the first pass of the contrast agent where each dynamic CE-PV MRA acquisition is performed within one breath-hold (BH). Subsequently, the proposed CE-PV-MRA protocol is started using a Look-Locker sequence and the proposed ECG-triggered free breathing (FB) CE-PV-MRA sequence. The Look-Locker sequence is used to estimate the optimal inversion time (TI) to null myocardial tissue. This optimal TI is then set as inversion time of the proposed ECG-triggered CE-PV-MRA sequence.

order to synchronize the beginning of the second conventional breath-hold 3D CE-PV MRA acquisition (Dynamic #2) with the first pass of the contrast bolus, a real time sequence was initiated at the time of the contrast agent administration (single bolus injection at 2 mL/s). A single slice was acquired in the coronal orientation using a GRE sequence with the following parameters: TR/TE/α = 3 ms/ 0.87 ms/40°, FOV = 530 × 530 mm^2, voxel size = 2.1 × 4.1 mm^2, slice thickness = 80 mm, and temporal resolution = 390 ms. The real time acquisition was stopped upon arrival of the contrast media into the right ventricle and followed by breath-holding instructions and the conventional first pass breath-hold 3D CE-PV MRA (Dynamic #2).

After completion of the conventional first pass breath-hold 3D CE-PV MRA protocol, a Look Locker sequence [37] was acquired and followed by the proposed accelerated free-breathing ECG-triggered 3D CE-PV MRA, acquired at ~3 minutes after contrast administration. This sequence used an inversion recovery steady-state free precession (SSFP) sequence with the following parameters: TR/TE/α = 4.1 ms/2 ms/90°, FOV = 320 × 320 × 90 mm^3, voxel size = 1.5 × 1.5 × 1.5 mm^3, fat saturation using SPIR, and acquisition window = 140 ms, frequency, phase, and slice encoding directions = (FH, RL, AP, respectively). K-space segments were acquired at every RR interval. The inversion time was selected to null myocardial tissue and was estimated from the prior Look Locker sequence. Data were acquired at the mid rest diastolic period which was identified from a cine scan acquired before contrast injection. The sequence was respiratory gated (gating window = 7 mm) and tracked (factor = 0.4 [38,39]) using a pencil beam navigator positioned on the right hemi diaphragm. The position of the pencil beam navigator was slightly shifted away from the dome of the right hemi-diaphragm towards the right hand side of the patient to minimize the intersection between the navigator beam and the PVs and resulting PV inflow artifacts. An acceleration rate of 5 with respect to the elliptical window

(acceleration rate of 6.3 with respect to the whole k-space) was employed using a prospective random undersampling pattern [40] (as illustrated in Figure 2). This sampling scheme acquires the full k-space center lines (32 × 19 lines in k_y-k_z) and randomly discards outer k-space lines to reach an acceleration factor of 5. A radial re-ordering of the k-space data was used to minimize the k-space jumps and to reduce eddy current artifacts [40]. Note that the same random undersampling pattern was used in all subjects. The average scan time of the proposed sequence was 90 seconds assuming a 100% gating efficiency and 60 beats/minute.

The CS reconstruction was performed using an advanced B_1-weighted CS reconstruction technique [41] which iteratively alternate between thresholding of the combined coil image using the low-dimensional-structure self-learning and thresholding reconstruction (LOST) [40] and enforcement of data consistency. The reconstruction has been performed offline in the first 2/3 of the patients and then online in the remaining patients using an online in-house reconstruction tool [42]. The average reconstruction time was ~1 h per case.

Data analysis

Quantitative analysis of the PV sharpness was performed as illustrated in Figure 3. Inner and outer contours of each PV were first manually drawn in the sagittal plane using our in-house platform (MedIACARE) developed in Matlab [43,44]. Each point of the outer contour was then paired with the closest point of the inner contour to generate a virtual segment crossing the PV border. The intensity profile of each segment was then used to measure the PV sharpness as described in [45,46]. The intensity profile along each segment was extracted. Bilinear interpolation was used to increase the sampling density of intensity profiles to 10 points/mm. For each intensity profile, the minimum intensity (I_{min}) and maximum intensity (I_{max}) were measured and two thresholds (T_{min}, T_{max}) were defined as $T_{min} = I_{min} + (I_{max}-I_{min}) \times 0.2$ and $T_{max} = I_{min} +$

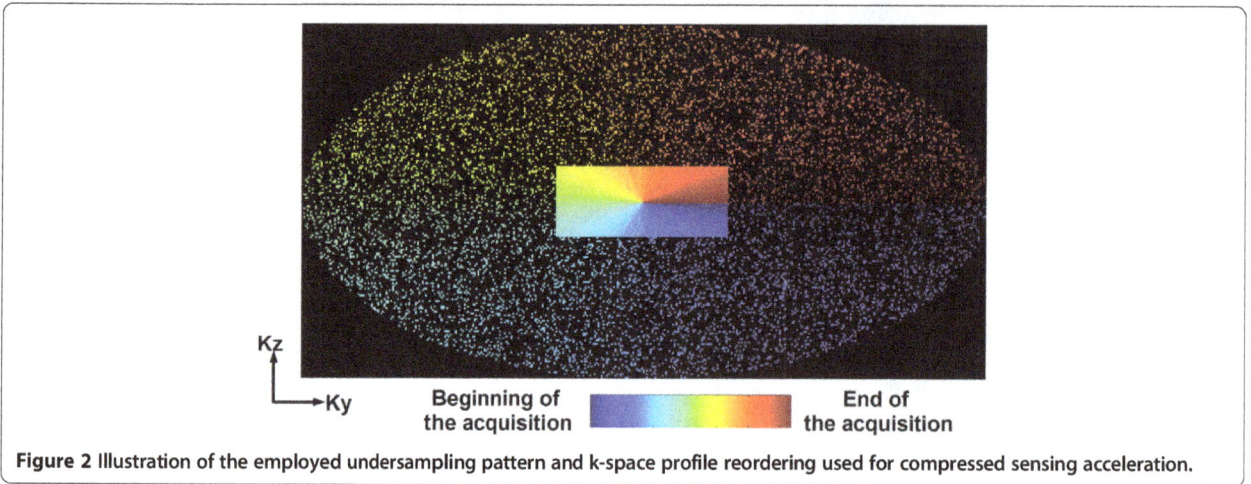

Figure 2 Illustration of the employed undersampling pattern and k-space profile reordering used for compressed sensing acceleration.

$(I_{max}-I_{min}) \times 0.8$. The length (L) of the signal transition between these two thresholds was then measured and the sharpness was defined as $1/L$. The sharpness measured over each segments was averaged and used as an overall sharpness measure of the PV.

Subjective qualitative analysis was performed to compare the conventional and the proposed CE-PV MRA sequences. All data were exported in the DICOM format and were loaded in the OsiriX platform (OsiriX 5.7.1; The OsiriX Fondation; Geneva, Swizerland) for image visualization and analysis. Data were visually assessed by an experienced cardiologist (>15 years of experience) who was blinded from the acquisition scheme and patient information. Overall image quality was assessed using a four point scale as: 1: poor image quality (PVs are not visible); 2: fair image quality (some artifacts prevent a clear delineation of all PVs), 3: good image quality (all PV are clearly defined); 4: excellent image quality (all the PVs are clearly defined and sharp).

Statistical analysis

Paired t-test was used to test the null hypothesis that the difference of quantitative PV sharpness between both

approaches is zero. Wilcoxon signed rank test was used to test the null hypothesis that the difference of overall image quality scores between the conventional and the proposed CE-PV MRA sequences was zero. Statistical significance threshold was defined for all tests at $p <0.05$.

Results

Figure 4 shows example of PV MRA data acquired in a 63 year-old patient, referred to CMR for assessment of PV/LA anatomy prior to a PVI procedures. Images acquired with the conventional CE-PV MRA protocol (Figure 4a) and the proposed free breathing ECG-triggered CE-PV MRA protocol (Figure 4b) are shown in the axial orientation as well as in two coronal views crossing the left PVs, and the right PVs, respectively. Blurring

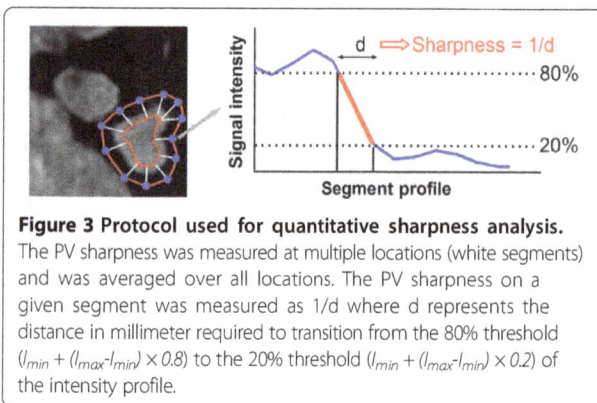

Figure 3 Protocol used for quantitative sharpness analysis. The PV sharpness was measured at multiple locations (white segments) and was averaged over all locations. The PV sharpness on a given segment was measured as 1/d where d represents the distance in millimeter required to transition from the 80% threshold $(I_{min} + (I_{max}-I_{min}) \times 0.8)$ to the 20% threshold $(I_{min} + (I_{max}-I_{min}) \times 0.2)$ of the intensity profile.

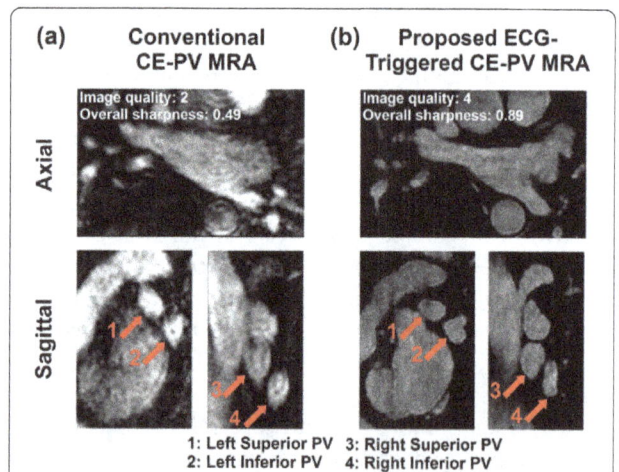

1: Left Superior PV   3: Right Superior PV
2: Left Inferior PV   4: Right Inferior PV

Figure 4 Conventional (a) and proposed (b) CE-PV MRA obtained in a 63 year-old patient, referred to CMR for assessment of PV/LA anatomy prior to a pulmonary vein isolation procedure. The conventional CE-PV MRA sequence led to blurring artifacts. PV sharpness and image quality were substantially improved with the ECG-triggered CE-PV MRA sequence.

artifacts and reduced PV sharpness is observed in images acquired with the conventional CE-PV MRA sequence (see arrows). The ECG-triggered CE-PV MRA sequence provided improved PV sharpness (0.89 vs. 0.49) and image quality (4 vs. 2).

Figure 5 shows another example of PV MRA data acquired in a 48 year-old patient acquired for assessment of PV/LA anatomy prior to PVI. Due to inaccurate acquisition timing, image acquired with the conventional CE-PV MRA protocol provided low contrast and poor image quality. The proposed ECG-triggered CE-PV MRA sequence resulted in substantial improvement of both PV sharpness (0.90 vs. 0.66) and image quality (4 vs. 2).

Table 1 shows the quantitative analysis of PV sharpness obtained with the conventional CE-PV MRA protocol and the proposed ECG-triggered CE-PV MRA protocol. Over all PVs, the proposed approach provided consistent increased sharpness (0.73 ± 0.09 vs. 0.51 ± 0.07 for the conventional CE-PV MRA protocol, $p < 0.001$). These differences were also found statistically significant for all individual PV ($p < 0.002$). There was no statistical difference between the sharpness of the right PVs and left PVs using the conventional approach (0.50 ± 0.08 vs. 0.53 ± 0.09, $p = 0.17$). However, higher sharpness was measured in the left PVs when compared to the right PVs using the proposed approach (0.70 ± 0.09 vs. 0.75 ± 0.10, $p = 0.04$).

Table 2 shows the qualitative analysis of overall image quality. With the conventional CE-PV MRA protocol, 1 dataset received a score of 1, 3 datasets received a score of 2, 4 datasets received a score of 3, and 11 datasets

Table 1 PV sharpness obtained with the conventional first pass non ECG-triggered CE-PV MRA (conventional CE-PV MRA) and the proposed free breathing ECG-triggered CE-PV MRA (proposed CE-PV MRA)

	Sharpness (mm^{-1})		
	Conventional CE-PV MRA	Proposed CE-PV MRA	P value
Left superior PV	0.51 ± 0.12	0.75 ± 0.14	P < 0.001
Left inferior PV	0.54 ± 0.10	0.75 ± 0.10	P < 0.001
Right superior PV	0.48 ± 0.1	0.72 ± 0.10	P < 0.001
Right inferior PV	0.52 ± 0.07	0.69 ± 0.10	P = 0.002
All PVs	0.51 ± 0.07	0.73 ± 0.09	P < 0.001

The proposed CE-PV MRA protocol led to increased sharpness of all PVs.

received a score of 4 (15 datasets (79%) received an overall image quality score ≥3 (good or excellent)). With the proposed ECG-triggered CE-PV MRA protocol, none of dataset received a score of 1, 3 datasets received a score of 2, 3 datasets received a score of 3, and 13 datasets received a score of 4 (16 datasets (84%) received an overall image quality score ≥3 (good or excellent)). In the four datasets which received an overall quality score ≤2 using the conventional CE-PV MRA protocol, the proposed ECG-triggered CE-PV MRA protocol provided an overall image quality score of 4. In the three datasets which received an overall quality score ≤2 using the proposed CE-PV MRA protocol, the conventional ECG-triggered CE-PV MRA protocol provided an overall image quality score of 4. Furthermore, at least one dataset (among the two sequences) received an image quality score of 4 in all subjects. The image quality of the proposed technique was superior, equal, and inferior than the conventional CE-PV MRA technique in 8, 6, and 5 cases, respectively. Overall, there were no statistically significant differences in image quality scores between the two techniques (3.5 ± 0.8 vs. 3.3 ± 0.9 using the conventional CE-PV MRA protocol, $p > 0.05$). The acquisition time of the proposed sequence was 212 ± 65 s which corresponded to a gating efficiency of $44 \pm 12\%$ with a heart rate of 62 ± 10 bpm.

Discussion

In this study, we demonstrated the feasibility of a five-time accelerated free-breathing ECG-triggered CE-PV MRA acquisition using CS. The method was successfully validated in a patient cohort. This approach has higher

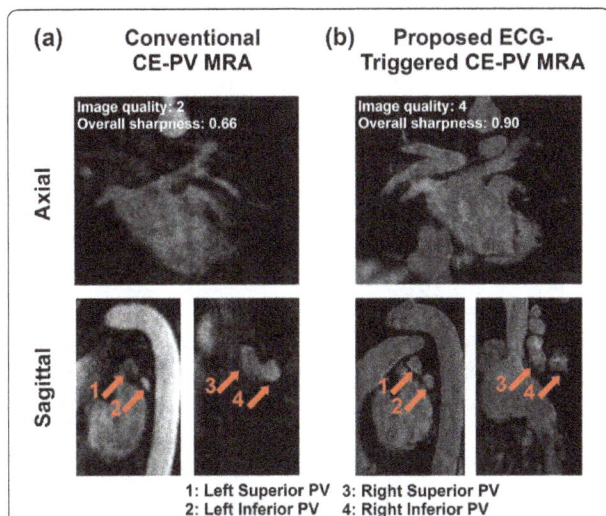

(a) Conventional CE-PV MRA   **(b) Proposed ECG-Triggered CE-PV MRA**

Axial / Sagittal

Image quality: 2 / Overall sharpness: 0.66
Image quality: 4 / Overall sharpness: 0.90

1: Left Superior PV   3: Right Superior PV
2: Left Inferior PV   4: Right Inferior PV

Figure 5 Conventional (a) and proposed (b) CE-PV MRA sequences acquired in a 48 year-old patient, referred to CMR for assessment of PV/LA anatomy prior to a pulmonary vein isolation procedure. Low contrast and poor image quality were obtained with the conventional CE-PV MRA sequence due to inaccurate acquisition timing. Improved PV sharpness and image quality were achieved using the proposed ECG-triggered CE-PV MRA sequence.

Table 2 Qualitative analysis of overall image quality

	Conventional CE-PV-MRA	Proposed CE-PV-MRA	P value
Overall image quality	3.3 ± 0.9	3.5 ± 0.8	0.63

Although differences between both approaches did not reach statistical significance, there was a tendency towards increased overall image quality using the proposed CE-PV-MRA protocol.

acceleration rate than previous free-breathing ECG-triggered CE-PV MRA studies [27-29]. Increased PV sharpness was obtained with the proposed approach when compared to a conventional first pass non ECG-triggered CE-PV MRA protocol. There were no differences in subjective image quality scores between the two techniques.

In this study, we used CS as acceleration technique. Other acceleration approaches such as parallel imaging have been previously used for ECG-triggered CE-PV MRA [27,28]. These approaches used lower acceleration factor of 2. Although parallel imaging has been used with higher rate for breath-hold non-contrast thoracic MRA [47,48], its feasibility for free breathing CE-PV MRA has not been shown yet. Furthermore, due to noise penalty induced by the g-factor maps, parallel imaging has been shown to result in higher noise level than compressed sensing [41]. Our CS reconstruction used a B_1-weighted technique [41] which exploits the sparsity of similar voxel blocks in a 3D volume. Other CS reconstructions have been proposed based on total variation (TV) [32,49], wavelet domain [50], or a combination of TV and wavelet domains [33,51]. However, these techniques were not evaluated in this study.

A radial k-space profile reordering was used for the acquisition of the randomly under-sampled k-space. Although this technique minimizes jumps during each segment acquisition, it increases the sensitivity to k-space weighting induced artifacts since the k-space center lines are acquired over the entire acquisition. Advanced profile reordering techniques which first acquire all k-space center lines over the first heart beats [52,35] may reduce the sensitivity of our approach to k-space weighting induced artifacts and should be investigated in future work.

A CS acceleration factor of 5 was used in this study after performing a pilot study to evaluate overall image quality by changing the acceleration rate from 3 to 6. Several factors could impact the maximum acceleration factor such as baseline SNR, imaging resolution and hardware. In our previous study using 5 channel cardiac coil [34], we found that an acceleration rate of 3 provide excellent image quality. Using 32-channel coil allows us to perform a B_1-weighted LOST reconstruction that enabled to acquire data with acceleration as high as 6 [41]. Furthermore, imaging sequence will impact the maximum achievable acceleration rate. For example LGE has lower baseline SNR because of use of an inversion pulse, therefore, lower acceleration factor can be used, while non-contrast coronary CMR which has better SNR can be acquired with higher acceleration.

In this study, we used 0.1 mmol/kg of gadobenate dimeglumine and data acquisition was performed in the following ~3 min. There will be some changes in the contrast media in the blood during the acquisition time, which will result in signal falloff and extra weighting on k-space. We

have previously studied the changes in T_1 after gadobenate dimeglumine contrast injection [53] and our data demonstrated that the changes are relatively small for the period of time required for the proposed sequence. Nevertheless, to mitigate the effect of the contrast wash-out, this sequence was designed to minimize the overall scan time using a high acceleration factor combined with a data acquisition at every RR interval. The use of alternate R-wave acquisition would reduce the impact of RR variations on the sequence but would increase the overall scan time by a factor of two. In this study, we decided to privilege the minimization of the contrast wash out effect at the cost of increased sensitivity to RR variations.

The inversion time was adjusted for each patient using a prior Look Locker acquisition and the selected inversion time was kept constant throughout the entire duration of the proposed ECG-triggered CE-PV MRA scan. Although the optimal inversion time variation is higher during the first minutes following the contrast administration [53], a satisfactory nulling of the myocardial signal was achieved in most patients. However, this effect could lead to artifacts in patients with very low gating efficiency which would result in prolonged acquisitions. Advanced k-space profile reordering, as previously discussed, may decrease the sensitivity of the method to the time variation of the optimal inversion time. Adaptive adjustment of the inversion time during the acquisition as initially proposed for late gadolinium enhancement (LGE) imaging [54] could be a valuable option for these patients.

In this study, the respiratory navigator was slightly shifted away from the dome of the right hemi-diaphragm to minimize PV inflow artifacts. Nevertheless, the efficiency of this strategy could be decreased in the presence of certain orientation/anatomies of the heart, as suggested by the slightly lower sharpness measurements obtained in the right PVs. Several approaches have been recently proposed to reduce PV inflow artifacts by modifying the timing of the navigator restore pulse [55] or the timing of the actual navigator signal acquisition [39]. However, these methods were not used in our study.

The proposed sequence is also independent of the breath-hold ability of the patient and does not require any specific breathing pattern. This approach is thus well suitable and compatible with a contrast-enhanced CMR clinical exam. Furthermore, conventional first pass CE-PV MRA may fail with inaccurate first pass timing prediction or in patients with inability to sustain a 20–25 seconds breath-hold. Therefore, our approach represents a valuable CE- alternative PV MRA protocol which could be immediately run when the conventional first pass CE-PV MRA protocol fails.

The proposed sequence has been designed for patients being imaged in sinus rhythm since the majority of patients with paroxysmal AF are most of the time in sinus rhythm during MR imaging. Since all patients in this study were in sinus rhythm at the time of imaging, the impact of AF event on image quality was not quantified. However, the presence of AF event during imaging is expected to create substantial motion/blurring artifacts using the proposed sequence. Further studies are warranted to evaluate this approach in patients being imaged during AF events.

In the methodology used for sharpness quantification, it is difficult to ensure that all lines joining the inner and outer contours were perpendicular to the PV border. Therefore, this may have led to reduced PV sharpness measurements. However, since the same methodology has been used for the analysis of all the data, the potential bias induced between both techniques should have been kept to the minimum.

Despite the PV sharpness improvement achieved using the proposed approach, no statistical difference was obtained in term of qualitative scores between both sequences. This could be explained by several factors. First the narrow score scale combined with the small patient cohort may have limited the assessment of differences between the two approaches. Furthermore, despite the overall higher level of blurring artifact in conventional images, the reader still felt confident in assessing the PVs anatomy in most cases, therefore reducing the spread of the subjective scores.

This study has several limitations. Our patient population was small and could have limited the assessment of differences for qualitative metrics. Both signal to noise ratio (SNR) and contrast to noise ratio (CNR) were not examined in our study due to non-linear LOST reconstruction. The qualitative analysis was only performed by one cardiologist. However, based on his extensive experience in reading of clinical CMR images including PV MRA images, the potential scoring approximation should have been kept to the minimum. Finally, the benefit of the proposed approach for the planning and guidance of PVI procedures as well as the detection of potential postprocedural complications was not evaluated.

Conclusions

CS-accelerated free-breathing ECG-triggered 3D CE-PV MRA allows evaluation of PV anatomy with improved sharpness compared to conventional non-ECG gated first-pass 3D CE-PV MRA. This technique may be a valuable alternative for patients in which the first pass CE-PV MRA fails due to inaccurate first pass timing or inability of the patient to perform a 20–25 seconds breath-hold.

Abbrevations

AF: Atrial fibrillation; CE: Contrast enhanced; CNR: Contrast to noise ratio; CMR: Cardiovascular magnetic resonance; CS: Compressed sensing; ECG: Electrocardiograms; FOV: Field of view; GRE: Gradient recalled echo; HIPAA: Health insurance portability and accountability act; LA: Left atrium; LGE: Late gadolinium enhancement; LOST: Low-dimensional-structure self-learning and thresholding reconstruction; MDCT: Multi-detector computed tomography; MRA: Magnetic resonance angiography; CMR: Cardiovascular magnetic resonance; PV: Pulmonary vein; PVI: Pulmonary vein isolation; SENSE: Sensitivity encoding; SNR: Signal to noise ratio; SSFP: Steady-state free precession; TE: Time of echo; TR: Time of repetition; TI: Inversion time.

Competing interests

MA and RN have a patent for Method for Image Reconstruction using Low-dimensional-structure Self-learning and Thresholding.

Authors' contributions

SR participated in the study design and coordination, carried out the CMR data acquisition, data reconstruction, data analysis and drafted the manuscript. MF carried out the subjective analysis of the CMR data. TB developed the prospective acquisition scheme on the scanner. MA conceived the employed data reconstruction. KVK, BG, and SB participated in CMR data acquisition. RN conceived the study, participated in its design and coordination and helped to draft the manuscript. All authors read and approved the final manuscript.

Acknowledgments

Supported by NIH R01EB008743-01A2.

References

1. Go AS, Hylek EM, Phillips KA, Chang Y, Henault LE, Selby JV, Singer DE. **Prevalence of diagnosed atrial fibrillation in adults: national implications for rhythm management and stroke prevention: the AnTicoagulation and Risk Factors in Atrial Fibrillation (ATRIA) Study.** *JAMA.* 2001; 285(18):2370–75.

2. Haissaguerre M, Jais P, Shah DC, Takahashi A, Hocini M, Quiniou G, Garrigue S, Le Mouroux A, Le Metayer P, Clementy J. **Spontaneous initiation of atrial fibrillation by ectopic beats originating in the pulmonary veins.** *N Engl J Med.* 1998; 339(10):659–66.

3. Calkins H, Kuck KH, Cappato R, Brugada J, Camm AJ, Chen SA, Crijns HJ, Damiano RJ Jr, Davies DW, DiMarco J, Edgerton J, Ellenbogen K, Ezekowitz MD, Haines DE, Haissaguerre M, Hindricks G, Iesaka Y, Jackman W, Jalife J, Jais P, Kalman J, Keane D, Kim YH, Kirchhof P, Klein G, Kottkamp H, Kumagai K, Lindsay BD, Mansour M, Marchlinski FE, McCarthy PM, Mont JL, Morady F, Nademanee K, Nakagawa H, Natale A, Nattel S, Packer DL, Pappone C, Prystowsky E, Raviele A, Reddy V, Ruskin JN, Shemin RJ, Tsao HM, Wilber D. **2012 HRS/EHRA/ECAS Expert Consensus Statement on Catheter and Surgical Ablation of Atrial Fibrillation: recommendations for patient selection, procedural techniques, patient management and follow-up, definitions, endpoints, and research trial design.** *Europace.* 2012; 14(4):528–606.

4. Tops LF, Bax JJ, Zeppenfeld K, Jongbloed MR, Lamb HJ, van der Wall EE, Schalij MJ. **Fusion of multislice computed tomography imaging with three-dimensional electroanatomic mapping to guide radiofrequency catheter ablation procedures.** *Heart Rhythm.* 2005; 2(10):1076–81.

5. Dong J, Dickfeld T, Dalal D, Cheema A, Vasamreddy CR, Henrikson CA, Marine JE, Halperin HR, Berger RD, Lima JA, Calkins H. **Initial experience in the use of integrated electroanatomic mapping with three-dimensional MR/CT images to guide catheter ablation of atrial fibrillation.** *J Cardiovasc Electrophysiol.* 2006; 17(5):459–66.

6. Dill T, Neumann T, Ekinci O, Breidenbach C, John A, Erdogan A, Bachmann G, Hamm CW, Pitschner HF. **Pulmonary vein diameter reduction after radiofrequency catheter ablation for paroxysmal atrial fibrillation evaluated by contrast-enhanced three-dimensional magnetic resonance imaging.** *Circulation.* 2003; 107(6):845–50.

7. Meng J, Peters DC, Hsing JM, Chuang ML, Chan J, Fish A, Josephson ME, Manning WJ. **Late gadolinium enhancement of the esophagus is common on cardiac MR several months after pulmonary vein isolation: preliminary observations.** *Pacing Clin Electrophysiol.* 2010; 33(6):661–66.

8. Badger TJ, Adjei-Poku YA, Burgon NS, Kalvaitis S, Shaaban A, Sommers DN, Blauer JJ, Fish EN, Akoum N, Haslem TS, Kholmovski EG, MacLeod RS, Adler DG, Marrouche NF. **Initial experience of assessing esophageal tissue injury**

and recovery using delayed-enhancement MRI after atrial fibrillation ablation. *Circ Arrhythm Electrophysiol.* 2009; 2(6):620–25.

9. Ames A, Stevenson WG. Cardiology patient page. Catheter ablation of atrial fibrillation. *Circulation.* 2006; 113(13):e666–668.

10. Syed MA, Peters DC, Rashid H, Arai AE. Pulmonary vein imaging: comparison of 3D magnetic resonance angiography with 2D cine MRI for characterizing anatomy and size. *J Cardiovasc Magn Reson.* 2005; 7(2):355–60.

11. Mansour M, Holmvang G, Sosnovik D, Migrino R, Abbara S, Ruskin J, Keane D. Assessment of pulmonary vein anatomic variability by magnetic resonance imaging: implications for catheter ablation techniques for atrial fibrillation. *J Cardiovasc Electrophysiol.* 2004; 15(4):387–93.

12. Wittkampf FH, Vonken EJ, Derksen R, Loh P, Velthuis B, Wever EF, Boersma LV, Rensing BJ, Cramer MJ. Pulmonary vein ostium geometry: analysis by magnetic resonance angiography. *Circulation.* 2003; 107(1):21–3.

13. Mansour M, Refaat M, Heist EK, Mela T, Cury R, Holmvang G, Ruskin JN. Three-dimensional anatomy of the left atrium by magnetic resonance angiography: implications for catheter ablation for atrial fibrillation. *J Cardiovasc Electrophysiol.* 2006; 17(7):719–23.

14. Kato R, Lickfett L, Meininger G, Dickfeld T, Wu R, Juang G, Angkeow P, LaCorte J, Bluemke D, Berger R, Halperin HR, Calkins H. Pulmonary vein anatomy in patients undergoing catheter ablation of atrial fibrillation: lessons learned by use of magnetic resonance imaging. *Circulation.* 2003; 107(15):2004–10.

15. Tsao HM, Yu WC, Cheng HC, Wu MH, Tai CT, Lin WS, Ding YA, Chang MS, Chen SA. Pulmonary vein dilation in patients with atrial fibrillation: detection by magnetic resonance imaging. *J Cardiovasc Electrophysiol.* 2001; 12(7):809–13.

16. Francois CJ, Tuite D, Deshpande V, Jerecic R, Weale P, Carr JC. Pulmonary vein imaging with unenhanced three-dimensional balanced steady-state free precession MR angiography: initial clinical evaluation. *Radiology.* 2009; 250(3):932–39.

17. Krishnam MS, Tomasian A, Malik S, Singhal A, Sassani A, Laub G, Finn JP, Ruehm S. Three-dimensional imaging of pulmonary veins by a novel steady-state free-precession magnetic resonance angiography technique without the use of intravenous contrast agent: initial experience. *Invest Radiol.* 2009; 44(8):447–53.

18. Hu P, Chuang ML, Kissinger KV, Goddu B, Goepfert LA, Rofsky NM, Manning WJ, Nezafat R. Non-contrast-enhanced pulmonary vein MRI with a spatially selective slab inversion preparation sequence. *Magn Reson Med.* 2010; 63(2):530–36.

19. Akcakaya M, Hu P, Chuang ML, Hauser TH, Ngo LH, Manning WJ, Tarokh V, Nezafat R. Accelerated noncontrast-enhanced pulmonary vein MRA with distributed compressed sensing. *J Magn Reson Imaging.* 2011; 33(5):1248–55.

20. Hauser TH, Yeon SB, Kissinger KV, Josephson ME, Manning WJ. Variation in pulmonary vein size during the cardiac cycle: implications for non-electrocardiogram-gated imaging. *Am Heart J.* 2006; 152(5):974 e971-976.

21. Kim RJ, Wu E, Rafael A, Chen EL, Parker MA, Simonetti O, Klocke FJ, Bonow RO, Judd RM. The use of contrast-enhanced magnetic resonance imaging to identify reversible myocardial dysfunction. *N Engl J Med.* 2000; 343(20):1445–53.

22. Simonetti OP, Kim RJ, Fieno DS, Hillenbrand HB, Wu E, Bundy JM, Finn JP, Judd RM. An improved MR imaging technique for the visualization of myocardial infarction. *Radiology.* 2001; 218(1):215–23.

23. McGann CJ, Kholmovski EG, Oakes RS, Blauer JJ, Daccarett M, Segerson N, Airey KJ, Akoum N, Fish E, Badger TJ, DiBella EV, Parker D, MacLeod RS, Marrouche NF. New magnetic resonance imaging-based method for defining the extent of left atrial wall injury after the ablation of atrial fibrillation. *J Am Coll Cardiol.* 2008; 52(15):1263–71.

24. Taclas JE, Nezafat R, Wylie JV, Josephson ME, Hsing J, Manning WJ, Peters DC. Relationship between intended sites of RF ablation and post-procedural scar in AF patients, using late gadolinium enhancement cardiovascular magnetic resonance. *Heart Rhythm.* 2010; 7(4):489–96.

25. Peters DC, Wylie JV, Hauser TH, Nezafat R, Han Y, Woo JJ, Taclas J, Kissinger KV, Goddu B, Josephson ME, Manning WJ. Recurrence of atrial fibrillation correlates with the extent of post-procedural late gadolinium enhancement: a pilot study. *JACC Cardiovasc Imaging.* 2009; 2(3):308–16.

26. Depa M, Sabuncu MR, Holmvang G, Nezafat R, Schmidt EJ, Golland P: "Robust atlas-based segmentation of highly variable anatomy: Left atrium segmentation," in MICCAI Workshop on Statistical Atlases and Computational Models of the Heart: Mapping Structure and Function (STACOM). 2010. p 85–94.

27. Fahlenkamp UL, Lembcke A, Roesler R, Schwenke C, Huppertz A, Streitparth F, Taupitz M, Hamm B, Wagner M. ECG-gated imaging of the left atrium and pulmonary veins: Intra-individual comparison of CTA and MRA. *Clin Radiol.* 2013; 68(10):1059–64.

28. Wagner M, Rief M, Asbach P, Vogtmann T, Huppertz A, Beling M, Butler C, Laule M, Warmuth C, Taupitz M, Hamm B, Lembcke A. Gadofosveset trisodium-enhanced magnetic resonance angiography of the left atrium–a feasibility study. *Eur J Radiol.* 2010; 75(2):166–72.

29. Allgayer C, Zellweger MJ, Sticherling C, Haller S, Weber O, Buser PT, Bremerich J. Optimization of imaging before pulmonary vein isolation by radiofrequency ablation: breath-held ungated versus ECG/breath-gated MRA. *Eur Radiol.* 2008; 18(12):2879–84.

30. Ohno Y, Adachi S, Motoyama A, Kusumoto M, Hatabu H, Sugimura K, Kono M. Multiphase ECG-triggered 3D contrast-enhanced MR angiography: utility for evaluation of hilar and mediastinal invasion of bronchogenic carcinoma. *J Magn Reson Imaging.* 2001; 13(2):215–24.

31. Wang Y, Riederer SJ, Ehman RL. Respiratory motion of the heart: kinematics and the implications for the spatial resolution in coronary imaging. *Magn Reson Med.* 1995; 33(5):713–19.

32. Block KT, Uecker M, Frahm J. Undersampled radial MRI with multiple coils. Iterative image reconstruction using a total variation constraint. *Magn Reson Med.* 2007; 57(6):1086–98.

33. Lustig M, Donoho D, Pauly JM, Sparse MRI. The application of compressed sensing for rapid MR imaging. *Magn Reson Med.* 2007; 58(6):1182–95.

34. Akcakaya M, Rayatzadeh H, Basha TA, Hong SN, Chan RH, Kissinger KV, Hauser TH, Josephson ME, Manning WJ, Nezafat R. Accelerated late gadolinium enhancement cardiac MR imaging with isotropic spatial resolution using compressed sensing: initial experience. *Radiology.* 2012; 264(3):691–99.

35. Roujol S, Basha TA, Akcakaya M, Foppa M, Chan RH, Kissinger KV, Goddu B, Berg S, Manning WJ, Nezafat R. 3D late gadolinium enhancement in a single prolonged breath-hold using supplemental oxygenation and hyperventilation. *Magn Reson Med.* 2014; 72(3):850–57.

36. Akcakaya M, Basha TA, Chan RH, Rayatzadeh H, Kissinger KV, Goddu B, Goepfert LA, Manning WJ, Nezafat R. Accelerated contrast-enhanced whole-heart coronary MRI using low-dimensional-structure self-learning and thresholding. *Magn Reson Med.* 2012; 67(5):1434–43.

37. Look DC, Locker DR. Time saving in measurement of NMR and EPR relaxation times. *Rev Sci Instrum.* 1970; 41(2):250–51.

38. Moghari MH, Goddu B, Kissinger KV, Goepfert L, Manning WJ, Nezafat R. *Estimation of Respiratory Tracking Factor between Pulmonary Vein and Right Hemi-Diaphragm For Free-breathing PV LGE.* Montreal, QC: ISMRM; 2011: p. 4552.

39. Moghari MH, Peters DC, Smink J, Goepfert L, Kissinger KV, Goddu B, Hauser TH, Josephson ME, Manning WJ, Nezafat R. Pulmonary vein inflow artifact reduction for free-breathing left atrium late gadolinium enhancement. *Magn Reson Med.* 2011; 66(1):180–86.

40. Akcakaya M, Basha TA, Goddu B, Goepfert LA, Kissinger KV, Tarokh V, Manning WJ, Nezafat R. Low-dimensional-structure self-learning and thresholding: regularization beyond compressed sensing for MRI reconstruction. *Magn Reson Med.* 2011; 66(3):756–67.

41. Akcakaya M, Basha TA, Chan RH, Manning WJ, Nezafat R. Accelerated isotropic sub-millimeter whole-heart coronary MRI: Compressed sensing versus parallel imaging. *Magn Reson Med.* 2014; 71(2):815–22.

42. Basha TA, Roujol S, Kissinger KV, Goddu B, Nezafat R. Software platform for flexible automated reconstruction of CMR data in a clinically feasible workflow. *J Cardiovasc Magn Reson.* 2014; 16(Suppl 1):W9.

43. Roujol S, Basha TA, Tan A, Khanna V, Chan RH, Moghari MH, Rayatzadeh H, Shaw JL, Josephson ME, Nezafat R. Improved multimodality data fusion of late gadolinium enhancement MRI to left ventricular voltage maps in ventricular tachycardia ablation. *IEEE Trans Biomed Eng.* 2013; 60(5):1308–17.

44. Roujol S, Basha TA, Tan AY, Anter E, Buxton AE, Josephson ME, Nezafat R. Feasibility of real time integration of high-resolution scar images with invasive electrograms in electro-anatomical mapping system in patients undergoing ventricular tachycardia ablation. *J Cardiovasc Magn Reson.* 2013; 15(Suppl 1):E94.

45. Larson AC, Kellman P, Arai A, Hirsch GA, McVeigh E, Li D, Simonetti OP. Preliminary investigation of respiratory self-gating for free-breathing segmented cine MRI. *Magn Reson Med.* 2005; **53**(1):159–68.

46. Shea SM, Kroeker RM, Deshpande V, Laub G, Zheng J, Finn JP, Li D. Coronary artery imaging: 3D segmented k-space data acquisition with multiple breath-holds and real-time slab following. *J Magn Reson Imaging.* 2001; **13**(2):301–07.

47. Lim RP, Winchester PA, Bruno MT, Xu J, Storey P, McGorty K, Sodickson DK, Srichai MB. Highly accelerated single breath-hold noncontrast thoracic MRA: evaluation in a clinical population. *Invest Radiol.* 2013; **48**(3):145–51.

48. Xu J, McGorty KA, Lim RP, Bruno M, Babb JS, Srichai MB, Kim D, Sodickson DK. Single breathhold noncontrast thoracic MRA using highly accelerated parallel imaging with a 32-element coil array. *J Magn Reson Imaging.* 2012; **35**(4):963–68.

49. Trzasko J, Manduca A. Highly undersampled magnetic resonance image reconstruction via homotopic I(0) -minimization. *IEEE Trans Med Imaging.* 2009; **28**(1):106–21.

50. Akcakaya M, Nam S, Hu P, Moghari MH, Ngo LH, Tarokh V, Manning WJ, Nezafat R. Compressed sensing with wavelet domain dependencies for coronary MRI: a retrospective study. *IEEE Trans Med Imaging.* 2011; **30**(5):1090–99.

51. Lustig M, Pauly JM. SPIRiT: Iterative self-consistent parallel imaging reconstruction from arbitrary k-space. *Magn Reson Med.* 2010; **64**(2):457–71.

52. Moghari MH, Akcakaya M, O'Connor A, Basha TA, Casanova M, Stanton D, Goepfert L, Kissinger KV, Goddu B, Chuang ML, Tarokh V, Manning WJ, Nezafat R. Compressed-sensing motion compensation (CosMo): a joint prospective-retrospective respiratory navigator for coronary MRI. *Magn Reson Med.* 2011; **66**(6):1674–81.

54. Hu P, Chan J, Ngo LH, Smink J, Goddu B, Kissinger KV, Goepfert L, Hauser TH, Rofsky NM, Manning WJ, Nezafat R. Contrast-enhanced whole-heart coronary MRI with bolus infusion of gadobenate dimeglumine at 1.5 T. *Magn Reson Med.* 2011; **65**(2):392–98.

54. Kecskemeti S, Johnson K, Francois CJ, Schiebler ML, Unal O. Volumetric late gadolinium-enhanced myocardial imaging with retrospective inversion time selection. *J Magn Reson Imaging.* 2013; **38**(5):1276–82.

55. Keegan J, Drivas P, Firmin DN: Navigator artifact reduction in three-dimensional late gadolinium enhancement imaging of the atria. *Magn Reson Med* 2013, doi:10.1002/mrm.24967.

19

Computed tomography angiography vs 3 T black-blood cardiovascular magnetic resonance for identification of symptomatic carotid plaques

Jochen M Grimm[1,2*†], Andreas Schindler[1†], Florian Schwarz[1], Clemens C Cyran[1], Anna Bayer-Karpinska[3], Tobias Freilinger[4], Chun Yuan[5], Jennifer Linn[6], Miguel Trelles[7], Maximilian F Reiser[1], Konstantin Nikolaou[1] and Tobias Saam[1]

Abstract

Background: The purpose of this prospective study was to perform a head-to-head comparison of the two methods most frequently used for evaluation of carotid plaque characteristics: Multi-detector Computed Tomography Angiography (MDCTA) and black-blood 3 T-cardiovascular magnetic resonance (bb-CMR) with respect to their ability to identify symptomatic carotid plaques.

Methods: 22 stroke unit patients with unilateral symptomatic carotid disease and >50% stenosis by duplex ultrasound underwent MDCTA and bb-CMR (TOF, pre- and post-contrast fsT1w-, and fsT2w- sequences) within 15 days of symptom onset. Both symptomatic and contralateral asymptomatic sides were evaluated. By bb-CMR, plaque morphology, composition and prevalence of complicated AHA type VI lesions (AHA-LT6) were evaluated. By MDCTA, plaque type (non-calcified, mixed, calcified), plaque density in HU and presence of ulceration and/or thrombus were evaluated. Sensitivity (SE), specificity (SP), positive and negative predictive value (PPV, NPV) were calculated using a 2-by-2-table.

Results: To distinguish between symptomatic and asymptomatic plaques AHA-LT6 was the best CMR variable and presence/absence of plaque ulceration was the best CT variable, resulting in a SE, SP, PPV and NPV of 80%, 80%, 80% and 80% for AHA-LT6 as assessed by bb-CMR and 40%, 95%, 89% and 61% for plaque ulceration as assessed by MDCTA. The combined SE, SP, PPV and NPV of bb-CMR and MDCTA was 85%, 75%, 77% and 83%, respectively.

Conclusions: Bb-CMR is superior to MDCTA at identifying symptomatic carotid plaques, while MDCTA offers high specificity at the cost of low sensitivity. Results were only slightly improved over bb-CMR alone when combining both techniques.

Keywords: Plaque imaging, Ischemic stroke, Atherosclerosis, Symptomatic carotid plaque, CT, Cardiovascular magnetic resonance

* Correspondence: jochen.grimm@chuv.ch
†Equal contributors
[1]Institute for Clinical Radiology, Ludwig-Maximilians-University Hospital Munich, Munich, Germany
[2]Department of Medical Radiology, University Hospital and University of Lausanne, Lausanne, Switzerland
Full list of author information is available at the end of the article

Background

Extracranial large vessel disease is held responsible for cerebral ischemic insults in up to 20% of cases [1]. It has been shown that stenosis alone is not always a reliable marker in the assessment of a plaque's causality for stroke [2]. There is increasing evidence that plaque morphologic aspects should be taken into consideration to assess a plaque's vulnerability [3-5]. Accordingly, previous studies involving CT angiography or high-resolution cardiovascular magnetic resonance (CMR) have identified morphologic markers, representing plaque instability.

Using parallel imaging techniques and dedicated surface-coils 3 T high-resolution black-blood CMR (bb-CMR) is capable of reliably assessing plaque prevalence, morphology and composition, allowing lesion classification according to the modified AHA classification [6-10]. High-resolution plaque imaging with modern multi-detector CT angiography (MDCTA) delivers high spatial resolution and also allows reliable assessment of plaque prevalence, size, surface configuration and – to some extent – composition in plaques with a low grade of calcification [11,12].

Using CMR plaque imaging the plaque characteristics most closely associated with symptomatic plaques are incorporated into lesion type VI according to the modified AHA classification (AHA-LT6), comprised of its defining features ruptured fibrous cap, intraplaque hemorrhage and juxtaluminal hemorrhage/thrombus. Each of these features as well as the general classification as AHA-LT6 plaque have shown an association with ipsilateral ischemic cerebral events [13-15]. MDCTA is reported to have shown a correlation of plaque surface irregularities (e.g. ulceration), plaque density and degree of calcification with ipsilateral symptoms [16-19]. Thus, both MDCTA and CMR are able to detect differences in plaque characteristics between symptomatic and asymptomatic plaques.

The purpose of this prospective study was to perform a head-to-head comparison of MDCTA and bb-CMR with respect to their ability to identify symptomatic carotid plaques.

Methods

This study was performed in accordance with local regulatory legislation and approved by the institutional review board. The methods used in the study were in accordance with the ethical standards laid down in the Declarations of Helsinki. This study was conducted in collaboration with the stroke unit of the Department of Neurology of the Ludwig-Maximilians-University Munich in 2008–2010. All subjects gave written informed consent.

Patients

We examined 44 internal carotid arteries of 22 consecutive patients. Only subjects with acute ischemic stroke in the vascular area of an internal carotid artery with >50%

stenosis as determined by duplex sonography were included in this study. The percentage of carotid stenosis was obtained using the NASCET method [20]. Ischemic stroke was defined as an acute lesion on diffusion weighted brain MR images (DWI) with a corresponding acute neurological deficit of more than 24 hours duration. The symptomatic artery was defined as being ipsilateral to the DWI lesion. The carotid arteries contralateral to the affected brain hemisphere served as asymptomatic control group. All patients underwent extensive clinical workup (lab, brain CMR, brain CT combined with MDCTA of the carotids, duplex sonography of the cervical arteries, 24-hour ECG, transoesophageal echocardiography) to determine the etiology of the ischemic stroke. Inclusion and exclusion criteria are summarized in Table 1.

Data acquisition
CMR
Imaging of all subjects was performed using a 3.0-T scanner (Magnetom Verio, Siemens Healthcare, Erlangen, Germany). To improve image quality, a dedicated four-channel surface carotid coil (Machnet, Elde, Netherlands) was used. The carotid coil was combined with a head coil and a head holder that prevented involuntary head movement during the scans.

Both the symptomatic and asymptomatic carotid arteries were imaged using a previously presented multi-sequence-protocol (time-of-flight (TOF), T2-, and, pre- and post-

Table 1 Inclusion/Exclusion criteria

Inclusion criteria	Ischemic stroke (acute DWI[a] lesion and corresponding acute neurological deficit of >24 h duration) in the territory of the anterior or middle cerebral artery <15 days before both MDCTA[b] and black-blood carotid CMR[c]
	Stenosing (i.e. luminal obstruction > 50% according to NASCET[d] criteria) atherosclerotic plaque in the internal carotid artery of the symptomatic side as determined by duplex sonography
Exclusion criteria	Stroke etiology other than large vessel disease
	Bilateral infarcts on cerebral
	Known contraindications against CMR or MDCTA
	Allergy to contrast material
	Impaired renal function (glomerular filtration rate < 30 ml/min)
	Previous radiation therapy to head or neck
	Surgical procedure within 24 h before bb-CMR
	Previous interventional or surgical manipulation of the symptomatic carotid artery (e.g. stenting, endarterectomy)
	Insufficient image quality in bb-CMR or MDCTA

[a]DWI = diffusion-weighted imaging [b]MDCTA = multi detector computed tomography angiography [c]CMR = cardiovascular magnetic resonance.
[d]NASCET = North American Symptomatic Carotid Endarterectomy Trial.

contrast T1-weighted) [21], proton density weighted images were not evaluated due to limited additional value for the present study. Best in-plane resolution was 0.5×0.5 mm^2. Images were acquired in segments of 3.0 cm (2 mm slice-thickness $\times$ 15), centered on the carotid bifurcation. This coverage is usually sufficient to image the whole atherosclerotic carotid plaque [22]. Parallel imaging based on the generalized auto calibrating partially parallel acquisition (GRAPPA) algorithm was used for all sequences with a parallel acquisition technique (PAT) acceleration factor of 2. Post-contrast T1w images were acquired 5 minutes after injection of 0.1 mmol/kg (0.1 ml/kg) Gadolinium-DO3A-butrol (GADOVIST®, Bayer Schering, Leverkusen, Germany) over an intravenous catheter in an antecubital vein. Total scan time was 17:43 min.

CT angiography

As stroke patient assessment is performed by several units in our clinical center, scans were performed on various CT scanners: Bright Speed S (GE Healthcare), Aquilion (Toshiba), Somatom Definition Flash (Siemens), Somatom Definition AS + (Siemens), Sensation 64 (Siemens). All MDCTA images were obtained with coverage at least from the aortic arch to the cranium using the respective standard protocol parameters, notably a collimation of 0.625 mm or less. Non-ionic iodinated contrast material was applied intravenously adjusted to patient weight (Ultravist 370, Bayer Schering Pharma, Berlin, Germany, i.e. 0.35-0.50 g iodine per kg bodyweight at an injection rate of 4.5-6 ml/s followed by 100 ml saline at identical flow). Axial images were reconstructed to volume rendered (VR) images, which has been reported to improve depiction of carotid plaque ulceration if used additionally to axial scans [23]. Bone and soft tissue impairing the 360° view of the bifurcation were manually removed from the images. In order to prevent biases in the further reviewing process, anonymized images of the right and left carotid arteries were stored separately.

Image review

All images were reviewed by two radiologists with 4 and 11 years of experience blinded to the patient's clinical history. Classification was reached in consensus. Images of all patients' left carotid arteries were reviewed first, followed by all images of the right side, in random order.

Image quality of each examination was rated on a five-point scale (1 = very poor, 2 = poor, 3 = acceptable, 4 = good, 5 = excellent) and cases with image quality <3 were excluded. All following analyses were performed on axial images.

On CMR images area-measurements of lumen, wall, and components were obtained using the image analysis tool CASCADE (University of Washington, Seattle, US). T1w images were used for obtaining values for lumen,

vessel wall and total vessel area. The normalized wall index (NWI) was calculated by dividing the wall area by the total vessel area. Atherosclerotic tissue components (lipid-rich necrotic core, hemorrhage, fibrous tissue, calcification) were identified and quantified based on previously published criteria [24]. For definition of a complicated AHA-LT6 plaque according to the modified AHA classification [8], at least one of the following three criteria was required: ruptured fibrous cap, intraplaque hemorrhage or juxtaluminal hemorrhage/thrombus.

For MDCTA window settings were adjusted depending on image properties to optimize the delineation of plaque properties [19]. The relative content of calcification in the stenotic plaque (calcification/tissue <40% vs. >40%) was visually quantified and categorized. As a high grade of calcification can cause beam hardening artifacts and thus spoil measurements in adjacent tissue [25], tissue density was not measured in plaques containing calcifications >40%. MDCTA images were evaluated for presence of plaque, plaque density/plaque type, surface configuration, calcification and thrombus. Plaque type was categorized as non-calcified, mixed, and calcified. Calcification volume in mm^3 was determined using the standard plug-in on a Syngo MultiModality Workplace (software version VE36A, Siemens Healthcare, Erlangen, Germany).

Tissue attenuation was measured in representative non-calcified plaque regions using several manually drawn ellipsoid regions of interest (ROI) per axial slice encompassing at least approximately 75% of the plaque area. Depending on plaque size, 4 to 16 ROIs with an area of up to 2 mm^2 were drawn. During this procedure calcifications and the contrast enhanced lumen were carefully avoided. The average HU of the measured ROIs on each axial slice was recorded. From this, a mean representative HU-value for the whole plaque was calculated. Based on the mean plaque HU, plaque type was categorized as follows: non-calcified plaque associated with lipid-rich necrotic core <60 HU, mixed plaque associated with fibrous tissue 60–130 HU and calcified plaque >130 HU [26]. Plaques with calcification >40% were not measured and rated as calcified plaques. Outpouching of contrast material into or adjacent to the plaque of < 1 was considered a surface irregularity, whereas ≥1 mm was considered ulceration [27].

Data analysis

Area measurements for each artery are given as average, minimum or maximum absolute areas, as appropriate. Plaque components are calculated as percentages of the vessel wall. Categorical variables are presented as absolute frequencies, while continuous variables are presented as mean ± [SD]. Wilcoxon's signed-rank test was used to test differences for continuous variablesthe McNemar test was used to determine differences between categorical variables. Kruskal-Wallis test was used if more than two categories were present, e.g. degree of stenosis and of calcification. Statistical evaluation was performed using SPSS version 16.0 (IBM, Armonk, USA). A p-value of <0.05 was considered statistically significant. Sensitivity, specificity positive and negative predictive values as well as odds ratios were calculated using a 2-by-2 table.

Results

Patients

CT-Scans were of diagnostic quality in all subjects with a mean image quality of 4.3 [±0.65]. 20 out of 22 of the CMR examinations had an IQ ≥ 3 (90.9%) with a mean image quality of 4.2 [±0.62]. Two patients had to be excluded due to severe motion artifacts. Consequently, a total of 20 patients with 40 carotid arteries could be included and evaluated in the study. Table 2 shows general patient characteristics and cardiovascular risk factors.

CMR

CMR detected a total of 20 AHA-LT6 plaques, of which 16 (80%) were located on the symptomatic side and 4 (20%) on the asymptomatic side. This difference was statistically significant (p < 0.001). Of AHA-LT6 plaques, a ruptured fibrous cap was found more frequently on the symptomatic than the asymptomatic side (12/20 (60%) vs. 1/20 (5%); p < 0.001) (Table 3). With respect to the degree of stenosis, AHA-LT6 plaques were found in 14 out of 19 arteries (74%) with high degree stenosis (70-99% stenosis) and in 6 out of 11 arteries (55%) with low grade stenosis (50-69%; p = 0.43). No AHA-LT6 plaques were encountered in vessels with a stenosis <50%. The quantitative evaluation showed a larger normalized wall index (NWI 0.88 vs. 0.78p = 0.008), and a tendency towards a smaller luminal area for symptomatic plaques

Table 2 Demographics

Variable	Value (mean [±SD[a]] or N (%))
Age [years]	**69.9 [±8,8]**
Male sex	15 (75%)
Body mass index [kg/m^2]	26.0 [±2,5]
Cardiovascular risk factors	
Nicotine abuse	
Current	5 (25%)
Former	7 (35%)
Hypertension	14 (70%)
Diabetes	4 (20%)
Hypercholesterolemia	12 (60%)
Coronary artery disease	3 (15%)
Family history of cardiovascular disease	4 (20%)

[a]SD = Standard Deviation.

Table 3 Plaque characteristics

	Symptomatic side	Asymptomatic side	P-value
Vessel Stenosis			
< 50% [N(%)]	0	10 (50%)	<0.001
50 – 69% [N(%)]	8 (40%)	3 (15%)	0.16
70 – 99% [N(%)]	12 (60%)	7 (35%)	0.21
Qualitative CMR Plaque Characteristics			
AHA Lesion Type VI [N(%)]	16 (80%)	4 (20%)	<0.001
Thin/ruptured fibrous cap [N(%)]	12 (60%)	1 (5%)	<0.001
Intraplaque hemorrhage [N(%)]	9 (45%)	4 (20%)	n.s.
Juxtaluminal hemorrhage/ thrombus [N(%)]	6 (30%)	1 (5%)	n.s.
Quantitative CMR Plaque Characteristics			
Mean lumen area [mm^2]	6.5 ± 4.3	10.8 ± 7.5	0.05
Mean wall area [mm^2]	72.2 ± 28.3	64.6 ± 20.9	0.17
Mean total vessel area [mm^2]	111.1 ± 43.4	102.3 ± 36.4	0.27
NWI[a]	0.88 ± 0.07	0.78 ± 0.11	0.008
Lipid rich necrotic core [%]	24.5 ± 12.9	14.5 ± 14	0.08
Calcification [%]	3.6 ± 5.2	7.3 ± 6.3	0.03
Intraplaque hemorrhage [%]	11.4 ± 17	2.1 ± 4.5	0.03
MDCTA[b] Characteristics			
Plaque Type			
Non-calcified [N(%)]	12 (60%)	7 (35%)	n.s.
Mixed [N(%)]	5 (25%)	10 (50%)	n.s.
Calcified [N(%)]	3 (15%)	3 (15%)	n.s.
CT Calcification Volume [mm^3]	0.082	0.0735	n.s.

[a] NWI = normalized wall index.
[b]MDCTA = multi detector computed tomography angiography.

compared to the asymptomatic side (6.5 ± 4.3 mm^2 vs. 10.8 ± 7.5mm^2; p = 0.05). Plaque composition differed significantly between the symptomatic and asymptomatic side: The relative area of intraplaque hemorrhage was significantly larger on the symptomatic side (11.4 ± 17% vs. 2.1 ± 4.5%; p = 0.03) (Table 3). Relative area of calcification was smaller in the symptomatic group than in the asymptomatic group (3.6 ± 5.2% vs. 7.3 ± 6.3%; p = 0.03). No other statistically significant differences were found.

Figures 1, 2, and 3 show black-blood CMR and MDCTA imaging examples of symptomatic (Figures 1 and 2) and asymptomatic (Figure 3) carotid plaques.

Computed tomography

Vessels/plaque

Plaques were detected in all symptomatic vessels (20/20, 100%), while two vessels of the asymptomatic side showed no sign of atherosclerosis (18/20, 90%; p = 0.49). Plaque types on the symptomatic vs. asymptomatic side as

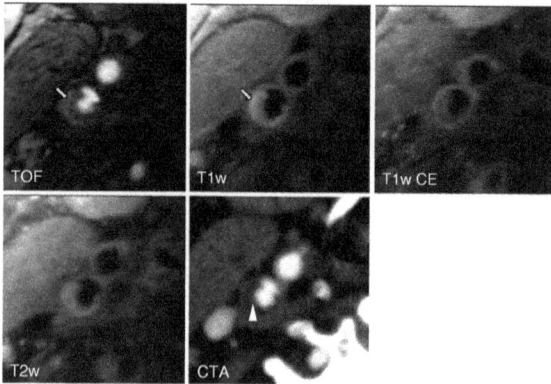

Figure 1 Shows axial TOF, T1 weighted pre- and post-contrast and T2 weighted high-resolution black-blood CMR and CTA (lower right) images of an ulcerated plaque in the right internal carotid artery of an 87-year old male patient with an acute ischemic stroke in the territory of the right middle cerebral artery. Note the clearly ulcerated plaque surface on both CMR and CTA images as well as the hypersignal of the plaque in TOF and T1 weighted images corresponding to intraplaque hemorrhage (arrow). A lack of contrast enhancement within the plaque indicates the presence of a lipid-rich necrotic core. CTA shows a non-calcified plaque with relatively hypodense plaque interior (mean plaque density = 34,5HUarrowhead).

detected by CT were distributed as follows: non-calcified plaque 12 (60%) vs. 7 (35%; p = 0.21) mixed plaque 5 (25%) vs. 10 (50%; p = 0.19) and calcified plaque 3 (15%) vs. 3 (15%; p = 1) (Table 3). Calcification volumes were not significantly different between the symptomatic (0.0820 ± 0.159 mm^3) and the asymptomatic (0.0735 ± 0.077 mm^3) side (p = 0.22). Degrees of stenosis on the symptomatic vs. asymptomatic side according to the NASCET criteria were distributed as follows: <50% stenosis 0 (0%) vs. 10 (50%; p < 0.001), 50-69% stenosis 8 (40%) vs. 3 (15%; p = 0.16) and 70-99% stenosis 12 (60%) vs. 7 (35%; p = 0.21). Kruskal-Wallis test for degree of stenosis yielded an adjusted H of 13.2, corresponding to a p-value of <0.001. Differences between groups were calculated using the McNemar test (Table 3). Stenosis <50% was only encountered in asymptomatic carotids. None of the vessels were occluded.

Surface

CT showed 8 vessels with ulceration on the symptomatic side (40%) and one (5%) in an asymptomatic internal carotid artery (p = 0.005). Multiple ulcerations within one vessel were not observed. In one case we found ulcers in both carotid arteries. The proportion of ulcerations in all arteries was not significantly different between 50-69% stenoses (3/11, 27%) compared to stenoses of 70-99% (6/19, 32%; p = 1).

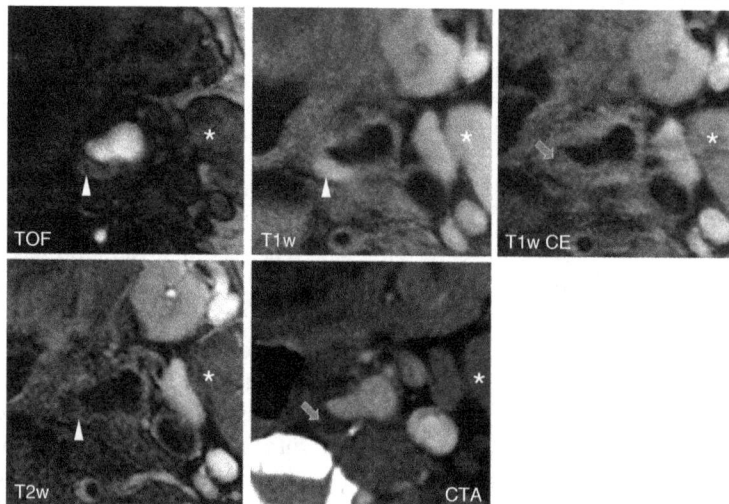

Figure 2 Shows axial TOF, T1 weighted pre and post contrast and T2 weighted high-resolution black-blood CMR and CTA (lower right) images of a plaque in the left internal carotid artery of a patient with an acute ischemic stroke on the left side. While both CMR and CT images fail to show a distinct surface defect, the fibrous cap is not entirely distinguishable and was therefore by definition classified as thin. The hyperintense signal within the plaque in TOF and T1 weighted images in combination with hypointense signal in the T2 weighted image corresponds to an intraplaque hemorrhage (arrowhead). The relative lack of contrast enhancement within the plaque indicates the presence of a lipid-rich necrotic core (arrow). Correspondingly, the CTA image shows a relatively hypodense plaque interior (mean plaque density = 65,1 HU). The hyperdense area in the dorsal wall of the plaque corresponds to a hypointense signal in the MR images and is consistent with a marginal calcification. *Sternocleid muscle.

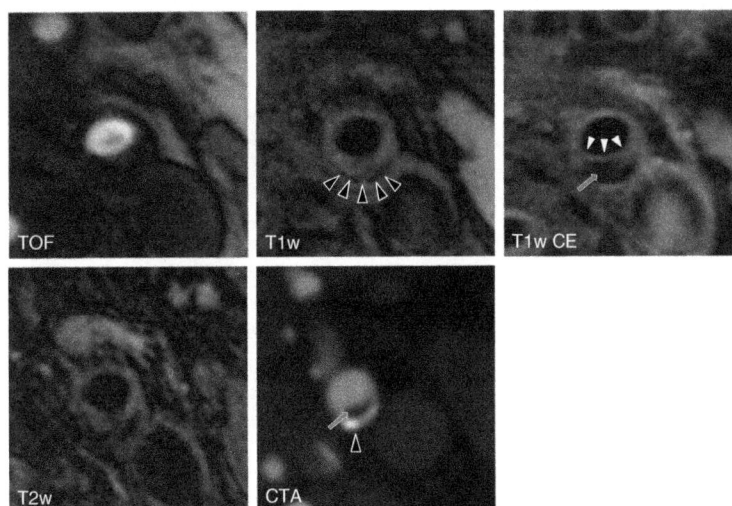

Figure 3 Shows axial TOF, T1 weighted pre- and post- contrast and T2 weighted high-resolution black-blood CMR and CTA (lower right) images of a stable carotid plaque on the asymptomatic left side in a 66 year old patient who had suffered from right hemispheric stroke. Both CMR and CTA images show the presence of an AHA lesion type 7 plaque in the dorsal wall of the left proximal internal carotid artery. After administration of contrast material the thick fibrous cap is delineated as a hyperintense rim in the T1 weighted contrast enhanced images, separating the plaque from the lumen (white arrowheads). Also note the hypointense signal of the plaque interior in the T1 weighted contrast enhanced image as well as the hypodense area in the CTA image corresponding to a large lipid-rich necrotic core (arrow), measured at 166 HU, probably due to blooming artifacts caused by its calcified portion. The hypointense rim in the peripheral plaque in all MR sequences and the corresponding hyperdense area in the CTA image indicate the presence of a calcification (black arrowheads).

Tissue density and calcification

Symptomatic plaques had a significantly lower density compared to asymptomatic plaques (48.9 ± 15.6 HU vs. 61.8 ± 15.6 HU; $p = 0.046$). Kruskal-Wallis and McNemar tests revealed no significant differences between symptomatic and asymptomatic plaques regarding presence of calcification. Calcification volume was not significantly different between symptomatic and asymptomatic plaques.

Thrombus

Using MDCTA we could observe the 'donut sign' - a filling defect within the lumen completely surrounded by contrast media indicating presence of a thrombus - in only one of the 20 symptomatic carotid arteries (5%) versus none in the asymptomatic arteries (0%).

Best predictors

AHA-LT6 as single predictor for the symptomatic side resulted in a sensitivity, specificity, PPV and a NPV of 80%,

80%, 80% and 80%, respectively, yielding an accuracy of 80% and an odds ratio of 16.0 (95% confidence interval: 2.8-108.9). With CMR, 4 out of 20 symptomatic plaques were not predicted correctly. In one of these 4 patients, MDCTA was able to detect an ulcerated plaque.

When a thin or ruptured fibrous cap was used as single predictor, sensitivity, specificity, PPV and NPV were 60%, 95%, 92% and 70%, respectively. The accuracy was calculated at 77.5% the odds ratio was 28.5 (95% confidence interval 3.2-257.5).

Using ulceration in MDCTA as single predictor for the symptomatic side led to a sensitivity, specificity, PPV and a NPV of 40%, 95%, 89% and 61%, accuracy of 67.5% and an odds ratio of 12.7 (95% confidence interval: 1.3-306).

Ulcer as detected in CT combined with AHA-LT6 Plaque in CMR led to a sensitivity of 85%, specificity of 75%, a PPV of 77% and a NPV of 83%, yielding an accuracy of 80% and an odds ratio of 17.0 (95% confidence interval: 2.8-121.2; Table 4).

Table 4 Best predictors for the symptomatic side

	Sensitivity	Specificity	PPV	NPV	Odds ratio
Ulceration (MDCTA[a])	40%	95%	89%	61%	12.7
AHA-LT6[b] (CMR[c])	80%	80%	80%	80%	16.0
Ulceration and AHA-LT6 (CTA + CMR)	85%	75%	77%	83%	17.0
Thin/ruptured fibrous cap	60%	95%	92%	70%	28.5

[a]MDCTA = multi detector computed tomography angiography.
[b]AHA-LT6 = American Heart Association lesion type VI.
[c]CMR = cardiovascular magnetic resonance.

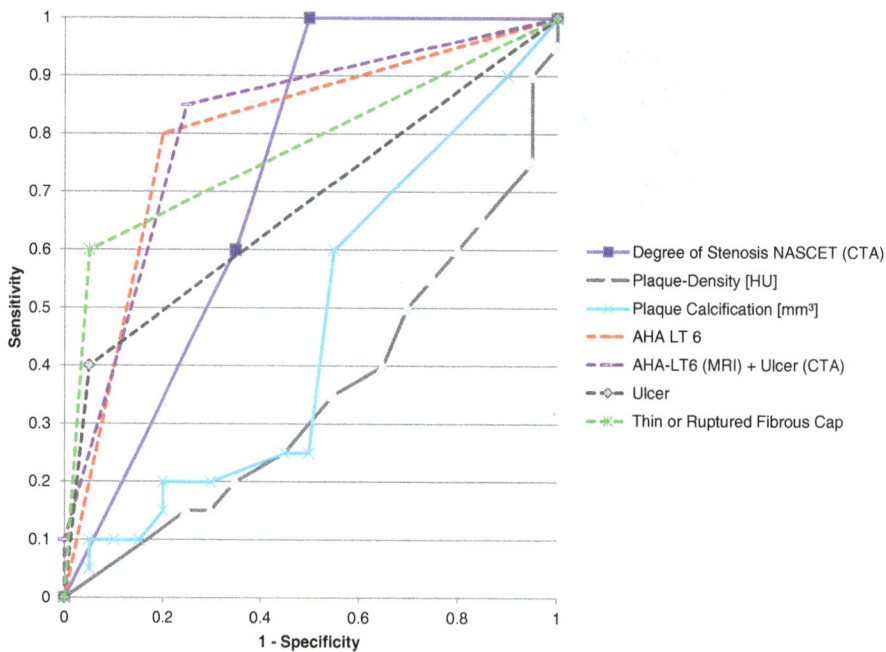

Figure 4 Shows the ROC graph of various variables. Lines are dotted where only one value was present. Note that especially AHA-LT6 with and without ulcer in CTA as well as thin or ruptured fibrous cap show high sensitivity and specificity, while plaque density in HU and volume of calcification are not suitable as predictors of the symptomatic side.

The ROC graph in Figure 4 gives an overview over the presented variables and their respective sensitivity and specificity.

Discussion

This study shows that both MDCTA and bb-CMR of the carotid arteries are able to detect differences between symptomatic and asymptomatic plaques in patients with ischemic large vessel stroke. CMR using AHA-LT6 as single criterion showed higher sensitivity, negative predictive value and accuracy than ulceration as the best MDCTA variable while the latter delivered a better specificity and positive predictive value but suffered from a low sensitivity. Even better specificity and positive predictive values were found when using a thin or ruptured fibrous cap as detected on bb-CMR as single predictor. Prediction of the symptomatic side was minimally enhanced when information from both MDCTA and CMR were combined.

AHA-LT6

Complicated AHA-LT6 plaques were more frequently encountered in symptomatic than in asymptomatic arteries (80% vs. 20%, p < 0.001). Consequently type III, IV, V and VII, which reflect clinically more stable plaques, were more common in asymptomatic vessels. These results are in line with findings of Saam et al. who found a statistically significant association between complicated AHA-LT6 carotid plaques and ipsilateral symptoms in a

cohort of 23 symptomatic patients who underwent CMR-plaque imaging [13]. This makes AHA-LT6 a useful parameter for risk assessment in atherosclerotic carotid plaques. In our study, as a single criterion, the presence of an AHA-LT6 plaque proved to be the best overall predictor for the symptomatic side.

We noted a greater frequency of AHA-LT6 plaques in high degree stenoses compared to low degree stenoses. Even though not statistically significant, this result is in line with findings of previous studies [28,29], which report an increasing prevalence of vulnerable plaques with increasing degree of stenosis.

Ulceration

Former studies could show that ulceration of the carotid arteries is associated with cerebral lesions and is encountered more frequently in symptomatic patients [17,30-32]. The present study found ulcerations with a prevalence of 40% in symptomatic carotid arteries and in 5% of the asymptomatic arteries. Overall prevalence of ulceration was 32% in high grade stenoses (70-99%), 27% in low grade stenoses (50-69%) and 0% in non-stenosed arteries. The reported prevalence of plaque ulceration in our study is similar to the NASCET study, which reported ulcerations in 35% of vessels with a stenosis >70% as detected by DSA [33].

In our study, using ulceration in MDCTA as the sole predictor for the symptomatic side led to a relatively low sensitivity but a high specificity. The lower sensitivity may be explained by the fact that other mechanisms that are hard to detect in MDCTA, such as rupture of the fibrous cap or intraplaque hemorrhage potentially followed by thrombus formation and consequent embolisation may also cause cerebrovascular incidents.

Other factors

While other plaque properties analyzed in this study failed to reach the predictive power of AHA-LT6 or plaque ulceration, they may still be useful for plaque characterization and general risk assessment.

Analysis of the plaque density showed that plaques on the symptomatic side had significantly lower HU values than asymptomatic plaques. This may be due to higher lipid content and confirms the findings of other studies by Saba et al. [30] and Serfaty et al. [25] which both found a statistically significant association between fatty plaque or decreased plaque density and neurological symptoms in cohorts of 112 and 141 patients. Trelles et al. similarly found a greater thickness of the non-calcified plaque component in AHA-LT6 plaques in a study on 51 stroke patients [34]. These results are also in line with previous observations in coronary plaques which suggested that plaques with a large lipid-rich/necrotic core strongly correlate with formation of thrombi and plaque disruption [35]. Despite these differences in HU, a reliable cut-off point to distinguish symptomatic from asymptomatic plaques has not yet been determined [19].

Juxtaluminal hemorrhage/thrombus impose a high risk of distal embolization and thus thrombotic occlusion of a distal vessel. In a previous histological study with 241 patients Fisher et al. observed that thrombus is highly associated with ipsilateral symptoms and plaque ulceration (p < 0.005) [33]. Using MDCTA we could identify a fresh thrombus ("donut sign") in only one carotid artery (2.5%). CMR, however, showed juxtaluminal hemorrhage/thrombus in 30% of the symptomatic and 5% of the asymptomatic arteries. Our study thus shows that for detection of juxtaluminal hemorrhage/thrombus CMR is more sensitive than MDCTA, a fact that may be attributed to MDCTA's comparatively poor soft tissue contrast and its inability to identify the fibrous cap and intraplaque hemorrhage. In 6 out of 7 cases thrombi detected by CMR were associated with a rupture of the fibrous cap. This supports the thesis that thrombi evolve from surface defects of plaques presenting thrombogenic components.

In our study a thin or ruptured fibrous cap itself was closely associated with the symptomatic side (OR 28.5). This may be attributed to thrombogenic potency of surface defects of the fibrous cap with subsequent formation of unstable thrombi, potentially causing embolism. Our results indicate that a thin or ruptured fibrous cap may be a more accurate predictor than juxtaluminal hemorrhage/thrombus. Compared to AHA-LT6, a thin

or ruptured fibrous cap as single predictor showed superior specificity and positive predictive value, while sensitivity and negative predictive value were inferior. Because of its high specificity and positive predictive value a thin or ruptured fibrous cap may be a factor to be considered separately.

Bb-CMR or MDCTA?

Based on the data of our study bb-CMR is better suited than MDCTA to identify symptomatic carotid plaques. This is mainly owed to the better detection of subtle plaque features on bb-CMR. In order to further assess the potential of bb-CMR, several prospective studies, such as the CAPIAS trial (NCT01284933) [36] or the PARISK study (NCT01208025) are currently under way which examine the ability of carotid bb-CMR to predict recurrence of ischemic stroke in patients with less than 70% stenosis.

While the diagnostic value of bb-CMR regarding the characterization of carotid plaques cannot reasonably be disputed, it is still not routinely applied in many centers. This may be attributed to a generally lower availability of suitable CMR equipment and longer scan times of bb-CMR compared to MDCTA, requiring a higher degree of patient cooperation. Another limiting factor for carotid CMR in the acute setting is the narrow time window for treating acute strokes, so examination times need to be kept reasonably short. It needs to be noted that the use of a dedicated carotid coil, which is not available at every center, enhances MR image quality. However, with careful design of the examination and its sequence parameters, image quality should be sufficient to determine the major plaque features even without such a dedicated coil.

On the other hand, MDCTA requires application of a considerable amount of ionizing radiation and, more importantly, iodinated contrast agent with the known adverse effects, especially in the patient population with cardiovascular risk factors. Logistically, bb-CMR of the carotids can be performed immediately following brain CMR with reasonable extension of the examination time, which will at least in part be compensated by avoiding a transfer of the patient between the CT and CMR device.

Limitations

One limitation of this study is the use of different CT scanners, so that examination parameters are not completely identical. We chose to include examinations from various CT scanners to increase the number of patients and accounted for possible differences in image acquisition parameters by applying a uniform image quality score to all images.

Furthermore, our study followed a cross sectional design by examining patients who were already symptomatic. To assess the predictive value of different plaque characteristics regarding the risk of future cerebrovascular events, longitudinal studies are necessary. It should be noted that our study population contains a comparatively large number of vessels with high degree stenoses. This is owed to the inclusion criteria requiring ≥50% stenosis in the artery ipsilateral to the ischemic stroke and does not represent the prevalence of high degree stenosis in the general population. It needs to be noted that we performed all tests on subjects of a symptomatic population where by definition the prevalence of symptomatic carotid plaques is 100%. This may influence the absolute validity of sensitivity, specificity, positive and negative predictive values for the reported plaque features at predicting the symptomatic side. It should, however, not significantly impair the comparability of the different predictors with each other.

3D sequences were not part of this study. While these might have increased the arterial coverage or decreased examination times, we chose to not apply them in this study because they are less well validated and may provide less spatial in-plane resolution. Furthermore, coverage of the 2D sequences used was sufficient to depict the entire plaque in each case so that it seemed safe to use the previously established 2D protocol, which has proven to deliver excellent image quality while being robust and reliable.

We did not use contrast enhanced MR angiography (CEMRA) because we performed perfusion imaging of the plaques, which was not evaluated for this study. Evaluation of CEMRA might have increased the sensitivity of CMR to detect surface irregularities in carotid plaques. However, several studies have shown that ulcerations are an unreliable predictor of patient's symptoms and we therefore believe that while CEMRA might have further accentuated the superiority of CMR, this would not have significantly changed our conclusion.

Conclusions

Bb-CMR is superior to MDCTA at detecting symptomatic plaques. Predictive power of CMR using AHA-LT6 is only slightly enhanced if combined with ulceration from MDCTA. Presence of a thin or ruptured fibrous cap on MR images may be a useful individual property for predicting the presence of symptoms due to its excellent specificity and positive predictive value. Although MDCTA has a lower sensitivity to identify the symptomatic side, it does offer some insights into plaque vulnerability and remains useful in patients who cannot undergo CMR.

Competing interests
JMG – Travel and meeting expenses by Fumedica not related to the study presented.
AS – Dr. Schindler reports no disclosures.
FS – Grants and Speakers Bureau Services not related to the study presented.
CCC – Grants by Bayer Healthcare and Novartis AGSpeakers Bureau Bayer Healthcare, all not related to the study presented.
AB – Grants and Speakers Bureau Services not related to the study presented.

TF – Grants and Speakers Bureau Services not related to the study presented.
CY – Consultancy for Bristol Myers Squibb Medical Imaging and Philips HealthcareGrants from US National Institutes of Health and Philips healthcare, all not related to the study presented.
JL – Dr. Linn reports no disclosures.
MT – Dr. Trelles reports no disclosures.
MFR – Editor in Chief of "European Radiology".
KN – Various speakers bureau services not related to this study.
TS – Grants by DFG, Diamed Medizintechnik, Pfizerpayment for lectures and service on Speakers Bureaus by Glaxo Smith Kline, MSD Merck Sharp & Dohme GmbH, all not related to the study presented.

Authors' contributions
JMG participated in data acquisition, interpretation, statistical evaluation, draft and revision of the manuscript. AS participated in patient and data acquisition, statistical evaluation, data interpretation, draft and revision of the manuscript. FS participated in designing the study and evaluating the data as well as revising the manuscript. CCC participated in patient and data acquisition and revising the manuscript. AB participated in evaluating the data and revising the manuscript. TF participated in evaluating the data and revising the manusctipt. CY participated in evaluating the data and revising the manuscript. JL participated in evaluating the data and revising the manuscript. MT participated in statistical evaluation, and data interpretation as well as revision of the manuscript. MFR participated in designing the study and revising the manuscript. KN participated in designing the study and revising the manuscript. TS participated in designing the study, acquiring and evaluating the data, and revising the manuscript. All authors read and approved the final manuscript.

Author details
[1]Institute for Clinical Radiology, Ludwig-Maximilians-University Hospital Munich, Munich, Germany. [2]Department of Medical Radiology, University Hospital and University of Lausanne, Lausanne, Switzerland. [3]Institute for Stroke and Dementia Research, Ludwig-Maximilians-University Hospital Munich, Munich, Germany. [4]Department of Neurology and Hertie Institute for Clinical Brain Research, University of Tuebingen, Tuebingen, Germany. [5]Department of Radiology, University of Washington School of Medicine, Seattle, USA. [6]Department of Neuroradiology, Ludwig-Maximilians-University Hospital Munich, Munich, Germany. [7]Department of Radiology, University of Texas Medical Branch, Galveston, USA.

References
1. Sacco RL, Kargman DE, Gu Q, Zamanillo MC. Race-ethnicity and determinants of intracranial atherosclerotic cerebral infarction. The northern manhattan stroke study. Stroke. 1995; 26:14–20.
2. Lindsay AC, Biasiolli L, Lee JM, Kylintireas I, MacIntosh BJ, Watt H, Jezzard P, Robson MD, Neubauer S, Handa A, Kennedy J, Choudhury RP. Plaque features associated with increased cerebral infarction after minor stroke and TIA: a prospective, case–control, 3-T carotid artery MR imaging study. J Am Coll Cardiol Img. 2012; 5:388–96.
3. Park AE, McCarthy WJ, Pearce WH, Matsumura JS, Yao JS. Carotid plaque morphology correlates with presenting symptomatology. J Vasc Surg. 1998; 27:872–78. discussion 878–879.
4. Ballotta E, Da Giau G, Renon L. Carotid plaque gross morphology and clinical presentation: a prospective study of 457 carotid artery specimens. J Surg Res. 2000; 89:78–84.
5. Wasserman BA, Wityk RJ, Trout HH 3rd, Virmani R. Low-grade carotid stenosis: looking beyond the lumen with MRI. Stroke. 2005; 36:2504–13.
6. Saam T, Cai JM, Cai YQ, An NY, Kampschulte A, Xu D, Kerwin WS, Takaya N, Polissar NL, Hatsukami TS, Yuan C. Carotid plaque composition differs between ethno-racial groups: an MRI pilot study comparing mainland Chinese and American Caucasian patients. Arterioscler Thromb Vasc Biol. 2005; 25:611–16.
7. Hatsukami TS, Ross R, Polissar NL, Yuan C. Visualization of fibrous cap thickness and rupture in human atherosclerotic carotid plaque in vivo with high-resolution magnetic resonance imaging. Circulation. 2000; 102:959–64.

8. Cai JM, Hatsukami TS, Ferguson MS, Small R, Polissar NL, Yuan C. Classification of human carotid atherosclerotic lesions with in vivo multicontrast magnetic resonance imaging. *Circulation.* 2002; 106:1368–73.

9. Yuan C, Mitsumori LM, Ferguson MS, Polissar NL, Echelard D, Ortiz G, Small R, Davies JW, Kerwin WS, Hatsukami TS. In vivo accuracy of multispectral magnetic resonance imaging for identifying lipid-rich necrotic cores and intraplaque hemorrhage in advanced human carotid plaques. *Circulation.* 2001; 104:2051–56.

10. Cai J, Hatsukami TS, Ferguson MS, Kerwin WS, Saam T, Chu B, Takaya N, Polissar NL, Yuan C. In vivo quantitative measurement of intact fibrous cap and lipid-rich necrotic core size in atherosclerotic carotid plaque: comparison of high-resolution, contrast-enhanced magnetic resonance imaging and histology. *Circulation.* 2005; 112:3437–44.

11. Randoux B, Marro B, Koskas F, Duyme M, Sahel M, Zouaoui A, Marsault C. Carotid artery stenosis: prospective comparison of CT, three-dimensional gadolinium-enhanced MR, and conventional angiography. *Radiology.* 2001; 220:179–85.

12. Koelemay MJ, Nederkoorn PJ, Reitsma JB, Majoie CB. Systematic review of computed tomographic angiography for assessment of carotid artery disease. *Stroke.* 2004; 35:2306–12.

13. Saam T, Cai J, Ma L, Cai YQ, Ferguson MS, Polissar NL, Hatsukami TS, Yuan C. Comparison of symptomatic and asymptomatic atherosclerotic carotid plaque features with in vivo MR imaging. *Radiology.* 2006; 240:464–72.

14. Parmar JP, Rogers WJ, Mugler JP 3rd, Baskurt E, Altes TA, Nandalur KR, Stukenborg GJ, Phillips CD, Hagspiel KD, Matsumoto AH, Dake MD, Kramer CM. Magnetic resonance imaging of carotid atherosclerotic plaque in clinically suspected acute transient ischemic attack and acute ischemic stroke. *Circulation.* 2010; 122:2031–38.

15. Saam T, Hetterich H, Hoffmann V, Yuan C, Dichgans M, Poppert H, Koeppel T, Hoffmann U, Reiser MF, Bamberg F. Meta-analysis and systematic review of the predictive value of carotid plaque hemorrhage on cerebrovascular events by magnetic resonance imaging. *J Am Coll Cardiol.* 2013; 62:1081–91.

16. Wintermark M, Jawadi SS, Rapp JH, Tihan T, Tong E, Glidden DV, Abedin S, Schaeffer S, Acevedo-Bolton G, Boudignon B, Orwoll B, Pan X, Saloner D. High-resolution CT imaging of carotid artery atherosclerotic plaques. *AJNR Am J Neuroradiol.* 2008; 29:875–82.

17. Saba L, Caddeo G, Sanfilippo R, Montisci R, Mallarini G. CT and ultrasound in the study of ulcerated carotid plaque compared with surgical results: potentialities and advantages of multidetector row CT angiography. *AJNR Am J Neuroradiol.* 2007; 28:1061–66.

18. de Weert TT, Ouhlous M, Meijering E, Zondervan PE, Hendriks JM, van Sambeek MR, Dippel DW, van der Lugt A. In vivo characterization and quantification of atherosclerotic carotid plaque components with multidetector computed tomography and histopathological correlation. *Arterioscler Thromb Vasc Biol.* 2006; 26:2366–72.

19. U-King-Im JM, Fox AJ, Aviv RI, Howard P, Yeung R, Moody AR, Symons SP. Characterization of carotid plaque hemorrhage: a CT angiography and MR intraplaque hemorrhage study. *Stroke.* 2010; 41:1623–29.

20. Eliasziw M, Streifler JY, Fox AJ, Hachinski VC, Ferguson GG, Barnett HJ. Significance of plaque ulceration in symptomatic patients with high-grade carotid stenosis. North American Symptomatic Carotid Endarterectomy Trial. *Stroke.* 1994; 25:304–08.

21. Saam T, Raya JG, Cyran CC, Bochmann K, Meimarakis G, Dietrich O, Clevert DA, Frey U, Yuan C, Hatsukami TS, Werf A, Reiser MF, Nikolaou K. High resolution carotid black-blood 3T MR with parallel imaging and dedicated 4-channel surface coils. *J Cardiovasc Magn Reson.* 2009; 11:41.

22. Chu B, Zhao XQ, Saam T, Yarnykh VL, Kerwin WS, Flemming KD, Huston J 3rd, Insull W Jr, Morrisett JD, Rand SD, DeMarco KJ, Polissar NL, Balu N, Cai J, Kampschulte A, Hatsukami TS, Yuan C. Feasibility of in vivo, multicontrast-weighted MR imaging of carotid atherosclerosis for multicenter studies. *J Magn Reson Imaging.* 2005; 21:809–17.

23. Saba L, Caddeo G, Sanfilippo R, Montisci R, Mallarini G. Efficacy and sensitivity of axial scans and different reconstruction methods in the study of the ulcerated carotid plaque using multidetector-row CT angiography: comparison with surgical results. *AJNR Am J Neuroradiol.* 2007; 28:716–23.

24. Saam T, Ferguson MS, Yarnykh VL, Takaya N, Xu D, Polissar NL, Hatsukami TS, Yuan C. Quantitative evaluation of carotid plaque composition by in vivo MRI. *Arterioscler Thromb Vasc Biol.* 2005; 25:234–39.

25. Serfaty JM, Nonent M, Nighoghossian N, Rouhart F, Derex L, Rotaru C, Chirossel P, Thabut G, Guias B, Heautot JF, Gouny P, de la Vega A, Pachai C, Ecochard R, Villard J, Douek PC; CARMEDAS Study Group. Plaque density on CT, a potential marker of ischemic stroke. *Neurology.* 2006; 66:118–20.

26. de Weert TT, de Monye C, Meijering E, Booij R, Niessen WJ, Dippel DW, van der Lugt A. Assessment of atherosclerotic carotid plaque volume with multidetector computed tomography angiography. *Int J Cardiovasc Imaging.* 2008; 24:751–59.

27. Saba L, Sanfilippo R, Sannia S, Anzidei M, Montisci R, Mallarini G, Suri JS. Association between carotid artery plaque volume, composition, and ulceration: a retrospective assessment with MDCT. *AJR Am J Roentgenol.* 2012; 199:151–56.

28. Saam T, Underhill HR, Chu B, Takaya N, Cai J, Polissar NL, Yuan C, Hatsukami TS. Prevalence of American Heart Association type VI carotid atherosclerotic lesions identified by magnetic resonance imaging for different levels of stenosis as measured by duplex ultrasound. *J Am Coll Cardiol.* 2008; 51:1014–21.

29. Demarco JK, Ota H, Underhill HR, Zhu DC, Reeves MJ, Potchen MJ, Majid A, Collar A, Talsma JA, Potru S, Oikawa M, Dong L, Zhao X, Yarnykh VL, Yuan C. MR carotid plaque imaging and contrast-enhanced MR angiography identifies lesions associated with recent ipsilateral thromboembolic symptoms: an in vivo study at 3T. *AJNR Am J Neuroradiol.* 2010; 31:1395–402.

30. Saba L, Montisci R, Sanfilippo R, Mallarini G. Multidetector row CT of the brain and carotid artery: a correlative analysis. *Clin Radiol.* 2009; 64:767–78.

31. Golledge J, Greenhalgh RM, Davies AH. The symptomatic carotid plaque. *Stroke.* 2000; 31:774–81.

32. Sitzer M, Muller W, Siebler M, Hort W, Kniemeyer HW, Jancke L, Steinmetz H. Plaque ulceration and lumen thrombus are the main sources of cerebral microemboli in high-grade internal carotid artery stenosis. *Stroke.* 1995; 26:1231–33.

33. Eliasziw M, Streifler JY, Fox AJ, Hachinski VC, Ferguson GG, Barnett HJM. Significance of Plaque Ulceration in Symptomatic Patients with High-Grade Carotid Stenosis. *Stroke.* 1994; 25:304–08.

34. Trelles M, Eberhardt KM, Buchholz M, Schindler A, Bayer-Karpinska A, Dichgans M, Reiser MF, Nikolaou K, Saam T. CTA for Screening of Complicated Atherosclerotic Carotid Plaque–American Heart Association Type VI Lesions as Defined by MRI. *AJNR Am J Neuroradiol.* 2013; 34(12):2331–7.

35. Falk E, Shah PK, Fuster V. Coronary plaque disruption. *Circulation.* 1995; 92:657–71.

36. Bayer-Karpinska A, Schwarz F, Wollenweber FA, Poppert H, Boeckh-Behrens T, Becker A, Clevert DA, Nikolaou K, Opherk C, Dichgans M, Saam T. The carotid plaque imaging in acute stroke (CAPIAS) study: protocol and initial baseline data. *BMC Neurol.* 2013; 13:201.

Permissions

All chapters in this book were first published in JCMR, by BioMed Central; hereby published with permission under the Creative Commons Attribution License or equivalent. Every chapter published in this book has been scrutinized by our experts. Their significance has been extensively debated. The topics covered herein carry significant findings which will fuel the growth of the discipline. They may even be implemented as practical applications or may be referred to as a beginning point for another development.

The contributors of this book come from diverse backgrounds, making this book a truly international effort. This book will bring forth new frontiers with its revolutionizing research information and detailed analysis of the nascent developments around the world.

We would like to thank all the contributing authors for lending their expertise to make the book truly unique. They have played a crucial role in the development of this book. Without their invaluable contributions this book wouldn't have been possible. They have made vital efforts to compile up to date information on the varied aspects of this subject to make this book a valuable addition to the collection of many professionals and students.

This book was conceptualized with the vision of imparting up-to-date information and advanced data in this field. To ensure the same, a matchless editorial board was set up. Every individual on the board went through rigorous rounds of assessment to prove their worth. After which they invested a large part of their time researching and compiling the most relevant data for our readers.

The editorial board has been involved in producing this book since its inception. They have spent rigorous hours researching and exploring the diverse topics which have resulted in the successful publishing of this book. They have passed on their knowledge of decades through this book. To expedite this challenging task, the publisher supported the team at every step. A small team of assistant editors was also appointed to further simplify the editing procedure and attain best results for the readers.

Apart from the editorial board, the designing team has also invested a significant amount of their time in understanding the subject and creating the most relevant covers. They scrutinized every image to scout for the most suitable representation of the subject and create an appropriate cover for the book.

The publishing team has been an ardent support to the editorial, designing and production team. Their endless efforts to recruit the best for this project, has resulted in the accomplishment of this book. They are a veteran in the field of academics and their pool of knowledge is as vast as their experience in printing. Their expertise and guidance has proved useful at every step. Their uncompromising quality standards have made this book an exceptional effort. Their encouragement from time to time has been an inspiration for everyone.

The publisher and the editorial board hope that this book will prove to be a valuable piece of knowledge for researchers, students, practitioners and scholars across the globe.

List of Contributors

Karine Moschetti, David Favre, Christophe Pinget and Jean-Blaise Wasserfallen
Institute of Health Economics and Management (IEMS), University of Lausanne, Route de Chavannes 31, VIDY, 1015 Lausanne, Switzerland

Jean-Blaise Wasserfallen, Christophe Pinget and Karine Moschetti
Technology Assessment Unit (UET), University Hospital (CHUV), Lausanne, Switzerland

Guenter Pilz
Klinik Agatharied, Akademisches Lehrkrankenhaus der LMU Munich, Hausham, Germany

Steffen E Petersen
National Institute for Health Research Cardiovascular Biomedical Research Unit at Barts, Queen Mary University of London, London, UK

Anja Wagner
Comprehensive Cardiology of Stamford and Greenwich, Stamford, CT 06902, USA

Juerg Schwitter
Cardiac MR Center, University Hospital (CHUV), Lausanne, Switzerland

Shazia T. Hussain
Papworth Hospital NHS trust, Papworth Everard, Papworth Everard, Cambridgeshire, UK
Cardiology Department, Papworth Hospital, Papworth Everard CB23 3RE, UK

Amedeo Chiribiri
King's College London BHF Centre of Excellence, NIHR Biomedical Research Centre and Welcome Trust and EPSRC Medical Engineering Centre at Guy's and St. Thomas' NHS Foundation Trust, Division of Imaging Sciences, The Rayne Institute, London, UK

Geraint Morton
Portsmouth Hospitals NHS trust, Portsmouth, UK

Nuno Bettencourt
Centro Hospitalar de Vila Nova de Gaia/Espinho, EPE, Vila Nova de Gaia, Portugal

Andreas Schuster
Department of Cardiology and Pulmonology and German Centre for Cardiovascular Research, Göttingen, Germany

Matthias Paul
Luzerner Kantonsspital, 6000 Luzern 16, Switzerland

Divaka Perera
King's College London BHF Centre of Excellence, NIHR Biomedical Research Centre at Guy's and St. Thomas' NHS Foundation Trust, Cardiovascular Division, The Rayne Institute, London, UK

Eike Nagel
DZHK Centre for Cardiovascular Imaging, University Hospital Frankfurt/Main, Frankfurt/Main, Germany

Animesh Tandon, Lorraine James, Gerald F. Greil and Tarique Hussain
Department of Pediatrics, University of Texas Southwestern Medical Center, 5323 Harry Hines Blvd, Dallas 75390, Texas, USA

Gerald F. Greil and Animesh Tandon
Department of Radiology, University of Texas Southwestern Medical Center, 5323 Harry Hines Blvd, Dallas 75390, Texas, USA

Amanda Potersnak, Gerald F. Greil, Lorraine James, Animesh Tandon and Tarique Hussain
Pediatric Cardiology, Children's Medical Center Dallas, 1935 Medical District Dr, Dallas 75235, Texas, USA

Markus Henningsson and René M. Botnar
Department of Imaging and Biomedical Engineering, King's College London, London, UK

René M. Botnar
Pontificia Universidad Católica de Chile, Escuela de Ingeniería, Santiago, Chile

Jamal N. Khan, Sheraz A. Nazir, Anthony H. Gershlick and Gerry P. McCann
Department of Cardiovascular Sciences, University of Leicester and the NIHR

Leicester Cardiovascular Biomedical Research Unit, University Hospitals of Leicester NHS Trust, Glenfield Hospital, Leicester, UK Research, Leeds Institute of Cardiovascular and

Daniel Blackman and John P. Greenwood
Multidisciplinary Cardiovascular Research Centre and The Division of Cardiovascular and Diabetes Research, Leeds Institute of Cardiovascular and Metabolic Medicine, University of Leeds, Leeds, UK

Joyce Wong, Thiagarajah Sasikaran and Miles Dalby
Harefield Hospital, Royal Brompton and Harefield Foundation Trust, NIHR Cardiovascular Biomedical Research Unit, Middlesex, UK

Charles Peebles and Nick Curzen
University Hospital Southampton NHS Foundation Trust and University of Southampton, Southampton, UK

Simon Hetherington
Kettering General Hospital, Kettering NN16 8UZ, UK

Damian J. Kelly
Royal Derby Hospital, Derby, UK

Arne Ring
Leicester Clinical Trials Unit, University of Leicester, UK and Department of Mathematical Statistics and Actuarial Science, University of Leicester, University of the Free State, Bloemfontein, South Africa

Marcus Flather
Norfolk and Norwich University Hospitals NHS Foundation Trust and Norwich Medical School, University of East Anglia, Norwich, UK

Howard Swanton
The Heart Hospital, University College London Hospitals, London, UK

Allison G. Hays, Micaela Iantorno, Monica Mukherjee, Gary Gerstenblith and Robert G. Weiss
Department of Medicine, Division of Cardiology, Johns Hopkins University, 600 N Wolfe St., Baltimore, MD 21287, USA

Matthias Stuber, Michael Schär and Robert G. Weiss
Department of Radiology, Division of Magnetic Resonance Research, Johns Hopkins University, 600 N. Wolfe St., Baltimore, MD 21287, USA

Robert R. Edelman, Robert I. Silvers, Kiran H. Thakrar, Mark D. Metzl, Jose Nazari and Ioannis Koktzoglou
Department of Radiology, NorthShore University HealthSystem, 2650 Ridge Avenue, Evanston, IL 60201, USA

Robert R. Edelman
Feinberg School of Medicine, Northwestern University, Chicago, USA

Robert I. Silvers, Kiran H. Thakrar, Mark D. Metzl and Ioannis Koktzoglou and Jose Nazari
The University of Chicago Pritzker School of Medicine, Chicago, USA

Shivraman Giri
Siemens Medical Solutions USA, Inc., Chicago, USA

Markus Henningsson, Joy Shome, Konstantinos Bratis, Miguel Silva Vieira, Eike Nagel and Rene M. Botnar
Division of Biomedical Engineering and Imaging Sciences, King's College London, London, UK

Eike Nagel
Institute for Experimental and Translational Cardiovascular Imaging, Goethe University, Frankfurt/Main, Germany

DZHK (German Centre for Cardiovascular Research, Standort RheinMain), Berlin, Germany

Rene M. Botnar
Escuela de Ingeniería, Pontificia Universidad Católica de Chile, Santiago, Chile

Florian von Knobelsdorff-Brenkenhoff
Department of Cardiology, Clinic Agatharied, Ludwig-Maximilians-University Munich, Norbert-Kerkel-Platz, 83734 Hausham, Germany

Matthias Stuber
Department of Radiology, Centre Hospitalier Universitaire Vaudois, Center for Biomedical Imaging (CIBM), University of Lausanne, Lausanne, Switzerland

Florian von Knobelsdorff-Brenkenhoff and Jeanette Schulz-Menger
Charité – Universitätsmedizin Berlin, corporate member of Freie Universität Berlin, Humboldt-Universität zu Berlin, and Berlin Institute of Health, DZHK (German Centre for Cardiovascular Research), partner site Berlin, Berlin, Germany

Working Group Cardiovascular Magnetic Resonance, Experimental and Clinical Research Center, a joint cooperation between the Charité Medical Faculty and the Max-Delbrueck Center for Molecular Medicine and HELIOS Klinikum Berlin Buch, Department of Cardiology and Nephrology, Berlin, Germany

R. van Dijk, M. van Assen, R. Vliegenthart and M. Oudkerk
Center for Medical Imaging, University Medical Center Groningen, University of Groningen, Hanzeplein 1 EB 45, Groningen, The Netherlands

R. Vliegenthart
Department of Radiology, University Medical Center Groningen, University of Groningen, Groningen, The Netherlands

P. van der Harst and R. van Dijk
Department of Cardiology, University Medical Center Groningen, University of Groningen, Groningen, The Netherlands

G. H. de Bock
Department of Epidemiology, University Medical Center Groningen, University of Groningen, Groningen, The Netherlands

Giulia Ginami, Radhouene Neji, Imran Rashid, Amedeo Chiribiri, Tevfik F. Ismail, René M. Botnar and Claudia Prieto
School of Biomedical Engineering and Imaging Sciences, King's College London, St Thomas' Hospital (Lambeth Wing), Westminster Bridge Rd, London SE1 7EH, UK

Radhouene Neji
MR Research Collaborations, Siemens Healthcare Limited, Sir William Siemens Square Frimley, Camberley GU16 8QD, UK

René M. Botnar and Claudia Prieto
Escuela de Ingeniería, Pontificia Universidad Católica de Chile, Vicuna Mackenna, 4860 Santiago, Chile

Kim-Lien Nguyen, Eun-Ah Park, Takegawa Yoshida and Peng Hu
Diagnostic Cardiovascular Imaging Laboratory, Department of Radiological Sciences, David Geffen School of Medicine at UCLA, Los Angeles, California, USA

Kim-Lien Nguyen
Division of Cardiology, David Geffen School of Medicine at UCLA and VA Greater Los Angeles Healthcare System, Los Angeles, California, USA

Kim-Lien Nguyen, Peng Hu and J. Paul Finn
Physics and Biology in Medicine Interdepartmental Graduate Program, Department of Radiological Sciences, University of California at Los Angeles, Peter V. Ueberroth Building Suite 3371, 10945 Le Conte Ave, Los Angeles, CA 90095-7206, USA

Eun-Ah Park
Department of Radiology and The Institute of Radiation Medicine, Seoul National University Hospital, Seoul 110-744, South Korea

Mengnan Wang and Xiuhai Guo
Department of Neurology, Xuanwu Hospital, Capital Medical University, Beijing 100053, China

Qi Yang and Fang Wu
Department of Radiology, Xuanwu Hospital, Capital Medical University, Beijing 100053, China

Yujiao Yang
Department of Neurology, Sanbo Brain Hospital, Capital Medical University, Beijing 100093, China

Qi Yang, Zhaoyang Fan and Huijuan Miao and Debiao Li
Biomedical Imaging Research Institute, Cedars Sinai Medical Center, Los Angeles, CA 90048, USA

Xunming Ji
Department of Neurosurgery, Xuanwu Hospital, Capital Medical University, Beijing 100053, China

Ali Serhal, Pascale Aouad, James C. Carr and Robert R. Edelman
Radiology, Northwestern Memorial Hospital, Chicago, IL, USA

Ioannis Koktzoglou, Robert R. Edelman and Ali Serhal
Radiology, Northshore University HealthSystem, Walgreen Building, G534, 2650 Ridge Avenue, Evanston, IL 60201, USA

Ioannis Koktzoglou
Radiology, University of Chicago Pritzker School of Medicine, Chicago, IL, USA

Shivraman Giri
Siemens Healthineers, Chicago, IL, USA

Omar Morcos
Surgery, Northshore University HealthSystem, Evanston, IL, USA

Markus Henningsson
School of Biomedical Engineering and Imaging Sciences, King's College London, London, UK

Riad Abou Zahr, Adrian Dyer, Gerald F. Greil, Barbara Burkhardt, Animesh Tandon and Tarique Hussain
Departments of Pediatrics and Radiology, University of Texas Southwestern/Children's Health, Dallas, TX, USA

Ioannis Koktzoglou, Matthew T. Walker, Joel R. Meyer, Ian G. Murphy and Robert R. Edelman
Department of Radiology, NorthShore University HealthSystem, Evanston, USA

Ioannis Koktzoglou, Matthew T. Walker and Joel R. Meyer
University of Chicago Pritzker School of Medicine, Chicago, USA

Ian G. Murphy
Northwestern University Feinberg School of Medicine, Chicago, USA

David P Ripley, Manish Motwani, Petra Bijsterveld, Neil Maredia, Sven Plein and John P. Greenwood
Multidisciplinary Cardiovascular Research Centre (MCRC) and Leeds Institute of Cardiovascular and Metabolic Medicine, University of Leeds, Leeds, UK

Julia M. Brown, Jane Nixon and Colin C. Everett
Clinical Trials Research Unit, University of Leeds, Clinical Trials Research House, 71-75 Clarendon Rd, Leeds, UK

Jennifer A Steeden, Bejal Pandya and Vivek Muthurangu
UCL Centre for Cardiovascular Imaging, University College London, 30 Guildford Street, London WC1N 1EH, UK

Bejal Pandya
The Heart Hospital, University College London Hospital Foundation Trust, London W1G 8PH, UK

Oliver Tann and Vivek Muthurangu
Cardiorespiratory Unit, Great Ormond Street Hospital for Children, London WC1N 3JH, UK

Sébastien Roujol, Murilo Foppa, Tamer A Basha, Mehmet Akçakaya, Kraig V Kissinger, Beth Goddu, Sophie Berg and Reza Nezafat
Department of Medicine (Cardiovascular Division), Beth Israel Deaconess Medical Center and Harvard Medical School, 330 Brookline Ave, Boston, MA 02215, USA

Jochen M Grimm, Andreas Schindler, Florian Schwarz, Clemens C Cyran, Maximilian F Reiser, Konstantin Nikolaou and Tobias Saam
Institute for Clinical Radiology, Ludwig-Maximilians-University Hospital Munich, Munich, Germany

Jochen M Grimm
Department of Medical Radiology, University Hospital and University of Lausanne, Lausanne, Switzerland

Anna Bayer-Karpinska
Institute for Stroke and Dementia Research, Ludwig-Maximilians-University Hospital Munich, Munich, Germany

Tobias Freilinger
Department of Neurology and Hertie Institute for Clinical Brain Research, University of Tuebingen, Tuebingen, Germany

Chun Yuan
Department of Radiology, University of Washington School of Medicine, Seattle, USA

Jennifer Linn
Department of Neuroradiology, Ludwig-Maximilians-University Hospital Munich, Munich, Germany

Miguel Trelles
Department of Radiology, University of Texas Medical Branch, Galveston, USA

Index